THE POSTURE PRINCIPLES

Dr. Krista Burns
Dr. Mark Wade

Editor, Dr. Dan Murphy

CONTENTS

FOREWORD

The Posture Principles

The Posture Principles by Krista and Mark could not have made its launch onto the healthcare platform at a better time. Never before in the history of healthcare has the importance of posture been as critical to the health and wellbeing of peoples around the world as it is today. For many of us, in earlier days our posture was defined by the number of times that our parents told us to "sit up straight". Of course, along those same lines we were also told to go outside and play and not return until dinner was served or we were otherwise called.

Until more recently, posture was not considered a player in the healthcare spectrum. Rather it was perceived as a trait of laziness or not having been properly mannered. The order in which Dr. Krista and Dr. Mark have organized this book gives the reader an understanding of "why" posture is important as well as "how" we came to develop our posture and "what" can now be done. Deviations from upright posture significantly alter the health and function of multiple body systems including the immune, cardiovascular, endocrine, digestive, and nervous.

As we proceed through the pages of this book, we are not only gifted with the understandings of posture and its relationship to health, but also given ample strategies to improve and restore posture. It is these clinical pearls that will impart value to the practitioner. For it is the practitioner who must influence the lifestyle of the patient with sufficient direction, inspiration, and motivation to create change in their daily activities. With that commitment, there must be solid value in the application, outcome, and results. This book is written in such a format as to guide the reader toward becoming an expert in posture assessment, corrections, and home-based exercises.

Chronic time in seated positions, sedentary lifestyles, viewing screens on multiple devices have all contributed to reduced tonus of the spine and proximal limb musculature. This alteration in tone has led the way for flexor-extensor imbalances and the onslaught of faulty postural patterns from forward head posture, upper and lower crossed syndromes, weakened core, to impaired gait and balance.

The chronic mismatch of sensory input from peripheral joints and muscles to higher centers of postural regulation has contributed to deterioration in corticobasal and vestibulo-cerebellar loops for volitional movement and spinal stabilization, and thus the growing clinical prevalence of movement disorders, cognitive impairment, tremors, and persistent pain syndromes. Forward head posture, rolled shoulders, and sitting have now been well documented in the scientific indexed literature as contributing to lowered oxygenation levels, reduced vital capacity of the lungs, sluggishness of the bowel, and poorer conscious awareness of limb placement and control.

Healthcare advances are continuing to reflect upon the postural model. Posture itself does not reflect a disease or pathological entity. However, it does represent an understanding of function and a potential precursor to disease or pathology. The process of chronic sitting has come to be known as a disease entity. Low postural tone with hypertonicity of flexor muscle groups alters normal joint kinematics and neurologic reception, which is associated with a variety of orthopedic and musculoskeletal conditions.

Understanding posture will be integral to healthcare approaches going forward. This book by Dr. Mark and Dr. Krista is well written, organized, referenced, and relevant. I expect that this will be a go-to book in the area of the science of posture with clinical applications. The reader is sure to gain insight into human function and form as well as the neurologic processes involved.

It is a pleasure to write this foreword and a greater pleasure to reflect on the lives that will be positively influenced based upon the work of these two dedicated, passionate, and committed individuals.

Michael W. Hall, DC, FIACN
Chiropractic Neurologist
Executive Director, NeuroLIFE Institute
Life University

INTRODUCTION

Welcome to the American Posture Institute

The mission of the American Posture Institute (API) is to be the world's leading professional resource for posture related information, products, and correction systems. The Certified Posture Expert (CPX) certification course is dedicated to providing healthcare professionals with the most modern and in-depth knowledge of postural correction systems.

Posturology is a scientific exploration of how the body stabilizes and orients itself in space while static and performing dynamic movements. This textbook will enlighten healthcare professionals on postural theoretic concepts, anatomy, and physiology specific to the posture system, how to perform a thorough posture analysis evaluating for common postural distortion patterns, and techniques for postural correction that can be immediately implemented into practice.

Proper posture is a fundamental component of health and wellness. Healthcare professionals from all disciplines agree that proper postural alignment, human biomechanics, and functional correction contribute to overall better health. The American Posture Institute emphasizes the understanding and application of intentional human design.

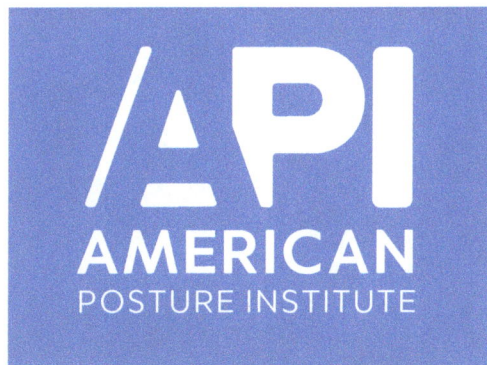

"Posture By Design, Not By Circumstance" is a proactive model empowering human beings to live with healthful intentions, not by the circumstances of their environment. As individuals learn to take control of their posture, they overcome environmental obstacles limiting their human potential and optimize their life performance.

Posture is a blue ocean market strategy for healthcare professionals to optimize their time, energy, and services. The CPX certification has provided experts worldwide with the tools they need to become a Certified Posture Expert and implement postural correction into their current healthcare protocols.

This will be an exciting journey of higher education as you develop the knowledge and expertise of postural correction. Your community needs you. Fulfill this need by providing the best service on the market. Through the implementation of the American Posture Institute's innovative postural correction system into your clinical practice, you will become recognized as the Go-To Posture Expert in your community.

Module 1

THEORY AND PRINCIPLES OF POSTURAL CORRECTION

INTRODUCTION: WHAT IS POSTURE?

The purpose of Module 1 is to define posture, learn the theoretical concepts of posture as a component of optimal health and wellbeing, and identify the physical and social determinants of posture. Throughout this module we will explore many theoretical concepts of posture that will serve as the foundation for your learning. In following the modules, you will learn the anatomy and physiology of the posture system, how to analyze postural distortion patterns, and how to utilize this information for postural correction purposes.

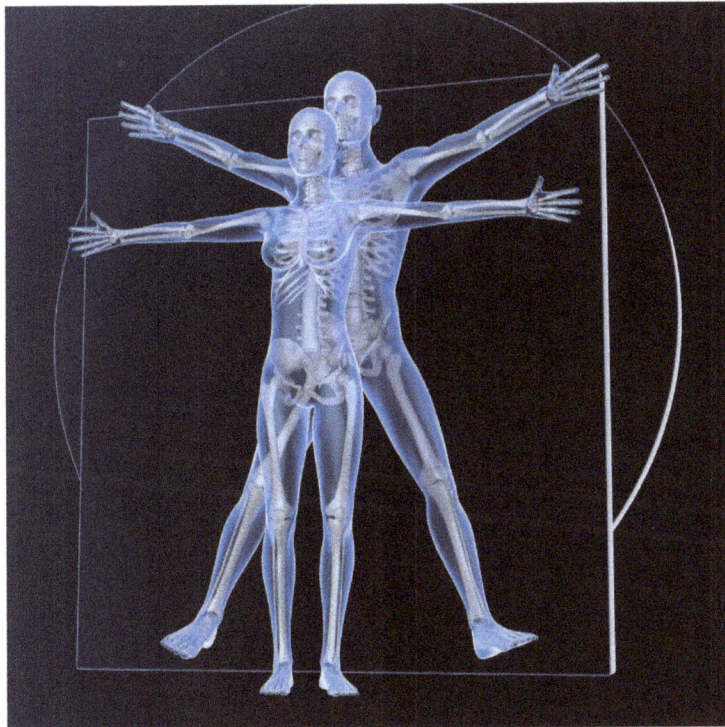

The American Posture Institute defines posturology as the scientific study of the body's static and dynamic alignment as it stabilizes itself in space against gravity and other forces. Posturology is a science; it is a method for analyzing the design of the body and how the body aligns itself in relationship to the surrounding environment.

Posture is the framework of human design while upright, static, and moving. Postural balance is the ability to maintain the body in an upright position against gravity. Postural fitness is the ability to maintain resilient static and dynamic posture during your activities of daily living.

Webster's Dictionary defines posture as "the position or bearing of the body whether characteristic or assumed for a special purpose."

The Oxford Dictionary defines posture as "a particular position of the body. The characteristic way in which someone holds their body when standing or sitting."

Dorland's Medical Dictionary defines posture as "the awareness of the position of the body or its parts in space, a combination of sense of equilibrium and kinesthesia, called also position S."

Our posture is the adaptation of our body to the environment in which we live. Everybody has a posture that defines the framework of his or her body's design. An individual's posture is either good or bad, there is no in between.

"Good" posture is synonymous with fluid bodily movements, supple balance against gravity, and efficient muscle utilization. "Bad" posture on the other hand is associated with dysfunctional movement patterns, weak balance-ability, and distorted body alignment.

The Posture Committee of the American Academy of Orthopedic Surgeons differentiates "good" and "bad" postural presentations.

> "Good posture is the state of muscular and skeletal balance which protects the supporting structures of the body against injury or progressive deformity irrespective of the attitude (erect, lying, squatting, or stooping) in which these structures are working or resting. Under such conditions the muscles will function most efficiently and the optimum positions are afforded for the thoracic and abdominal organs.
>
> "Poor posture is a faulty relationship of the various parts of the body which produces increased strain on the supporting structures and in which there is less efficient balance of the body over its base of support."

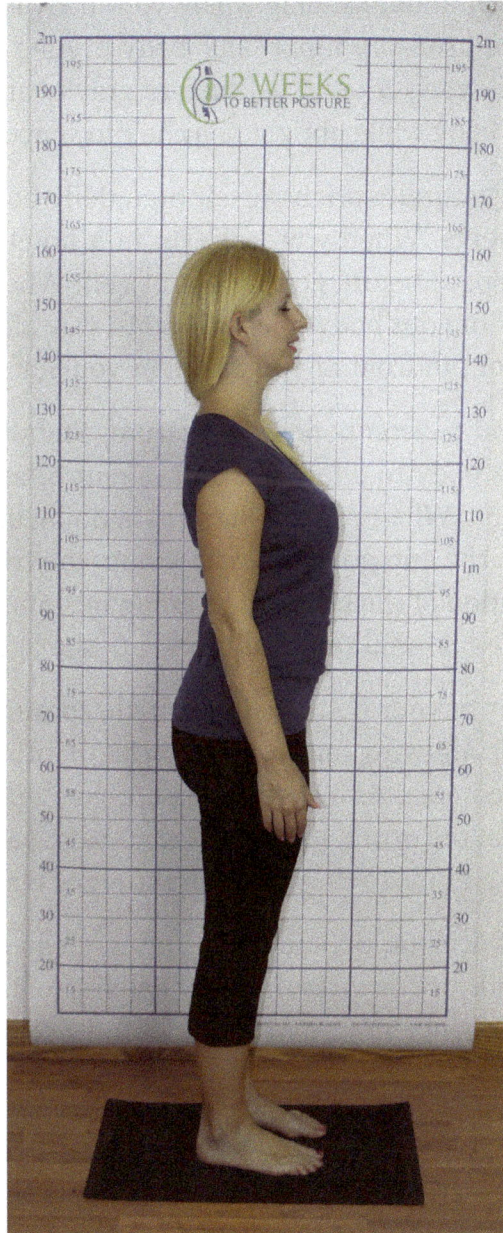

Posture is organized into two subcomponents based upon the sensory input received from the environment and the functional response of the body to this feedback. The body is in a constant state of receiving input, interpreting the input, and then balancing or moving the body accordingly. The two subcomponents of postural control are orientation and stabilization.

Orientation is the process of understanding where your body is in space, or proprioception, due to environmental sensory input. Our body orients in space by recognizing forceful factors within the world around us, such as gravity and modes of support like the ground to support the body while upright or a chair to support the body while seated.

Think of how your body naturally orients itself on a daily basis due to sensory input from changing environments. When you wake up in a hotel or an unfamiliar place, you orient your body in space before getting out of bed. When you dive into a swimming pool the framework of your body orients itself to stay afloat. If you are unable to see, you put your hands out in front of you to orient yourself with the setting.

Stabilization is the second subcomponent of posture. Stabilization is the process of stiffening one part of the body to allow free movement of another body part within the normal range of motion. When you are in the gym doing biceps curls to strengthen your biceps, for example, the antagonist muscle group, the triceps, stabilizes the arm, allowing full range of motion of the biceps. The antagonist muscle group also prevents hyperextension beyond the normal range of motion of the agonist muscle group.

When you injure one part of your body, as in an ankle sprain, the body naturally stabilizes the injured area, allowing more movement of other parts of the foot to compensate for the injured area. As a Posture Expert, you will commonly see patients who present with postural distortion patterns due to back pain. They immobilize the injured area of the spine and move their body in different ways to stabilize the pain.

The fluid combination of orientation and stabilization creates a healthy posture with sturdy balance. Healthy posture restores the body's ability to move freely yet efficiently. Empower your clients to change their perception of the world around them and to be mindful of their posture to make long-term postural correction sustainable.

SECTION REVIEW

1. *Posture* is the framework of human design while upright, static, and moving

2. Posture is organized into two subcomponents: *orientation* and *stabilization*

POSTURE IS A FUNDAMENTAL ASPECT OF OPTIMAL HEALTH AND WELLNESS

There are five pillars of health, all of which are necessary to obtain an optimal level of health and wellbeing. For the purposes of this textbook, we will be focusing in great detail upon the fifth pillar of health: posture.

The Five Pillars of Health include:

- A proper diet to provide the body with energy, hydration, and the nutrients that are essential to maintaining life

- Regular exercise that combines aerobic training, strengthening exercises, and stretches to increase flexibility. Movement of the muscles, joints, and connective tissue promotes agility and better bodily function

- Adequate rest and relaxation to rejuvenate the body and prevent burnout or chronic fatigue

- Positive mental focus to fuel the mind with happiness, empowerment, and the ability to overcome mental stressors

- Postural hygiene to ensure proper alignment, balance, and optimal biomechanical function of the body within its environment

Exceptional posture professionals hold themselves accountable for recognizing whole postural distortion patterns and posture's overall effect on the health and function of the body. Two terms are vitally important for posture professionals: holism and reductionism. Holistic practitioners view the body as one entity. Reductionism then is the method of analyzing a complex system, such as the human body, by subdividing the body into its fundamental systems.

For effective postural correction, posture should be analyzed holistically. The Posture Expert will begin by identifying the level of the primary postural distortion, and its compensation pattern in relation to the rest of the body. Traditional postural diagnoses identify postural distortions in terms of individual pieces, not patterns that affect components among the entire kinetic chain. Module 2 will provide an in depth analysis of postural distortion patterns as they relate to the posture system. The Posture Expert will learn how to analyze the structure and the function of the posture quadrants and how they relate to one another.

Human beings are self-healing organisms that can adapt and overcome stressors in the environment. An aligned spine is an open channel for sensory and motor neurons to communicate with the brain. Proper spinal alignment allows all the body's systems, such as the respiratory, circulatory, digestive, or nervous systems, to function at their highest levels. An aligned body is a balanced body. Balanced bodies are in homeostasis within their environments. Homeostasis is orderliness among bodily systems to prevent bodily disorders.

Upright posture is the most intelligent posture among animals. Humans adapted this posture thousands of years ago as an evolutionary process. Natural posture is the alignment of the internal skeletal support each human is designed to have. If an upright posture is the most intelligent posture among living beings, then it makes sense that abnormalities driving the individual away from this posture (such as rounded shoulders and forward head posture) would cause physiologic imbalances to the system resulting in pathology and decreased function. Harrison and Troyanovich state, "…Abnormal spinal loads over time do cause pathologies" (2003).

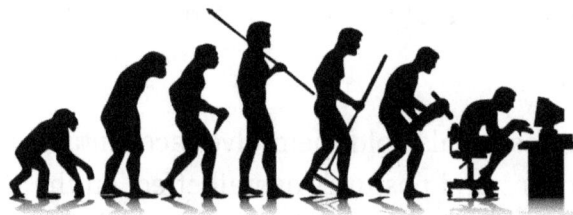

Lifespan is how long we live. "Wealthspan" is how long we live healthfully and well. Traditional allopathic medicine is superb at helping patients increase their lifespan by keeping patients alive in traumatic situations and teaching them basic physical hygiene necessary to prevent sickness from common pathogens. The goal to keep patients alive is important in our society.

However, keeping patients alive and teaching them how to thrive within their environment are two very different concepts. Intentional postural design increases the wealth of patients' lives by increasing their available energy expenditure to live and perform at a higher level of functional capacity.

Proper posture is important for all populations of people throughout the aging process of the life cycle. There is not a day that goes by in which having a symmetric structure of the body is not important. Proper postural design is one of the 5 pillars necessary to maintain optimal health, and should be evaluated throughout patients' lives for early detection of postural distortion patterns.

The American Posture Institute recommends that all individuals have their posture evaluated with posture imaging annually to evaluate for postural changes and to be proactive in the correction of postural faults. It is recommended that annual posture examinations begin at the age of six years old. The Posture Expert will have baseline posture images of their patients' development throughout their life cycle, helping them make accurate clinical decisions of the postural needs of their patients.

Six years of age is the age to begin annual postural analyses as this is when the majority of children begin attending school. When children begin attending school, they develop new habits among all aspects of their lives. By detecting postural distortion patterns early in life, the Posture Expert can discuss proper postural hygiene habits with the child and the parents as the child begins forming new lifestyle habits. The intention is to have posture by design, not by environmental circumstances of development.

SECTION REVIEW

1. *Upright* posture is the most intelligent posture among animals

2. *Wealthspan* is how long we live healthfully and well

POSTURAL DISTORTIONS, A MODERN DAY EPIDEMIC

Unhealthy postural presentations are such an epidemic in modern day society, health-care specialists commonly overlook the significance. Unhealthy posture has become the new "normal." Naturally aligned human beings have become the minority in our population, a true rarity. As a society, we rarely recognize unstable, sick postures, because they have become the new normal. Be advised that "normal" doesn't mean "healthy."

Loss of body consciousness is certainly a hidden downside of the convenience and power of the electronic age. And society is growing sicker and sicker for it. In the United States alone, 80% of people suffer from back pain at some point in their lives and seek necessary treatment (American Chiropractic Association, 2010).

The total cost of treating low back pain has superseded $100 billion per year in the United States, two-thirds of which is a result of lost wages and reduced productivity (Crow & Willis, 2009). The cost of treatment of painful musculoskeletal conditions is more expensive than the annual cost of chronic diseases such as diabetes, cancer, and heart disease.

Gaskin and Richard (2011) found that the total incremental annual cost of healthcare due to musculoskeletal pain was approximately $300 billion per year. The value of lost productivity due to musculoskeletal pain was then considered. This included days of work missed, hours of work lost, and lower wages. In consideration of the incremental healthcare costs and the loss of productivity, the total annual financial cost of musculoskeletal pain to society ranges from $560 to $635 billion.

The effects of poor posture are not just affecting adults later in life; rather, they are affecting children of young ages as well. Currently, 65% of school-aged children present with back pain due to postural distortion patterns, and children as young as 10 years old are demonstrating visible spinal degeneration on X-ray (Smith, 2003).

Kjaer et al. (2005) performed a research study analyzing MRIs. Their research indicated that of 439 13-year-old children who had an MRI of their lumbar spine, one third of them presented with lumbar disc degeneration. Neurodevelopmental problems are plaguing modern day children due to the disruption of a natural primal process. Children with poor posture develop into adults with even worse posture and develop sickly health conditions.

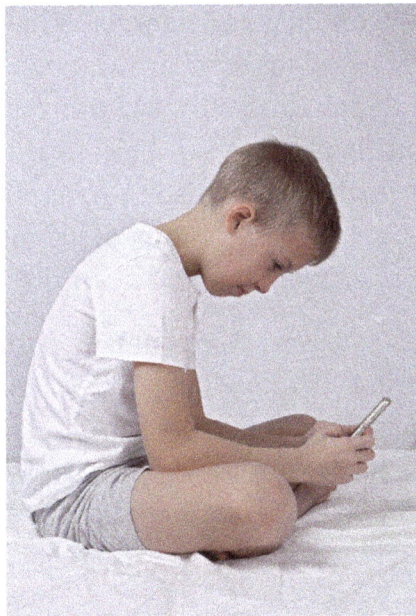

Modernization and technological advancement of our cultures, and the accompanying habits of being more sedentary and sitting poorly, have set new societal patterns in place. These patterns begin with school-aged children and carry on to adulthood, causing problems for millions of people. Poor posture then is not simply an aesthetical problem in our society; it is a modern-day epidemic affecting the lives of millions of people.

In a study conducted by Kado et al (2005), they evaluated the connection between posture and early mortality. The study evaluated 1,353 elderly participants. By evaluating the participants' kyphosis of the thoracic spine, the researchers were able to correlate an increase in early death among the elderly population. The researchers discovered that persons with a hyperkyphotic posture have a 144% greater rate of mortality. Therefore, as the posture weakens and begins to form this type of postural distortion pattern, the percentage of people dying before the normal lifespan is greatly increased.

Kado, Prenovost, and Crandall (2007) estimate that 20–40% of the adult population present with hyperkyphosis. It is noted that hyperkyphosis is highly prevalent among the adult population. However, it is often overlooked and misunderstood. Noted health effects of a hyperkyphotic spine are impaired pulmonary function, decreased physical function capabilities, and increased risk of spinal fractures.

Patients with hyperkyphotic postural distortion patterns commonly present with decreased height as they age due to spinal degeneration. The British Regional Heart Study found that men who lost 3cm in height were 64% more likely to die of a heart attack. Conducted over a 20-year timespan, the study also concluded that men lose an average height of 1.67cm throughout their life cycle. This height loss was associated with a 42% increased risk of heart attacks; this statistic also applied to men who had no prior history of cardiovascular disease. The prevention of height loss due to proper postural design is thus associated with decreased risk of heart disease in men as they age.

Also associated with aging individuals who present with postural distortion patterns is decreased balance and equilibrium. Kado et al. (2007) demonstrate the correlation of hyperkyphotic posture and injurious falls in older persons. Elderly individuals who present with hyperkyphosis are more likely to suffer from falls that can cause serious injuries. Unfortunately, these falls lead to hospitalization of patients, increasing the probability of developing a hospital-acquired illness leading to further health complications.

SECTION REVIEW

1. 80% of Americans suffer from *low back pain*

2. What postural distortion pattern is associated with early mortality and decreased balance? *Hyperkyphosis*

DETERMINANTS OF HEALTHY POSTURE AND WEAK POSTURE

Everyone presents with a unique posture. All human beings differ in size, height, weight distribution, body shape, muscle tone, joint function, congenital deformities, anatomical misalignments, and levels of bony degeneration. Although age and genetics play a role in the makeup of posture, their significance is minimal. For example, if elderly individuals practice good lifestyle habits such as daily postural exercises, they are much less likely to present with a weak, bent forward posture. Similarly, if someone is born with no serious postural deformities, but they do not practice healthy lifestyle habits, their posture is likely to degenerate more rapidly.

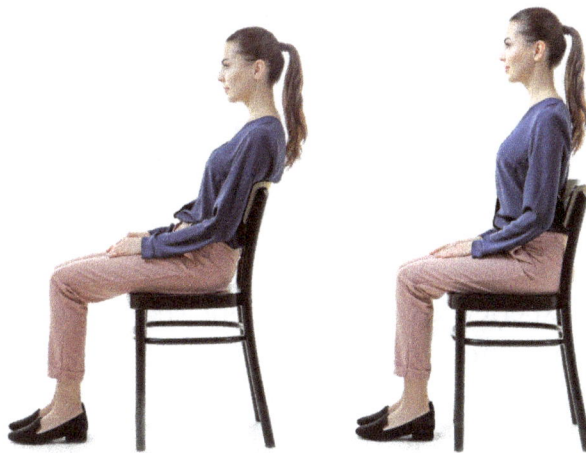

The primary determinant of posture is our lifestyle habits. However, societal assumptions tell us that age and genetics control our posture. Thus people are less empowered to take care of their bodies. Your posture is neither completely genetic, nor something you are stuck with for the rest of your life. Your posture, instead, is due to your lifestyle habits and how you orient and stabilize yourself in consideration of the conditions of your environment. This can be changed at any point of a patient's life that they are committed to improving their lifestyle design.

The high incidence of postural faults in adults is related to the tendency toward a highly specialized or repetitive pattern of activity. Habitual and repetitive movements, such as sitting in an office in front of a computer screen for hours on end, limit the flexibility and agility of movements and perceptual horizons. Repetitive motions are generally uniplanar motions that are so simple to perform they diminish bodily conscious awareness.

Performing complex movements contributes to intelligence, creativity, and intentional consciousness. Thus it is pertinent for Posture Experts to give patients multiplanar exercises to challenge their physiology and correct postural alignment.

Stress is the ultimate mechanism behind shaping biology. When natural life stressors affect the human body, they directly sculpt the way the body will develop, regardless of genetic predisposition. Stressors our current day humanity experiences, however, have changed dramatically. Humanity is beginning to de-evolve into a hunched over, sedentary species with no core musculature control. Flexibility is decreased, strength is diminished, and the functional capacity of humanity is suffering. Function has decreased, yet environmental stressors have increased.

Society lives in a state of stress, but this type of stress has changed greatly over time. While humans in the early stages of humanity experienced stress for survival purposes (such as encountering a dangerous animal while gathering food), the modern-day human experiences imposed environmental stressors putting the body into a state of sympathetic overdrive.

Animals in nature only experience this sympathetic stress in a life or death situation, and their response is movement oriented to flee from the situation. Modern-day humans, on the other hand, live in this heightened sympathetic state day in and day out. The evolved human responds to stress by remaining sedentary, causing a vicious cycle of degenerative physiological breakdown both structurally and functionally.

Posture derives from how a person moves, or in this modern-day society how they don't move. The behaviors that are repeated over time eventually become ingrained in your physiology, both healthy behaviors and unhealthy behaviors. How you use your body and are consciously present during your daily routine will change your posture. Healing your posture is a process of self-discovery from a mental and physical aspect. Maintaining healthy posture throughout the lifecycle requires a lifelong commitment to intelligent lifestyle habits.

Consider the 10 most common factors that are likely affecting your posture on a daily basis.

Ten Most Common Factors of Posture

1. **Repetitive occupational movements**. These are simple motions performed in the same plane of motion on a repetitive basis. Although these movements vary based upon occupation, they usually occur in the coronal (frontal) plane of the body. For example, a construction worker who hammers nails, a painter who paints walls using a roller, or a secretary typing on their computer. All of these occupational motions are uniplanar, repetitive, and occur in the frontal plane. Multiplanar motions are motions across multiple planes of movement to stimulate the posture system.

2. **Living a sedentary lifestyle**. Muscles, bones, and joints require movement to stay mobile. Aging individuals who are sedentary demonstrate muscles that atrophy and lose massive muscle fiber content, the mineral content of their bones decreases, connective tissues become less flexible, and joint motion becomes limited (American Academy of Orthopedic Surgeons, 2010). Movement keeps the joints and connective tissue more mobile and contributes to stronger muscles and higher bone density. Long periods of inactivity are related to loss in flexibility, osteoarthritis, and postural collapse.

3. **Prolonged sitting**. Prolonged sitting with postural collapse occurs when the patient slouches in their chair and sustains that position for an extended period of time. Improper seated posture includes forward head posture, a rounded thoracic spine, and anterior translation of the pelvis. The thoracic spine maintains a C-shape in this position rather than a healthy S-curve. Prolonged sitting is commonly associated with an occupational expectation of being seated at a desk or driving for long periods of time without taking a break.

4. **Flexor dominant posture.** Patients commonly present with flexor dominant posture, such as slouching the shoulders forward and forward head posture, while reading, watching TV, texting, typing on a computer, etc. As the head and shoulders are drawn forward, the chest drops anteriorly into flexion affecting respiration and often causing physical

symptoms such as neck pain and shoulder pain. This postural distortion pattern is becoming more prevalent in the technology era.

5. **Improper lifting and bag carrying**. Common improper lifting techniques are rounding the shoulders forward with a C-shaped spine and bending forward at the waist into flexion. Patients commonly keep their legs straight and the pressure of lifting is more prominent in the lumbar spine. Repetitive lifting with postural collapse is a common contributing factor to lumbar disc herniations, especially when patients are repetitively lifting heavy objects and twisting the spine. Carrying bags over the same shoulder each day also affects the alignment of the posture system. With the strap over one shoulder, the patient will commonly hunch that shoulder in a superior direction to prevent the bag from falling off their shoulder. Repetitive superior hunching of the shoulder girdle can lead to shoulder asymmetry and irregular muscular development.

6. **Sitting on your wallet**. This is a common cause of pelvic unleveling and sciatica, especially for men. Pelvic unleveling causes local postural distortion patterns and postural compensations in other areas of the posture system. When a patient is sitting on a wallet, the pressure can compress important tissues such as the sciatic nerve. The patient can easily prevent this from affecting their posture by putting their wallet in their front pocket instead of sitting on it in their back pocket.

7. **Physical trauma**. Physical traumas such as car accidents or sports injuries affect the posture system at the level of the injury, causing compensation patterns. The area of the injury is stabilized and the patient learns how to walk, move, and function with that body part stabilized. This compensation pattern can lead to prolonged body re-sequencing patterns while performing normal activities. The body becomes used to the new position, and without correction, the postural collapse can continue to get worse.

8. **Improper shoe support**. Wearing shoes that do not support the feet and distort natural weight distribution is a common problem. Wearing shoes that support balanced upright posture is important for sustaining proper posture while standing. When a person is wearing high heels, the weight of their body is distributed anteriorly and the gastrocnemius and the soleus muscles

are tightened. Shoes that do not support the natural arch of the foot can contribute to fallen arches and abnormal gait patterns.

9. **Shifted weight while standing**. After standing for a prolonged period of time, patients will commonly shift their weight to one side or another with the torso shifted over one hip. This shift in weight misaligns the posture, adding excessive weight to one side of the body. This shift in weight at the hip causes compensation patterns in the spine, feet, shoulders, and head.

10. **Improper sleep hygiene**. Sleeping on your stomach with the lumbar spine in extension and the cervical spine rotated can negatively impact posture, whereas sleeping on your back or side is much healthier. Abnormal sleeping posture is a common contributing factor to postural decline. Optimal sleeping positions are to sleep on the back or the side with the spine and hips in a neutral position. When the spine is flexed or extended during the night, excess pressure is absorbed. Pillow consideration is also important. The pillow should support a neutral cervical curve. With the use of excess pillows the neck is stressed in flexion throughout the course of the night.

SECTION REVIEW

1. The primary determinant of posture is our *lifestyle habits*

2. The 10 most common factors of posture:
   - Repetitive occupational movements
   - Living a sedentary lifestyle
   - Prolonged sitting
   - Flexor dominant posture
   - Improper lifting and bag carrying
   - Sitting on your wallet
   - Physical trauma
   - Improper shoe support
   - Shifted weight while standing
   - Improper sleep hygiene

POSTURE BY DESIGN, NOT BY CIRCUMSTANCE

We control the unique design of our posture by favorably responding to the circumstances of our environment. Everything in our reality functions within the natural laws of the environment. The person who can effectively incline their behaviors toward the physical laws of the universe is more likely to emerge as a healthy human. Inclining your behaviors toward the physical laws of the universe works by choosing natural solutions to health issues. Unnatural solutions break universal laws and drive the human organism away from their natural design.

The key to functional posture correction is finding a harmony of the body to work within the laws of the universe, not to fight them. Postural correction strategies are intended to reinforce the body's natural design and preserve the integrity of an elongated spine at all times. Good posture is a good habit that contributes to health and wellbeing. Once in good posture, the biomechanical structure and function of the body allow the person to maintain sturdy posture. Bad posture is a bad habit, beginning with the misuse of the capacities of the structure and function of the body.

Postural mindfulness is the moment-by-moment awareness of your body and how it is stabilized and moving. So much of what we do as human beings is reactive and subconscious. Have you ever had the experience of traveling in your car, on a road that you often take, and although you safely arrive at your destination, your travel experience was completely mindless? You can't recall what cars you passed, whether you stopped at stoplights or had the green to go. Mindless actions are habitual activities performed by instructions from the basal ganglion. Your body performs the actions from subconscious controls, merely responding to the conditions of the environment, instead of predicting and choosing actions.

If mindlessness is habitual, mindfulness is intentional. When you are intentional with postural correction strategies, you are successful in obtaining the results that you desire. Try being mindful right now. Think about your posture. If you are seated, how are you seated? Are you leaning back in your chair, or slumped forward? Are both feet touching the ground? Is your back straight, or weakly folded forward? Before being prompted to think about your posture, did you take notice of any of these cues? Likely you didn't.

Or if you did notice your posture, it was likely because you were in pain. When someone has acute back pain, for example, they are very mindful of the position of their spine so as to avoid triggering the onset of pain or discomfort. When in a sense of urgency, we become mindful to the needs of our body. Without this urgency, however, the majority of individuals neglect their posture altogether. To achieve postural correction results, your patients must be mindful of the position of their bodies in space as it interacts with their surrounding environment.

Recognition of posture creates neural pathways that support proper posture. Think of the word "recognition". "Re-cognition" means to become reactivated in your cognitive brain. When you recognize postural collapse, you become mindful of it, and can then strategize how to improve or prevent it. In later modules, we will discuss important cues to prompt postural mindfulness.

As a human race, our biological sustainability for good posture has weakened. Throughout history humans have evolved to adapt to the environment, for purposes of survival. With the ease of modern-day technology, however, survival is no longer a serious threat to humanity. Humans are de-evolving at the speed of technology. Our biological adaptations are bringing us further away from nature, in a state of undesirable physiologic function.

Human beings are by no means stronger, faster, or more conditioned for physical activity than other animals in nature. We have evolved, however, as the most intellectual species on the planet. The ability for the cortical brain to receive, process, and understand information that it receives separates humans from all other species. The ability to understand and choose, instead of just reacting to the environment, is a unique feature separating human beings from animals in terms of superiority.

Standing upright is the most intelligent posture of the modern-day animal kingdom. Over thousands of years of evolution, human beings have risen from being hunched over animals to upright humans with the ability to understand and choose how to coordinate their posture. With mindful intentions, we choose the position in which our postural framework sustains itself upright. To utilize our evolutionary strength, which is intellect, as a society, we need to intellectually develop better postural habits. If we don't, we will continue to de-evolve into a structure of lesser intelligence and lesser biologic sustainability.

SECTION REVIEW

1. If mindlessness is habitual, *mindfulness* is intentional

2. Humans are de-evolving at the speed of *technology*

THRIVING CHILDREN

A healthy change in societal patterns begins with changing the lifestyle habits of children. As children develop, they are influenced by the norms to which they are exposed. By educating children about the importance of proper postural design, society shifts toward a healthier population.

The new "normal" should be children learning how to interact with technology in a way that promotes healthy body structure instead of deteriorating their postural framework. Children thrive when they have better posture. Their postural presentation during the developmental stages of life predicts their ability to grow and develop with less pain, have more bodily confidence, and perform better at school.

Lifestyle habits for children are highly dependent upon how they hold their body upright while at school. Incorrect postural patterns that begin during the school-age years of life are more likely to persist as unhealthy lifestyle habits into adulthood. Postural training helps children prevent painful musculoskeletal conditions that are common during the developmental stages, such as neck and back pain. In fact, Mendez et al. (2001) demonstrated that postural hygiene programs are highly effective in preventing back pain.

Postural hygiene programs that provide participants with motivating strategies and actions to change their health are considered to be the most effective (Mendez, 2001). Simply telling a child to sit up straight without telling them why or how is considered ineffective. Research demonstrates that postural self-correction methods, such as "sitting up straight" when prompted, are ineffective in correcting posture. According to Stoliński and Kotwicki (2011), "Non-instructed school children straighten their back by introducing pathological lordosis in the lower thoracic spine, and only slightly correct upper thoracic kyphosis. Adults' commands of correcting posture may be not beneficial for the children."

School performance and back pain are significantly related, demonstrating the need for postural hygiene programs in schools. A study of 270 children found that children who reported having cervical and/or lumbar pain had poorer school performance than the children who were asymptomatic (Salminen, 1984). Salminen (1992) also found that low back pain was the third most common form of pain interfering with school-work and leisure activities. Of the children who experienced back pain, 35% reported disabling low back pain and were aware of recurrent or continual pain.

To improve school performance, children who maintain alert posture have the advantage over their classmates. Not only is upright posture the most intelligent posture, it also prevents neck and back pain which can distract students from their studies. The effects of back pain and postural distortion patterns are far more serious than just feeling uncomfortable at school. With persistent postural distortion patterns, there are many pathologic consequences that can prevent children from having a normal development. Thus, teaching children to be mindful of their postural habits will instill within them healthy lifestyle habits.

A common cause of postural distortion patterns in children is wearing backpacks that exceed the safe limit for postural health. Multiple research studies have demonstrated that when children carry backpacks that are too heavy, exceeding 10% of their bodyweight, they are more likely to develop musculoskeletal pain. The prevalence of schoolchildren carrying heavy backpacks is extremely high: 61.4% of children presented with backpacks that weigh more than 10% their body weight (Paloma Rodríguez-Oviedo et al., 2012).

Negrini, Carabalona, and Sibilla (1999) found that 34.8% of Italian schoolchildren carry more than 30% of their bodyweight at least once a week, exceeding lifting limits that are proposed for adults. Paloma Rodríguez-Oviedo et al. (2012) concluded that carrying heavy backpacks increases the risk of back pain in school-aged children by 50%, and possibly increases the risk of back pathology.

The U.S. Consumer Product Safety Commission estimates that hospitals and doctors in the United States annually treat more than 7,300 backpack-related injuries. Injuries range in severity from bruises to sprains and strains to the back and shoulders, and even fractures (American Chiropractic Association). The repetitive stress of excessive backpack weight is not to be taken lightly. The Federal Consumer Product Safety Commission calculated that carrying a 12lb backpack to and from school and lifting it 10 times a day for an entire school year puts a cumulative load on a child's spine of bodies of 21,600lb, the equivalent of six mid-sized cars.

The specific incidence and location of back pain due to backpack weight was identified by Trousler (1994): 41% of the population of children evaluated had lumbar spine pain, 34% had thoracic pain, and cervical pain was present in 26.5% of children. Cheung, C. et al. (2010) showed a correlation between the craniovertebral angle, backpack weights, and disability due to neck pain in school-aged children, indicating that children who carry backpacks with higher weight present with forward head posture which is directly related to disability due to neck pain.

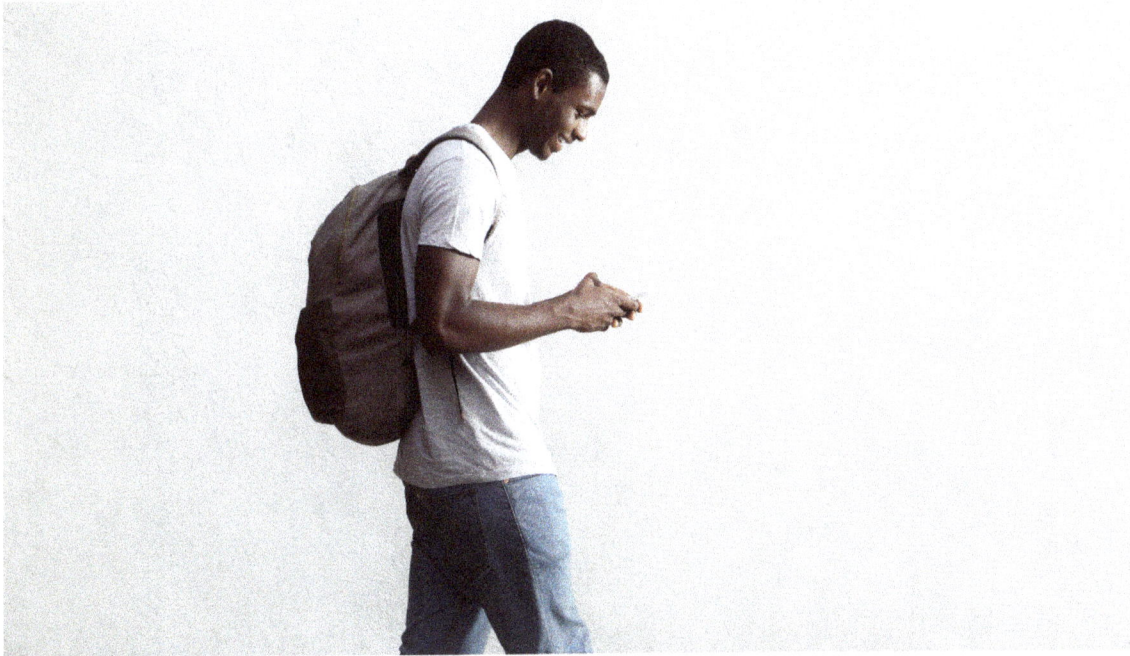

Preventive and educational activities should be implemented to reduce this injury associated with incorrect backpack use. This involves educating teachers, students, and parents. Parental knowledge of their child's backpack weight and contents was assessed by Forjuoh et al. (2011), identifying that of a population of students who carried backpacks weighing at least 10% of their body weights, 96% of parents had never checked their child's backpack weight, and 34% of parents had never checked the contents within the backpack.

Another factor that contributes greatly to postural decline in children is sitting with postural collapse, or weak posture. Sitting with improper posture is associated with back pain in children. Trousler (1994) determined that 41.6% of school-aged children experienced back pain while sitting in class—30% of these children experienced pain within one hour of sitting, and 70% after sitting for longer than one hour.

Children on average sit for 6–8 hours during a typical day at school. Not only should children be taught how to sit with proper posture, they should be given the equipment that supports them being seated in this posture. An inexpensive yet effective way to provide ergonomic equipment to children is the use of exercise balls instead of chairs. While seated on exercise balls, children have greater core activation and trunk stabilization and are able to move around with comfort while maintaining proper postural patterns.

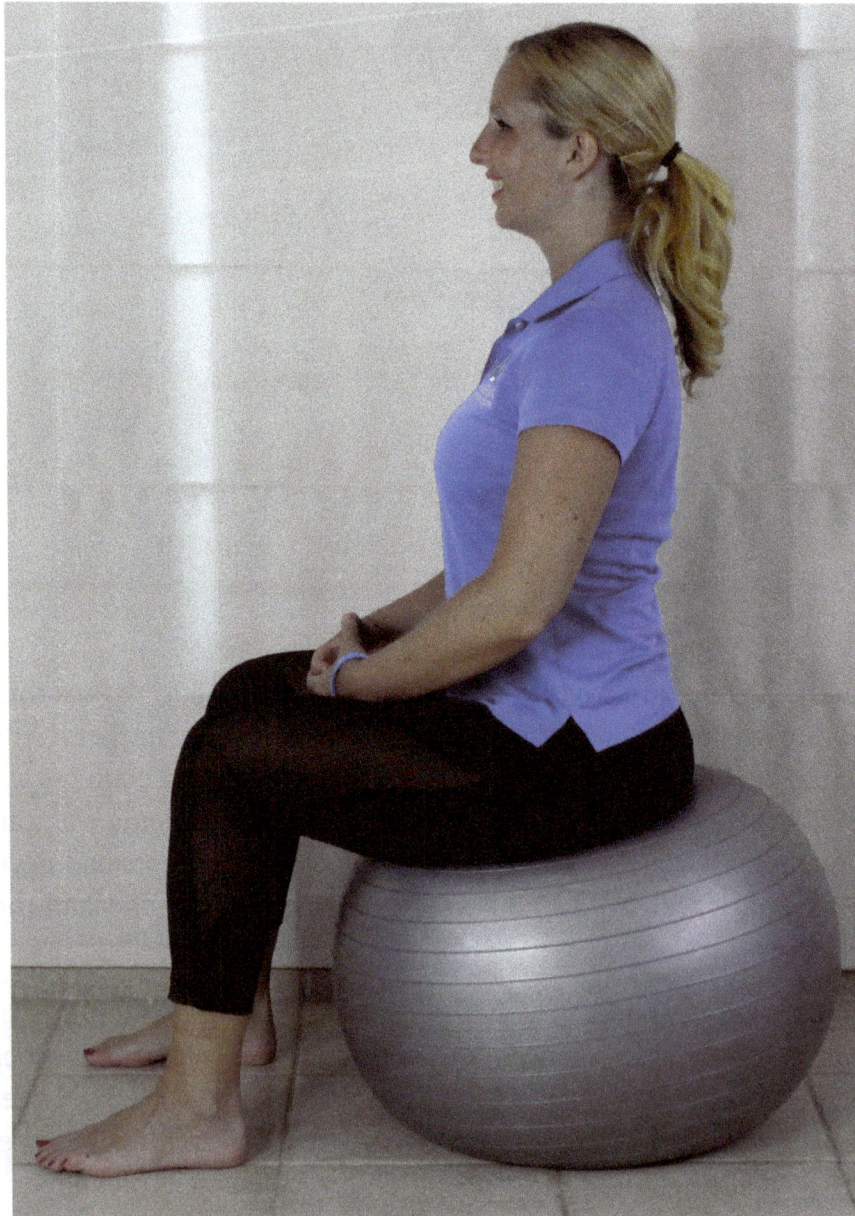

Schilling et al. (2004) demonstrated that the level of engagement was higher and in-seat behavior was better of children with autism spectrum disorder (ASD) when they were seated on exercise balls instead of regular school chairs. While seated on exercise balls, the children had better trunk stabilization, a demonstration of how the sensory-processing theory translates into effective practice in a classroom context. Better engagement and behavior of the children allowed teachers to provide more effective instruction. In 2003 Schilling also demonstrated that children diagnosed with Attention Deficit Hyperactive Disorder (ADHD) had better in-seat behavior and higher levels of productivity when seated on exercise balls.

This revolutionary concept, when applied to a larger population, can help school-aged children succeed in school and behave in socially appropriate ways when interacting with their classmates. Given the tools to maintain proper posture during school, children demonstrated the ability to thrive. In addition, the research demonstrated that both teachers and students preferred the exercise balls to normal school chairs.

SECTION REVIEW

1. Postural hygiene programs are highly effective in preventing *back pain*

2. A common cause of postural distortion patterns in children is wearing *backpacks* that exceed the safe limit for postural health

HOW SITTING IS MAKING YOU SICK

Many modern day workers spend the majority of their time seated. Sitting has been described as "the new smoking" due to the ill health effects associated with a sedentary lifestyle. Sitting is the structural equivalent of metabolic syndrome. Researchers have found that prolonged sitting increases the risk of developing chronic disease such as various types of cancer, heart disease, and type 2 diabetes.

According to Levine (2013) prolonged sitting causes the body's metabolic function to be inactive. The joints stop moving, the muscles aren't firing, and the heart rate slows.

> **"Then, the body's calorie-burning rate plummets to about one calorie per minute—a third of what it would be if you were walking. Insulin effectiveness drops and the risk of developing Type 2 diabetes rises. Fat and cholesterol levels rise too."**
>
> **Levine, 2013**

Sedentary behaviors are also linked to higher levels of depression in adults (Teychenne et al., 2010). Van Uffelen et al. (2013) conducted a research study evaluating the effects of sitting for more than 7 hours per day and symptoms of depression in women. They found that women who do not exercise and women who are seated more than 7 hours per day are 47% more likely to suffer from symptoms of depression. Women who sit for 7 hours per day and do not engage in physical activity are 3 times more likely to have depression than women who sit fewer than 4 hours per day.

Other research shows that people who are sitting in front of their computers for 5 hours or more per day have an increased risk of developing mental illness, depression, and insomnia. Tetsuya (2003) concluded that mental health and sleep-related symptoms were significantly higher in the research group that spent five hours or more in front of a computer screen.

The effects of prolonged sitting are so dramatic to the body that recent studies are showing that the effects of long-term sitting are not reversible through exercise (Drexler,

2014). Simply put, a 1-hour workout will not offset the effects of sitting for a standard 8-hour workday. Human beings were designed to be athletes. The human body was perfectly designed to perform dynamic movements, not to sit in a chair hour after hour, day after day.

The structural framework of the human body was created for survival in the environment in which we live and interact. Survival requires strength and endurance, which our musculature provides. Perceptual organs from the bottom of our feet to the top of the neck provide awareness of our body in relation to our surroundings. The human body was designed to perform complex movements, to resist physical stressors, to run fast, and to stay grounded and balanced against gravity. We were designed to be athletic, and yet we choose not to be. Our lifestyle doesn't require athleticism; rather it promotes mindless movements leading to laziness. Human posture is de-evolving at the speed of technology.

Prolonged sitting decreases metabolic function and increases pressure to the spine and posture system. While you are in a seated position, the pressure in the lower back is increased by about 1.7 times your body weight. And this is when you sit with proper posture. If you slouch, that pressure increases further. Research also shows that on average there is a 10% increase in forward head posture when sitting and working with a computer monitor (Szeto, 2002).

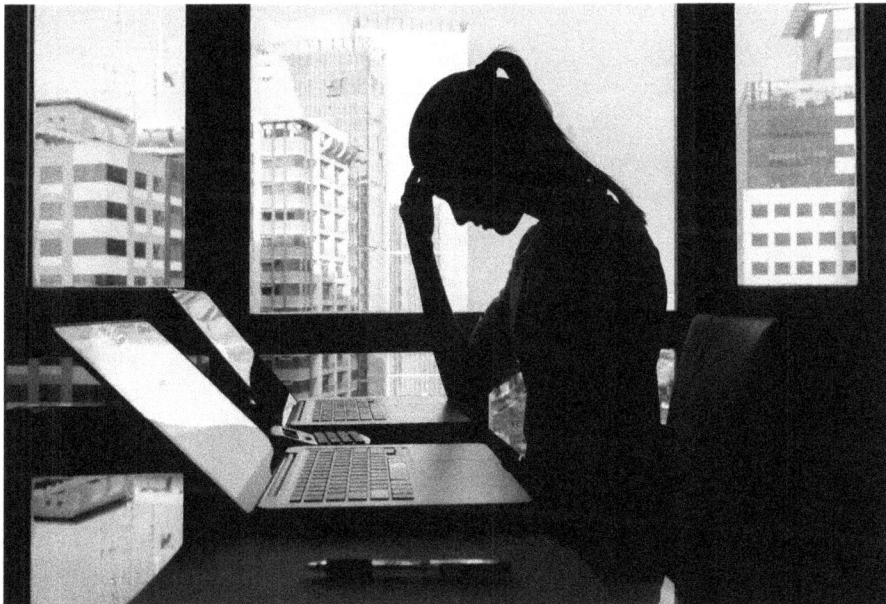

The spine is generally strong enough to tolerate the pressure of a slouched spine for about 20 minutes before the vertebral discs start to absorb the pressure. Thus, posture breaks are recommended at least once per hour. Posture breaks lengthen contracted muscles associated with sitting while stimulating inactive postural musculature.

If modern day occupations require prolonged sitting, as a society, how can we preserve our health while performing necessary job-related tasks? Vernikos (2005) states that it is not how many hours you're sitting that's bad for you, it is how often you interrupt that sitting position that is good for you. Vernikos (2005) states, "It's actually *the change in posture* that is the most powerful in terms of having a beneficial impact on your health, not the act of standing in and of itself."

Modern day occupations require prolonged sitting, but ultramodern occupations should not. To increase biologic sustainability of the human race, occupations and activities of daily living should promote dynamic, multi-dimensional movements of employees to stimulate changes in posture throughout the day. It is not just the job requirements that are important in stimulating proper postural habits, but also the equipment that employees utilize throughout their workday.

SECTION REVIEW

1. Women who do not exercise and women who are seated more than 7 hours per day are 47% more likely to suffer from symptoms of *depression*

2. Prolonged sitting decreases *metabolic function* and increases pressure to the spine and posture system

ERGONOMICS AND HUMAN FACTORS

To design your unique postural presentation, you should design efficiency in places where you spend the most amount of time. Design your home life and your workspace in a way that supports and strengthens your postural framework, not fights it. The terms "human factor engineering" and "ergonomics" have arisen in the research as highly effective ways of overcoming postural collapse in your typical daily settings.

The research is overwhelmingly in favor of the implementation of postural ergonomic programs in the workplace and your life space to improve health and vitality while preventing common musculoskeletal injuries. According to OSHA, poor posture at work results in 34% of all lost workday injuries and illnesses.

Human factor engineering is similar to ergonomics, but considers the component of psychological factors when employees are interacting with their environments. How they view their environment can change how they interact with it. Stichler (2013) claims that the ultimate design solution for effective workspaces is a combination of ergonomics and human factors engineering. This method considers the equipment that workers are using and the way in which they interact with it on a daily basis.

Although this is best practice for employee health and safety, 88% of managers surveyed had not heard of human factor engineering and 94% of managers had not studied the consequences of improper ergonomics (Shahraki and Bakar, 2004). This provides a great market opportunity for Posture Experts to engage with corporations.

According to the Environmental Health and Safety, the purpose of ergonomic design is to facilitate task performance, minimize fatigue and injury, overcome human limitations, and support humans to achieve operational objectives. In order to accomplish this purpose, it is recommended to consider the 4 key elements of ergonomic design: equipment, software design, workstation design, and training. As explained by Ferris (2013), the purpose of machines should be to maximize human effort, not to cause pain or discomfort.

The 4 key elements of ergonomic design are in fact essentially the basis of any workplace. The equipment is what is used to perform the work activity. Whether your patients' occupation is performing construction work or janitorial duties, there are specific pieces of equipment utilized to produce work.

Tools utilized repetitively in the workplace are essentially an extension of the human body, and thus should be designed with the human body in mind. The tools should be able to be utilized easily without causing additional strain to the body part. Software design should be user friendly and should not strain the eyes to see the computer screen. One of the most common ergonomic errors in the workplace is lack of adequate lighting, causing the worker to strain their neck forward to see the computer screen.

Workstation design is very important for employees and will be discussed in greater detail. For a visual indication of correctly designed ergonomic workplaces in which the employee is seated and in which the employee is standing, refer to the graphic.

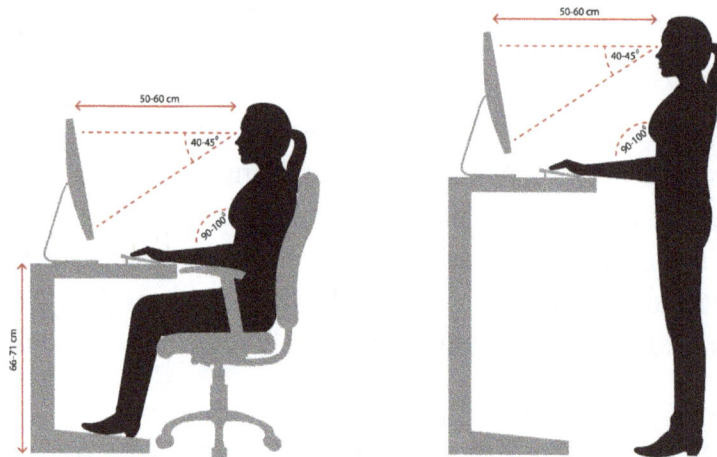

The final aspect of the 4 key elements of ergonomic design is training. Ergonomic equipment is essentially useless if the employee is not trained how to use it properly. All employees should be educated on proper ergonomics in the workplace with safety precautions for the utilization of work related equipment.

According to Harte et al. (2011), "The health and productivity of the employee workforces has a direct relationship to the health and the well-being of the organization" (p. 26). Healthy, pain-free employees are able to perform their jobs better and have a greater level of fulfillment for their work completed. Thus, postural correction programs in corporations should not be limited to a one-time occurrence. The literature suggests that continual postural ergonomic programs are more effective than one-time training sessions.

In addition, the health prevention programs of any corporation should be in alignment with the strategies and values of that particular company to improve longevity of the program. Generic corporate wellness programs can commonly miss important needs of specialized professions. Lawyers have different needs than bus drivers, and teachers have different needs than hair stylists.

The most effective long-term health programs emphasize proper posture and ergonomic education, a discussion of how to prevent injuries and avoid absenteeism among employees, health and wellness advice that employees can implement while they are at work, as well as continuous reinforcement of healthy behaviors. To reinforce healthy behaviors, management can implement rewards and praise for employees who implement the regular utilization of them.

Kelby (2014) explains 5 key factors for the success of ergonomic programs in corporations: to use a systems approach to ergonomics; incorporate ergonomics into the mission and vision of the organization; develop an effective business strategy with key stakeholders; build ergonomic performance standards into the job descriptions of employees; and continuously evaluate and improve the ergonomic program over time.

This research article also demonstrates the importance of implementing the mission and the values of the company into the Corporate Posture Program. By working directly with key stakeholders, the company will successfully implement the program at all levels of the corporation. When stakeholders value the importance of the program, the program will be at the forefront of importance for the corporation. Continuous evaluation of the program renders quality feedback for improvement.

The work tools and technology for employees to use have dramatically increased over recent years. Jobs are becoming more and more specialized. However, employees' postures are not evolving with the demands of modern day work. Lotz (2012) demonstrates that postural ergonomic programs are the way of the future for business.

Employers who consider employees' health needs will build a strong business. In the index report created by JustStand.org, it was demonstrated that 70% of full-time American employees highly dislike sitting for so long, but that they do it anyway because their jobs require it. In addition, 85% of employees report taking breaks during work due to pain and discomfort of sitting. This is an average loss of productivity ranging from 15 minutes to two hours per day among employees. Employees are very receptive to changes to a sedentary lifestyle, 95% saying they would prefer to be more active during their work hours (Lotz, 2012). By listening to employees, employers can learn about their needs and can structure the business to more appropriately match those needs.

Employers and employees benefit from ergonomic programs. According to the Department of Labor in the United States, an employer who implements an injury prevention program should expect a return on investment of up to 6 times the initial fees. A direct correlation has been demonstrated between safety of employees and increased financial gain for the company.

A study conducted by MacLeod (2009) demonstrated the benefits of implementing an ergonomics program with the employees of a die cast plant in Ohio. After implementing the program, the study measured that productivity increased 54%, absenteeism dropped 67%, workers' compensation cases dropped by 93%, and turnover went down by 94%.

MacLeod concluded the ways in which ergonomic programs benefit corporations. These include: decreased employee error, more accuracy due to better posture, less exertion, improved efficiency due to less motions, better heights and reaches, less fatigue, less downtime, human resource protection, waste reduction, new insight on operations, less limitations for elderly workers, improved morale, more employee involvement, improved labor, innovative engineering, progressive ergonomics, greater compatibility of products, improved human system interface, and greater employee understanding of how to work efficiently.

In 1995 the state of Oregon issued an ergonomics initiative to improve posture and ergonomic support for state employees in order to reduce work related musculoskeletal pain. The initiative included specialized ergonomic training for employees including educational meetings, exams for comprehension, and expert ergonomic recommendations of equipment to utilize. This initiative was re-evaluated 10 years later by Brace (2005). He concluded that the posture and ergonomic program demonstrated a significant decrease in money lost for musculoskeletal disorders of the hand, wrist, arm, and shoulder for the state of Oregon. This is a great example of how proper ergonomics benefit the employees—they presented with less injury and musculoskeletal pain, and it benefited the employers, in this case the state of Oregon, due to a decrease in the amount of money lost.

Laeser, Maxwell, and Hedge (1998) based their research on the concept that "keyboard and mouse placed on a standard desktop promote unhealthy posture, discomfort, lost productivity, and risk of musculoskeletal injury in adult office workers" (p. 1). If computer station positioning affects the posture of adults, they assumed it would be the same in school-aged children. Their study compared the posture of students who utilized an adjustable workstation with an adjustable keyboard versus those who utilized a standard computer workspace.

It was demonstrated that the students with proper ergonomic setup of their computers had better posture and higher scores on the Rapid Upper Limb Assessment. Brink et al. (2014) concluded that the most prevalent posture that students present with while seated at a computer is greater range of motion of the trunk, meaning that they tend to sit bent forward or reclining back. Increased neck flexion was also noted as significant. By changing the way in which schoolchildren interact with their environment, we can help them develop smarter postural habits from an early age.

Throughout Europe, the importance of reducing back pain among employees is also of high importance to employers. European best practices for preventing back pain in children and adults suggest two primary recommendations. The principal recommendation is for patients to engage in regular physical activity. Regular physical activity contributes to increased mobility, flexibility, and cardiovascular health. Sedentary muscles and joints become rigid and painful upon exertion. Regular physical activity helps prevent early onset of spinal degeneration.

The second recommendation for European best practices is the implementation of formal education programs teaching patients how to prevent and avoid back pain in their daily lives. Recognizing the triggers of back pain and learning how to overcome them is a fundamental aspect of injury prevention. This includes proper postural hygiene tips and developing an efficient ergonomic workspace to prevent back pain while at work.

The literature recommends the same best practices in preventing chronic neck pain. Primary prevention programs include regular physical activity and proper ergonomic habits at work. Primary care for individuals who present with neck pain is conservative spinal rehabilitation. Green (2008) found that chronic neck pain patients tend to utilize the healthcare system twice as often as normal patients. From a public health perspective, it is thus highly valid and relevant to recommend cervical pain prevention standards to patients.

In addition to preventing musculoskeletal disorders, postural ergonomic programs have also been noted in the literature to improve energy levels and prevent obesity. Riddle and Purvis (2004) demonstrated how posture affects energy levels. Poor posture slowly decreases amounts of energy. They demonstrate that when you slouch, your muscles utilize more energy to hold the body upright. In fact, just 15 minutes of reading or typing in an ergonomically inefficient position with poor posture exhausts the neck, shoulders and upper-back muscles.

Perry (2012) demonstrates how proper ergonomically designed workspaces can help fight obesity. He concludes that office ergonomics, standing more, and in-office wellness programs are effective controls for safety, injuries, illnesses, and obesity. To help reduce obesity, health experts need to recommend ways of increasing activity in non-exercise situations, such as at work. Having an adjustable workspace allows the employee to work while standing, but also to sit when necessary.

Proper ergonomic design is complex, but not difficult. There are easy alternatives to buying expensive ergonomic equipment (although the research demonstrates the investment is worth the value). Consider the 10 ergonomic essentials listed below, and then consider how these can be applied to specialized professions. Again, when you're evaluating a corporation, it is critical to consider the needs of those employees specific to their job requirements, the environment in which they work, and the mission and values that the corporation upholds.

Ten Ergonomic Essentials

1. **Comfortable work chair with proper spinal support**. The chair should be designed so that employees can keep their backs straight and elongated comfortably. The chair should be height adjustable so the feet of the employee touch the ground and their knees are not restricted under the desk. If the employees' feet do not touch the ground, they should place a footrest under their feet.

2. **The spine should always be supported**. If necessary, the employee can insert lumbar and cervical supports between their chair and their spine (supports are generally small cushions). The purpose of the cervical and lumbar supports is to support the natural curve of the spine while seated. The spine should make a nice "S" curve, not a rounded "C" curve.

3. **Computer screens and reading materials should be placed at eye-level**. Having the material at eye-level, the employee is able to maintain a neutral cervical curve. If they are forced to look up, their neck is in extension; if they are forced to look down, their neck is in flexion. Prolonged flexion or extension increases tension to the cervical spine and supporting musculature.

4. **Proper lighting and decreased noise pollution.** These allow the employee to concentrate and maintain a more deliberate focus. With limited visibility and/or a noisy environment, the employee must perform their job tasks in a highly distracting environment, stressing their system. In a workplace with inadequate lighting and/or noise pollution, the potential for human error, miscommunications, and injury is greater. The employee should be able to perform their work without squinting. If they are squinting, they are jutting their head forward, causing forward head posture. If they are unable to hear, they are leaning laterally toward the communication they are trying to hear.

5. **Comfortable mouse pad and keyboard placement.** The mouse and keyboard should be placed in a manner that does not strain the wrist and elbows. If they are placed too far forward, the employee is reaching for them with their upper extremity, whereas if they are too close, the employee is maintaining an awkward crunched posture. If the desk is too high, their wrists are in extension to type. Prolonged wrist extension can cause irritation to the median nerve, commonly seen as carpal tunnel syndrome (note: repetitive work activities performed with the hands, especially vibratory activities, increase the risk of carpal tunnel syndrome). Wrist rests are a good solution to prevent wrist pain. A wrist rest should be utilized with the keyboard and the mouse, allowing the employee to maintain neutral position of their wrists while working at their computer.

6. **Keep most commonly used items within an arm's reach away at elbow level**. Repetitive reaching causes strain to the upper extremity, can cause unnecessary rotation of the spine, and can compromise the important vasculature of the upper extremity. Repetitive reaching can

cause uneven muscular development as individuals tend to reach forward with their dominant hand. Commonly used items that are too close to the body cause the employee to scrunch their body, and feel cramped and crowded. This results in a closed posture. If their arms are too close to their body, they may be repetitively hitting their elbows on their sides. Commonly used tools should also be placed at elbow height. The arm then remains in a neutral position, not chronically flexed, extended, or stressed.

7. **Shoes with proper support**. Shoes with proper support are essential for employees, especially for employees who are on their feet for prolonged periods of time and who do a lot of walking, lifting, or physical activity. In certain high-risk jobs, protective shoes are necessary to protect the feet from injury. Proper shoe selection can help prevent foot pain and discomfort, as well as low back pain. Common foot problems due to hard floors and inadequate shoe support are blisters, callus formation, toe malformations, ankle sprains, fallen arches, bunions, shin splints, etc. Footwear should adequately support the natural design of the foot, and should fit properly. High heels cause unnatural muscular contraction of the lower leg muscles and shift the weight forward to the anterior aspect of the foot. Pointed shoes can cause strain to the toes; shoes with lack of adequate arch support can lead to fallen arches and common foot misalignments; shoes that are too tight can lead to blisters and calluses; shoes that are too loose can cause ankle sprains and instability on the job.

8. **Sitting on a posture cushion or exercise ball.** Posture cushions or exercise balls are the best option for sitting correctly at work. With an unstable surface, employees are constantly engaging their core muscles throughout the day to stay upright. The instability of the rounded surface doesn't allow you to be lazy and slouch, because if you do, you fall off. By engaging the inner core muscles to stay upright, employees are strengthening their postural muscles and supporting the natural alignment of their spine. Maintaining a "C" shaped curve of the spine is much more difficult on a wobble cushion or stability ball, thus maintaining proper posture becomes a natural habit. Movement is a key way to keep joints

healthy and prevent degeneration. In addition, sitting on an uneven surface day in and day out improves balance and proprioceptive activation, both of which are important components of posture and wellbeing.

9. **Adjustable workstations.** These are the best option for employees of all size dimensions. Adjustable workstations are the innovative vision of businesses, recognizing that with office ergonomics it is not a "one size fits all" mentality. Businesses with proper ergonomic equipment recognize that all employees have different body types, and they invest in adjustable equipment that meets the needs of the natural design of everyone's body type. Adjustable workstations allow the employee to perform their job-related tasks while sitting down or standing up. In this way, employees are prompted to stand up throughout the day and be more active. Being sedentary is not only contributing to back pain and lack of productivity of employees, but also the development of lifestyle related chronic diseases. An adjustable workstation allows employees to engage in good postural habits and stay productive.

10. **Posture breaks.** Posture breaks are another highly effective way of developing postural fitness at work. Posture breaks require little time but render healthy returns. They are effective because they engage the anti-gravity muscles that tend to be under-activated throughout the day. A posture break should be performed every hour for 20–30 seconds. The API Posture Break starts at the base of the spine. While seated at the edge of your chair, begin by engaging the transversus abdominis muscle by rolling your hips underneath you and flattening the lumbar curve. Elongate the spine, sitting tall. Roll the shoulders up, back, and down so they are not in a raised position. Straighten the upper extremity bringing your arms and hands wide. Arch your thoracic spine (keeping your core tight, don't collapse at the core), push your chest out, and bend back (at the point of the dorsal spine, not the lumbar spine). Arms stay wide. Feeling a stretch through the pectoral muscles and arms, bring the head back into extension. Hold the position for 15 seconds, or until you feel your proper posture collapse.

To remember to perform posture breaks, set a reminder at your workstation.

SECTION REVIEW

1. What are the four key elements of ergonomic design? *Equipment, software design, Workstation design,* and *Training*

2. The 10 ergonomic essentials:
   - Comfortable work chair with proper spinal support
   - The spine should always be supported
   - Computer screens and reading materials should be placed at eye-level
   - Proper lighting and decreased noise pollution
   - Comfortable mouse pad and keyboard placement
   - Keep most commonly used items within an arm's reach away at elbow level
   - Shoes with proper support
   - Sitting on a posture cushion or exercise ball
   - Adjustable workstations
   - Posture breaks

THE PAIN CYCLE AND UNDERLYING CAUSE OF PAIN AND DISEASE

Pain is a subjective nociceptive experience that individuals perceive when they interact with a stimulus that causes them some level of discomfort. Pain is subjective as different people perceive pain in different ways, and cope with the pain in different ways physically and mentally. Patients commonly describe pain as throbbing, stinging, shooting, sharp, dull, visceral, diffuse, localized, stabbing, sore, daunting, pins and needles, gnawing, burning, and aching. Each of these descriptions helps the Postural Specialist understand the source of the patient's pain.

Pain associated with tissue damage is algogenic. Tissue damage includes damage to the bone, viscera, soft tissue, or organs. This may occur post trauma.

Pain associated with nerve damage is neurogenic. Central pain syndrome is neurogenic pain originating in the central nervous system, commonly caused by tumors.

Peripheral pain is common among patients with poor postural presentations, and is often described as shooting pain, or a feeling of tingling or pins and needles in the upper and/or lower extremities. Chronic diseases such as diabetes, a virus such as post-herpetic neuralgia, inflammation such as is the case in Trigeminal neuralgia, and mechanical stress such as a spinal misalignment complex cause peripheral neuropathies.

Psychogenic pain is prolonged due to mental triggers of fear, nervousness, anxiety, doubt, or negativity. Psychological factors will vary from patient to patient but may have a significant effect on their perception of pain and the ability to heal. Psychological factors in painful situations heighten the emotional response of the patient, and may make them feel desperate, scared, or hopeless. Regardless of the psychogenic influence on the patient's perceived pain, as a Postural Specialist it is important to recognize the patient's needs (mentally and physically), but always proceed with treatment from an objective standpoint.

Posture injury is due to one of two occurrences of trauma: acute trauma or repetitive micro trauma. Repetitive micro trauma is the much more common presentation of patients seeking postural correction care. In cases of acute trauma, however, it is always important to view the body holistically, correcting the entire postural distortion pattern, not just the area of injury.

Repetitive motion injuries are due to the failure of tissues that occurs gradually over time as they are exposed to loads beyond their functional capacity. The cumulative effects of constant or repeated small stresses over a long period of time can be as significant as a sudden, severe stress. Plouvier et al. (2008) studied the most common factors of repetitive micro trauma for patients who present with low back pain. These factors include: repetitive bending or twisting, duration of exposure to pushing, pulling, or carrying heavy loads, and driving for prolonged periods.

Patients engaging in these activities for a duration of time were noted to have symptoms associated with chronic low back pain, lasting beyond the duration of exposure to the mechanical stress. Many participants of the study, for example, felt the effects of low back pain into retirement, after eliminating the repetitive stressors from their lifestyle.

Although the effects of repetitive micro trauma clearly cause postural degeneration over time, patients often don't understand the significance of micro trauma as they experience it at low pressures or for short durations. The body is dynamic and adaptable and compensates for micro injuries. The primary reason patients may not view micro trauma as being a severely debilitating factor to their health is because they learn to work around injury. If an injury occurs in one area, the body stabilizes that body part and recruits surrounding tissues to perform the intended movement or action. Musculoskeletal recruitment leads to compensatory postural distortion patterns.

Compensatory postural distortion patterns affect the entire kinetic chain of movement to some degree. Consider a patient with an acute ankle sprain. They stabilize the ankle, shifting the weight to the ball of the foot and the base of the phalanges, altering the kinetic chain of the injured leg, and also the non-injured leg. While the patient is standing and walking, the strong leg absorbs the additional weight distribution, causing a shift in the position of the hips and the load absorbed by the knee, ankle, and arches of the foot.

Now consider the effects of the spine. When a patient has low back pain, they often present with antalgic posture, in particular in acute situations. The antalgic posture is a stabilization mechanism of the body. Postural correction procedures are indicated to correct the compensatory antalgic pattern. If this is left uncorrected, neural pathways and habit feedback loops favoring antalgic posture of the kinetic chain will develop. Postural rehabilitation is more complex at this stage of chronicity.

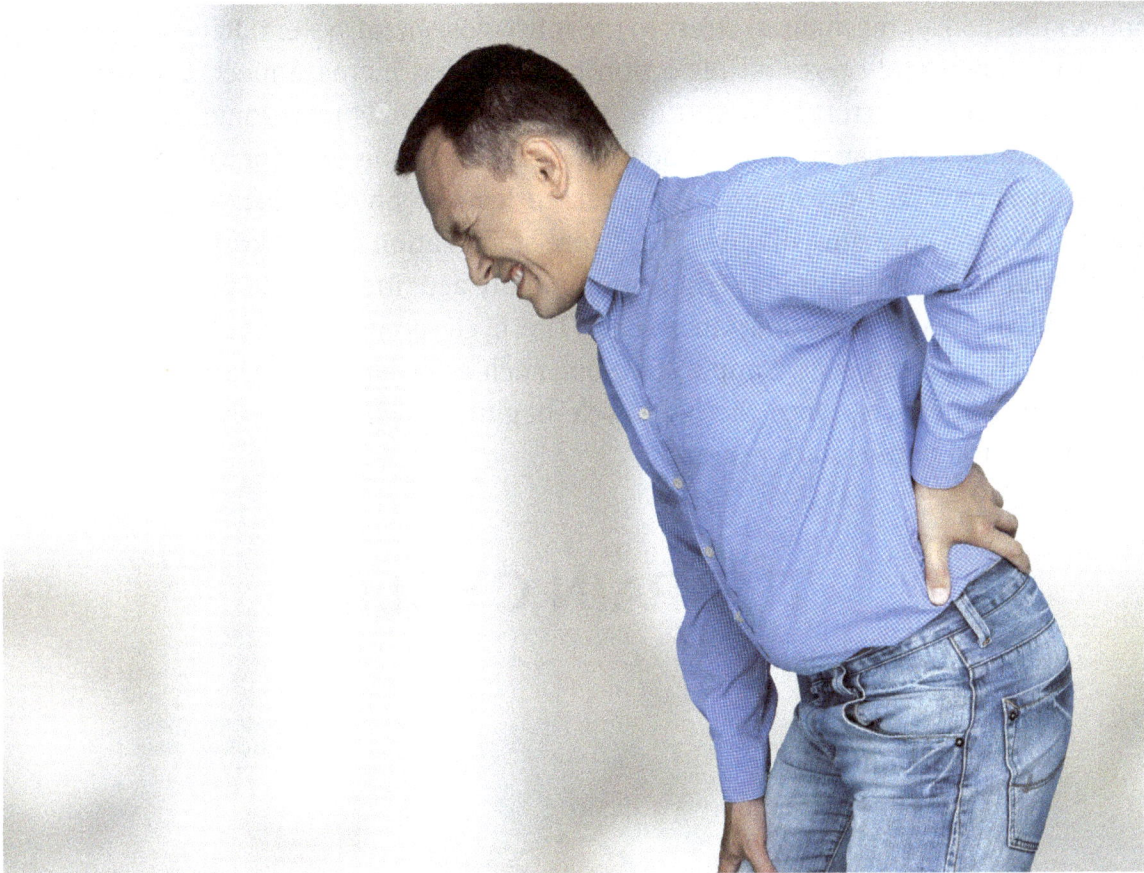

Patients presenting with back pain move differently. In a study conducted by Jones et al. (2011), neuromotor alterations to pain were noted which either represent movement patterns that have developed in response to pain or could reflect underlying impairments that may contribute to recurrent episodes of low back pain. Understanding the relationship between pain and how postural distortion patterns disrupt dynamic movements helps the Posture Expert make predictions of kinetic chain dysfunction compensation patterns.

Pettorossi and Schieppati (2014) explain that tonic cervical proprioceptive input may induce persistent influences on the subject's mental representation of space, creating plastic changes associated with motion patterns, motor responsiveness, and head position. Thus if a patient presents with cervical postural distortion patterns, their motion patterns and neural plasticity will be altered.

The pain cycle begins with repetitive micro trauma (that the patient may or may not notice) that causes mechanical stress to the musculoskeletal system. Repetitive injuries lead to compensatory postural distortion patterns that increase mechanical stress to the spine and supporting musculature. Poor posture leads to chronic pain patterns. The pain causes the patient to become more sedentary in an attempt to avoid activities that trigger pain and discomfort. A decreased level of physical activity leads to stiff joints and weak core musculature. Weak core stabilization causes greater postural degeneration and postural collapse in common daily activities. As the posture weakens, mechanical stress to the body increases. The cycle continues repeatedly until the patient actively intervenes. Simple stressors, such as occupational related habits, can trigger the pain cycle. Once the pain cycle begins, it will not resolve unless proper neural postural patterns are restored.

THE PAIN CYCLE

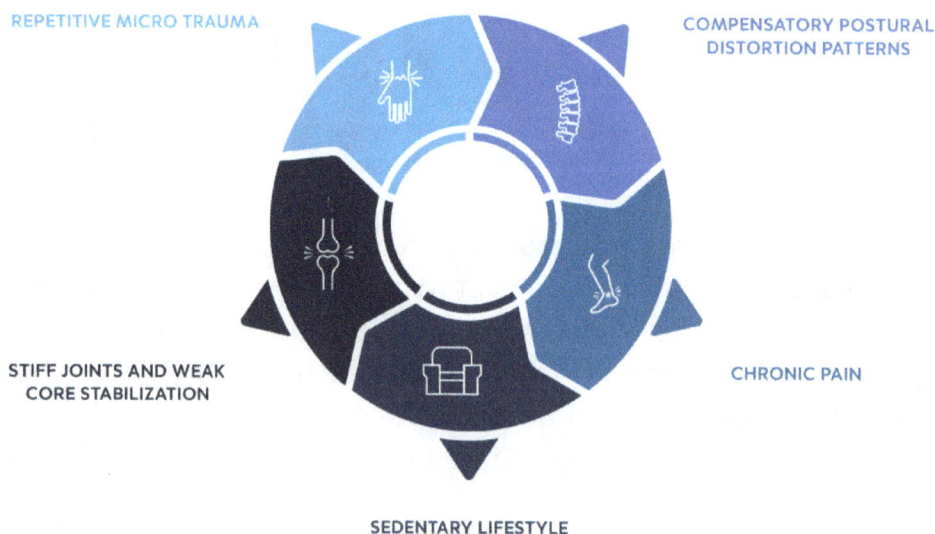

REPETITIVE MICRO TRAUMA

COMPENSATORY POSTURAL DISTORTION PATTERNS

STIFF JOINTS AND WEAK CORE STABILIZATION

CHRONIC PAIN

SEDENTARY LIFESTYLE

Patients who are caught in the chronic pain cycle are in desperate need of help. Posture Experts recognize the importance of correcting the entire postural distortion pattern that has developed, not just the area where the patient is experiencing pain. By correcting compensatory patterns, you are helping the patient prevent recurring postural collapse. Postural distortion patterns are a modern day epidemic. Consider the following statistics.

Chronic low back pain patients make up the majority of the population. According to Plouvier (2008), 55% of European workers have experienced back pain in the last year, 80% of Americans have experienced back pain at some point in their lives, and half of American workers experience symptoms associated with back pain each year. Musculoskeletal issues such as arthritis, low back pain, and repetitive motion injuries are the leading cause of absenteeism among employees (American Chiropractic Association, 2014).

According to the Global Burden of Disease, low back pain is the single leading cause of disability worldwide. At any given moment, 31 million Americans are suffering from low back pain, making it the second most common reason for visits to the doctor's office, outnumbered only by upper-respiratory infections.

SECTION REVIEW

1. Is pain subjective or objective? *Subjective*

2. The pain cycle begins with repetitive *micro trauma* that causes mechanical stress to the musculoskeletal system

UNDERSTANDING STATIC AND DYNAMIC POSTURE PATTERNS

Posture is how you orient the framework of your body to specific events and interactions in your daily life. Your responses to the environment program how your body moves and stabilizes itself upright. Posture constantly adjusts in space due to the internal environment of the individual, so the individual can interact with the outside world. This ongoing process frees up certain parts of the body, and stabilizes others in synchronicity so the body can move fluidly.

Proper posture in a changing world requires constant modification of the positions of your joints, bones, musculature, and connective tissue. Keeping the body mobile and flexible helps promote better postural adaptations.

As a Posture Expert, a very important concept to understand is that postural analyses should not just consider static postural presentations, but also dynamic. Humans are highly dynamic individuals, thus our posture is in constant motion to adapt to a changing environment.

Static posture refers to the alignment of your body when you are not moving. A static posture, for example, is your posture while sitting in a car or while sitting at work. Static implies lack of movement, or maintaining the same position of the body for a prolonged period of time. Static is not the same as sedentary, which implies inactivity. Often to maintain a static position, the body requires effort and muscle tone. Consider a static yoga pose. At a certain point, it is difficult to maintain static stability; the body may even begin to shake. It is more natural for the body to be in motion than to be static.

Although specialists argue if static posture actually exists, from the perspective of this book we will assume it does. We will consider the body to be static when it is not making large uniplanar or multiplanar movements. The argument is due to postural sway and cellular changes that constantly create minute movements. Human beings are dynamic; we are literally always moving.

We perceive ourselves as being still, but while we are standing "still," our nervous system is firing to postural muscles, making hundreds of small adjustments per second to keep us upright. The larger masses of the body, such as the head, are located far away from the base of support, the feet. The feet are small stabilizers of the mass of the body in terms of size. To adapt, the feet move to stay grounded underneath the body, or the body parts move to stay centered over the feet.

Dynamic posture refers to the alignment of the body in motion. It is how you carry yourself throughout life and interact with your environment. An example of dynamic posture is how you hold yourself upright while taking a walk, or while performing activities of daily living. To a more extreme level, this also refers to bodily alignment while playing sports or performing complex activities like ballet dancing.

Dynamic posture can be reactive in nature, or can be learned. For example, the body is constantly reacting to changing stimuli. This happens quickly, and often subconsciously to keep the body safe. If you are crossing the street and see a car coming quickly at you, your dynamic posture instantly changes from a comfortable walk to a quick run. Your posture innately adapts to the factors of the environment.

When you're learning a new skill, like playing tennis, the dynamic postures necessary to aggressively hit the ball across the court and anticipate the return of the ball most likely do not come naturally. These are examples of learned dynamic postures that tennis pros seek to master over the years. With intentional training, the learned dynamic postures become natural and rapid upon execution.

When you're evaluating patients, it is important to first understand proper static postures, and then learn how to correctly evaluate posture with movement. Proper static posture is the foundation for efficient dynamic posture. Just as a child learns to balance on two feet before learning to run, your patients should master strong static posture before focusing on dynamic posture.

Postural patterns are developed by factors of stress, time, and load. Everyone's unique posture has the ability to conform to the supporting surface symmetrically and with weight distributed equally through the load bearing surfaces. When walking, you generate about 2.5 times your body weight, and when running you generate 3.5 times. Your body absorbs this force in all articulations from the feet to the temporomandibular joint. Proper posture patterns are required to effectively absorb this force and adapt to the environment. Because there are over 300 articulating surfaces of the body, bodies may present with one of up to 300,000,000 different dynamic postural presentations (Harrison, 2000).

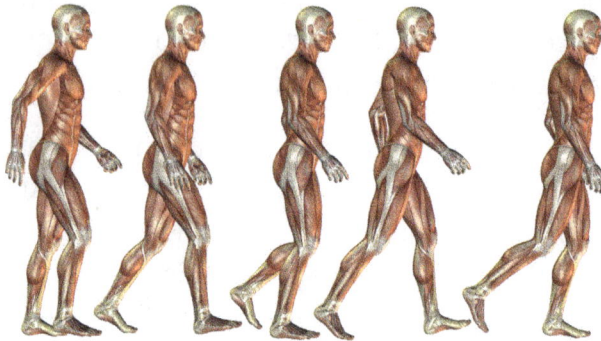

Stress plays a large role in shaping static or dynamic postures. Stress itself can be static and persistent or dynamic and repetitive. When discussing the pain cycle, we talked about sedentary patients and how sedentary individuals have heightened loads of mechanical stress. What about your active patients? Why is it that athletes experience injuries if they train hard to be strong and have quick dynamic postures?

Unfortunately, exercise fanatics who do the same dynamic exercises every day have just as much stress to their posture as someone who is sedentary. Repetitive motions with improper posture cause micro trauma to the tissues that can change postural patterns and be extremely debilitating to the athlete with time. Athletes should learn to master primal moves with good form before moving to more complex movements. Primal movements include cross-crawl mechanisms, squats, jumping and landing, falling forward and falling backward, planks, and pushups. Mastering these basic moves is prerequisite to improving dynamic posture.

From the perspective of a Posture Expert, primal movements are diagnostic. Watch your patients perform a squat and evaluate for postural collapse. Where in the kinetic chain is the collapse coming from: the position of the foot and ankle, weak musculature, inward or outward bending of the knee, a misalignment of the hip, weak gluteal muscles? Understanding the cause of postural collapse during basic dynamic movements and correcting the patient's form will greatly increase their ability to move with ease, prevent injury, and improve their athletic form. Proper static and dynamic posture is the foundation for a long, high-performance sports career.

The inability to perform basic movements with the correct posture leads to habitual postural collapse and faulty bodily alignment. Postural muscles supporting the framework of the body suffer consequences of weak posture. Depending upon the postural presentation of the patient, they will present with muscular patterns that have become adaptively shortened due to prolonged contraction and stretch weakness of other muscular groups due to prolonged elongation.

People who tend to sit for many hours with a rounded spine demonstrate stretch weakness of the thoracic and lumbar paraspinal musculature, and adaptive shortening of the hip flexor complex. The paravertebral muscles supporting the spine continue to weaken if this postural presentation continues, and the hip flexors continue to tighten with lack of physical activity.

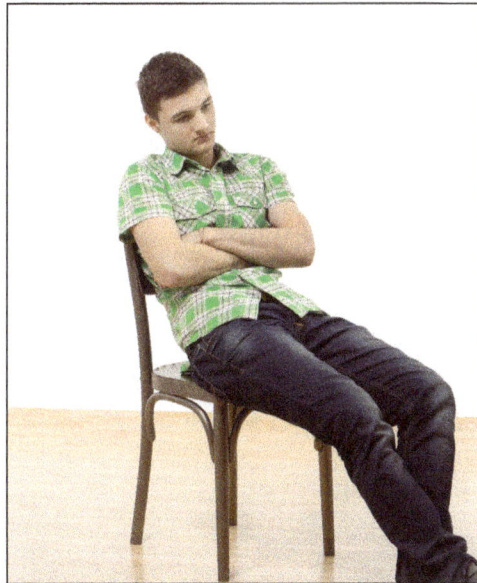

SECTION REVIEW

1. *Static* posture refers to the alignment of your body when you are not moving

2. *Dynamic* posture refers to the alignment of the body in motion

THE MOVEMENT HIERARCHY OF OPTIMAL HUMAN PERFORMANCE

When a person moves with precision, it is not by accident. The person has trained their body to be mobile and agile through proper joint biomechanics, neural balancing, and correct muscular recruitment patterns. With a strong postural framework of the body, humans move with the natural athleticism that we were designed to have. Posture principles are revolutionizing human movement to achieve optimal human performance.

Modern-day humans suffer from lack of agility because we are so sedentary. Consider an animal in nature: they are able to go from resting to running in a split second without injuring themselves. Human beings on the other hand would likely hurt themselves if they did this. Why? The modern day human framework is misaligned and inactive, creating postural immobility patterns. Even patients who are strong and workout regularly or flexible dancers and gymnasts run the risk of injury if they have asymmetric postural design.

There is a movement hierarchy predicting optimal human performance. This hierarchy includes the following components:

1. Proper spinal and pelvic alignment

2. Core control

3. Proper kinetic chain function

4. The application of proper movement principles to daily activities

Proper spinal and pelvic alignment is the base of the hierarchy, thus fundamental for optimal human performance. Proper spinal alignment should be evaluated, and postural distortion patterns should be corrected with a specific mode of postural correction: the Complete Posture Correction (which will be discussed in detail in Module 4). Postural correction strategies should be specific to the individual and not generalized. This requires balancing each part of the mobility system, including the joint mechanics, muscle recruitment patterns, and neural pathways, promoting balance and symmetry.

Core control is next on the hierarchy of optimal human performance. Core bracing is the ability to control the core musculature in order to stabilize the body upright against strong forces such as a blow to the abdomen or persistent forces such as gravity. The muscles of the core support the correct position of the spine. There are two ways to effectively utilize your core, both of which are utilized in different moments of time, specific to the activity. The first method is abdominal bracing, the second is abdominal hollowing (each is explained in detail in Module 2).

The next component of the movement hierarchy is the identification and elimination of kinetic chain dysfunctional compensation patterns to improve kinetic chain function. This includes correcting recruitment patterns of certain muscles and joints. This is accomplished by strengthening key postural muscles that have become weakened from chronic stretch, and lengthening musculature that has become adaptively shortened from chronic contraction. In Module 3 you will learn how to make accurate predictions of kinetic chain dysfunction with different presentations of postural decline. Although humans do not present with textbook postural cases, Posture Experts are highly trained to make predictions of postural distortion patterns limiting human performance, and then learn how to correct them.

Postural rehabilitation for the correction of kinetic chain dysfunction is based upon the ABCS of posture: Alignment, Balance, Core Control, and Stretching/Strengthening postural musculature. Alignment refers to proper articular alignment of the spinal column and pelvic girdle in relation to the other posture quadrants of the body. Balance refers to neurostructural balance: having symmetric structural balance and performing neurologically based training to maintain this balance. Core control again refers to strengthening core musculature to support the spine. Stretching and strengthening postural musculature refers to stretching tightened musculature and strengthening weak musculature causing postural collapse.

Once the body is in stable alignment, the application of proper movement principles into the daily lives of your patients is at the top of the hierarchy. Postural faults should be identified and corrected in a safe place so the patient can then apply proper movement principles to their daily activities. Proper movement principles prevent acute and repetitive use injuries limiting human function.

SECTION REVIEW

1. What are the components of the movement hierarchy of optimal human performance?
   - Proper spinal and pelvic alignment
   - Core control
   - Proper kinetic chain function
   - The application of proper movement principles to daily activities

2. What are the two forms of core control? *Abdominal bracing* and *abdominal hollowing*

POSTURAL FITNESS

When prompted, almost anyone can "sit up straight" or "have good posture." It is maintaining correct posture throughout the day that is difficult for the far majority of the population. The ability to maintain resilient static and dynamic posture during your activities of daily living is called postural fitness. Just as patients have to consistently workout to increase their level of physical fitness, it takes mindful commitment to postural correction to build postural fitness.

Do your patients have to be in shape to have good posture? Absolutely not. There is a posture program for everyone at all levels of physical and postural fitness. Everyone has the potential to design his or her unique posture to optimize human potential. They just need guidance. Patients will improve their human performance through compliance to their postural correction treatment plan. Posture, just like diet and exercise, is a natural biologic process that improves the function of the body when performed correctly. However, the contrary is also true. Lack of patient adherence to treatment plans prevents progress in achieving the ultimate goal of optimal human design.

Can someone be truly "fit," "healthy," or "flexible" if the bones of the spine are misaligned causing distorted muscle patterns, interruptions to the proper function of the nervous system, and improper alignment around the central axis? Being physically active while in a naturally aligned stance contributes to genuine fitness that can last well into advanced age. Real fitness merges mechanical alignment that is supported by deep core strength.

Patients lacking postural fitness tend to feel tightness in their muscles and rigidity in their joints. Lack of flexibility prevents the patient from having an open posture. Natural flexibility comes from an aligned structure. Muscles that are attached to aligned bones are more flexible, have less tension and strain, and can move bones with less fatigue.

Unnatural flexibility occurs in patients who do postural stretches to lengthen their muscles, but have not corrected the alignment of their body. Unnaturally flexible patients will feel better after they stretch, but the muscles will quickly become stiff and taut again because the body is misaligned. Patients with faulty alignment patterns lack the strength and stamina to sustain good postural presentation.

For a workout to benefit your posture, you must stay present in your body while exercising. Have your patients do dynamic movements that challenge their physiology. The only exercises worth doing are those that work with the body's design, not against it. Good exercise form is an elongated spine, a solidly anchored pelvis, a stable core, natural diaphragmatic breathing, flexible, efficient superficial muscles, and open, free moving joints. Dysfunctional movement patterns that are not initiated from the deep core put repeated stress on joints, creating imbalance, wearing down cartilage, and restricting full ranges of motion.

The contrary to postural fitness is postural aging. Everyone has a unique posture, and at any given moment patients are either working to increase postural fitness or accelerating postural aging. With natural aging, the bones themselves bend and collapse in the ways in which pressure and compressive forces have been applied to them. This is the basic principle of Wolff's Law. Muscles and connective tissues shorten or lengthen based upon the positions that they have maintained for prolonged periods of time.

Postural aging is accelerated or decelerated based upon the postural habits that your patients practice on a daily basis. The process of postural aging is accelerated as the body adapts to the postural inefficiencies of the external environment. The process is decelerated as patients create postural fitness habit loops. The postural age of your patients does not imply how old they are; it implies where they are on the spectrum of postural fitness.

SECTION REVIEW

1. The ability to maintain resilient static and dynamic posture during your activities of daily living is called *postural fitness*

2. The process of *postural aging* is accelerated as the body adapts to the postural inefficiencies of the external environment

CONFIDENCE AND BODY LANGUAGE

In addition to the health benefits of proper posture, the aesthetic appeal of proper posture is an additional benefit that patients will love. Remember, there are three primary motivating factors driving patients into healthcare offices. These consumer behaviors are to look better, move better, or feel better. Posture Experts have a favorable presence in the healthcare market as postural correction addresses each of these intrinsic needs of patients.

Posture is the expression of mind and body. How you feel inside is demonstrated by how you carry your body in space. The psychology and the physiology of your body are interrelated.

Consider the term "emotion". The word "e-motion" literally means "from movement", meaning that individuals have a sensory experience (a sensation) and create movement patterns from this sensation. Every day you see how people express e-motions. When someone is sad or timid, they have a slumped, closed posture with rounded shoulders.

When patients have confidence, are excited and happy, they present with an open posture: their shoulders pulled back, head up, and tight core musculature. The movement of opening your arms in the air with flexed fists demonstrates joy and victory, and opening your arms to embrace another person demonstrates love. Our natural human emotions are expressed through our physiologic posture.

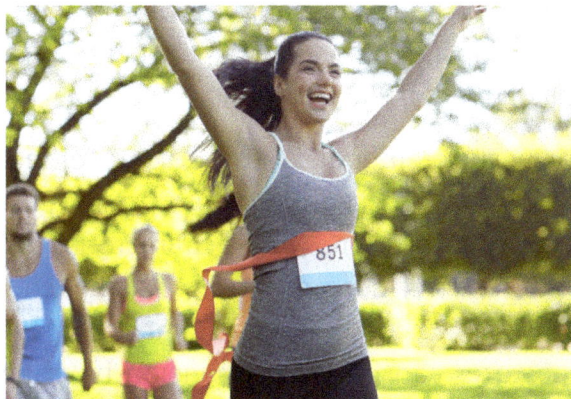

Proper posture demonstrates confidence and is attributed to a good appearance. Body language and appearance are important when interacting with others in society. In communication, 93% of it is non-verbal, meaning that *how* you present the information is often more important than the information presented. Proper posture contributes to better body language and non-verbal communication cues.

In addition to having more impactful communication, people who have symmetrical posture are considered to be more desirable human beings. Scheib, Gangestad and Thornhill (1999) demonstrate an association between body symmetry and higher sexual prowess, physical dominance, emotional stability, and fidelity.

An interesting research study was done at Harvard University regarding power postures. When the body is in an open power pose, the person not only looks more confident, but they actually are more confident. The research shows that holding a power pose for just 2 minutes at a time increases the levels of testosterone that the body produces, and decreases levels of cortisol. High testosterone levels are associated with power and dominance, whereas low cortisol levels are associated with decreased stress.

Patients can literally change their physiology to be more powerful with proper posture. According to Carney et al. (2010), power postures "cause neuroendocrine and behavioral changes [including] elevations in testosterone, decreases in cortisol, and increased feelings of power and tolerance for risk." Patients with proper posture embody self-confidence and power due to neuroendocrine changes in physiology

Posture extends into cognitive processing. Individuals who have a positive, upright posture have a higher level of self-perceived leadership. Arnette (2012) describes the psychologic connection of posture, indicating that body posture affects the cognitive and emotional state of patients. Patients presenting with aligned posture are more likely to see themselves as leaders than patients who present with timid posture. A higher perception of leadership also correlated to patients' demeanor during interviews, meetings, and when making important decisions.

Researchers found that posture embodies attitude and self-evaluation. Two groups of participants in this study were asked to sit with proper posture or with slumped posture and self-evaluate their best and worst characteristics. They concluded that people who present with an erect posture (straight spine, chest out, and shoulders back) had a more positive mentality with a confident self-image. According to Brinol et al. (2009), "body postures can impact persuasion by affecting the direction of thoughts" from negative to positive. The results concluded that the group sitting with correct posture viewed themselves with more positive characteristics than negative, while the group with bad posture found more negative characteristics than positive.

Your posture right now is literally an expression of not only how you feel mentally, but what chemicals your body is producing physiologically. Posture is more than skin deep. Your unique posture is not only a presentation of your mental and physical health and wellbeing now, but a prediction of sustainable wellness throughout the lifecycle.

SECTION REVIEW

1. Power postures have been shown to decrease hormonal levels of *cortisol* and to increase levels of *testosterone*

2. Researchers found that posture embodies attitude and *self-evaluation*

Module 2

THE PRINCIPAL ANATOMIC POSTURE QUADRANTS AND THEIR PHYSIOLOGIC FUNCTIONS

INTRODUCTION

Module 1 provided a clear understanding of the theoretical principles of posture and the determinants of healthy and weak postural presentations. Posture is a foundational component of a healthy lifestyle, affecting the manner in which humans move, feel, and present themselves. To improve postural presentation is to improve quality of controlled and balanced movements, relieving the body of unnecessary stressors. This helps patients feel better and function at a higher level of human performance.

From an aesthetic standpoint, a good postural presentation means core activation and the efficient utilization of postural muscles to stand up tall with an elongated spine and an anchored center of gravity. As the kinetic chain moves in synchronicity, the person moves with grace and confidence.

Patients' unique postural presentations are due to their lifestyle habits. The current posture epidemic has been demonstrated, showing the growing market need for talented Posture Experts to inspire change among their patients and to increase awareness of the emerging posture paradigm of health. Modern day stressors, dependence upon technology, occupational uniplanar repetitive movements, and an overall sedentary lifestyle of the majority of the population are triggering the postural degeneration cycle. These are the key contributing factors to the societal epidemic of weak posture.

Humans are de-evolving at the speed of technology. The most intelligent postural presentation in the animal kingdom is an upright human stance: the ability to efficiently resist gravity and perform precise movements with our upper extremity while staying grounded to the earth in a balanced bipedal position. Humans are dynamic beings, designed to move. With an increase in sedentary lifestyles throughout the world, commonly associated with occupations requiring humans to be seated all day, the level of postural intelligence worldwide is decreasing.

Patients are now presenting with postural collapse as their normal daily postural presentation. Postural collapse is indicated by forward head posture, anterior shoulder rotation, weak core activation, C-shaped thoracic spine with an increased lumbar lordosis (while standing), and unevenly balanced weight distribution over the hips, legs, and feet. Postural collapse is a closed, inefficient postural distortion pattern representing a lesser level of intellect among human beings. The human race is de-evolving in terms of physiological functionality; the evidence is all around you.

Each unique individual has the ability to improve their postural presentation, to improve their health. Changing the postural framework of the body is a natural biologic process that requires mindful intentions. The majority of individuals live their lives in a habitual, mindless state of self. They are unaware of their weak postural presentation until they reach a point of symptomatic pain and discomfort preventing them from doing their daily activities with ease. Instead of living habitually with poor posture, patients can be helped by Posture Experts to become mindful of how their body is holding itself upright in space, how the body is moving to perform actions, and how the body interacts with the environmental laws of the universe.

Increased mindfulness renders tremendous advantages in making long-term postural correction changes for patients. As posture becomes a conscious action, the patient makes intentional lifestyle decisions that support the design of the body, not weaken it. As the natural biologic process continues in the efficient posture cycle, the patient begins to develop postural fitness, or the ability to maintain resilient posture for prolonged periods of time without experiencing postural collapse. As postural fitness increases, the patient becomes healthier and more able to live well. Posture by mindful design, not by the circumstances of the environment—that is the goal of understanding and implementing the principles of posture.

Module 1 provided a strong theoretical foundation leading into Module 2. In Module 2 we will discuss the scientific principles of posture. Throughout this module, expect to gain a better understanding of the physiologic posture system with emphasis on The principal anatomic posture quadrants and their physiologic functions. The discussion will begin with the developmental stages of posture, ending with an emphasis on the effects of posture on the neurologic system, balance ability, and functional respiratory capacity.

DEVELOPMENTAL STAGES OF POSTURE

Now you have a clear understanding of the posture principles, Module 2 will discuss more specifically the anatomy and physiology of the posture system. The natural progression of this module thus begins with emphasis on the developmental stages of posture.

At what age does posture become important for your patients? Just as many developmental milestones begin in utero, so does postural development. The patterns that occur during pregnancy and during birth will lead an individual to develop a certain posture throughout their childhood and adolescent development, and thus throughout the rest of their lives. The posture maintained by the mother during pregnancy and during labor will also affect the postural development of the fetus.

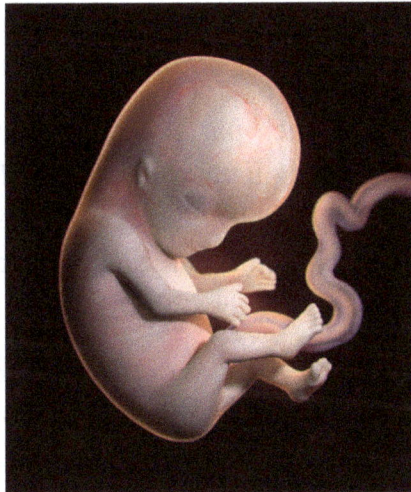

The fetus in the womb has a C-shaped curvature of the developing spine. The first curve that babies are born with is the thoracic kyphotic curve due to their postural position in the womb. The most common fetal presentation, especially in the final weeks of pregnancy, is the cephalad position.

The most compact position for the fetus is with the upper and lower extremities approximated, curling in opposing directions, causing a resultant rotation about the longitudinal axis. This rotational pattern stays with the fetus and baby through development into adulthood. After the baby is born, they will have a natural tendency to maintain the thoracic fetal position.

The ideal position for the baby pre-labor is with the baby's chin tucked under and its spine facing to the front of the mother's body. The labor process can be quite strenuous for the infant, particularly in the cervical spine.

According to Gutmann (1987), birth trauma remains an un-publicized and therefore significantly under-treated problem. Gutmann evaluated the prevalence of nerve dysfunction among newborn babies, concluding that 80% of newborns have nerve dysfunction after the birthing process. When Fryman (1992) evaluated 1,250 babies just 5 days after being born, he found that 95% of the babies evaluated presented with nerve dysfunction and cervical strain.

Cranial bones are often permanently modified by birth trauma before full ossification takes place. The majority of the cranial bones of the fetus are relatively flat plates consisting of one layer of primary cancellous bone with no serrations.

There are six fontanelles, one at each parietal angle, one at each mastoid, one at lambda in the occiput and one at bregma in the frontals. The base of the fetal skull is comprised of the occiput, made up of four flat cartilages and the temporal bones, each containing six separate cartilages. This anatomical presentation allows for a great deal of prenatal molding of the fetal skull (Pope, 2003).

The mechanism of labor refers to the changes of the fetus as it passes through the birth canal. The skull of the infant is highly vulnerable to forces of labor. Uterine contractions normally exert a pressure on the amniotic cavity, and subsequently on the fetus itself, varying from 4.5–26.5lb per square inch (Pope, 2003).

Since the occiput is typically the presenting anatomic part, it receives the most pressure. With the occipital presentation, the head must undergo several movements to accommodate the maternal bony pelvis. This process has been divided into seven movements: engagement, flexion, descent, rotation, extension, restitution, and expulsion. Expulsion is the final delivery of the fetus from the birth canal and includes delivery of the right shoulder and then the left shoulder.

The fetal skull must move against the resistance of the maternal symphysis. It is thought that this resistance is sufficient to keep the squamous portion of the occiput from achieving complete restitution (Fryman, 1992).

After delivery, most of the distortion of the fetal skull is corrected by the infant through crying, which balloons the skull, and by sucking, which flexes the sphenobasilar junction thus normalizing the pull of the intracranial membranes. There is an ongoing relationship of functional continuity between the distortions of the infant's head and the sacral base angle. The sacrum maintains the same tilt pattern as the occiput because the meninges of the spinal cord attach firmly to the foramen magnum, the second and third cervical vertebrae and the second sacral segment (Pope, 2003).

The mother's postural presentation during pregnancy and pre-labor health choices can reduce the strain of labor and reduce the incidence of infant birth trauma. Women who present with an aligned pelvis and straight spine demonstrate less pain and trauma during delivery.

As weight is added on to the front of the mother-to-be during pregnancy, common postural distortion patterns arise. With a shift in the center of gravity, the pregnant mother often leans back and juts the abdomen forward. Preparation for labor is greatly enhanced by sitting, standing, and squatting with proper posture, and knowing how to release the pelvic floor.

When the mother is in proper alignment, the core muscles function like a hammock that cradles the baby from below and helps hold the belly in place. After delivery, strengthening the transverse abdominis can repair the overstretched rectus abdominis muscles. As the transverse abdominis muscle tones, its horizontal fibers have a cinching effect on the waist.

Once the baby has been born, given the ability to thrive, the baby will begin to grow and develop physically and mentally, with 65% of neurological development occurring in the baby's first year of life (Chestnut, 2003). The need for an aligned spine during the first year of life is of utmost importance to improve the child's ability to create correct neural patterns. Nerve dysfunction during this period of life can alter their developmental skills.

Statistics demonstrate that 47.9% of children land on their head at least once in the first year of life, experiencing stress to the head and cervical spine. Babies will continue to challenge their physiology as they grow. It is estimated that the average child will experience 2,500 falls before the age of 7 (Del Rosso, 2004).

As the baby begins to grow, the ability to maintain an erect posture is shaped through the development of the anterior lumbar curvature and the anterior cervical curvature. The first curve that babies develop is the thoracic kyphotic curve. As they begin to gain control of their head, the baby will develop the cervical lordotic curvature. With further development, the baby gains the ability to crawl and eventually walk, shaping the lumbar lordotic curvature.

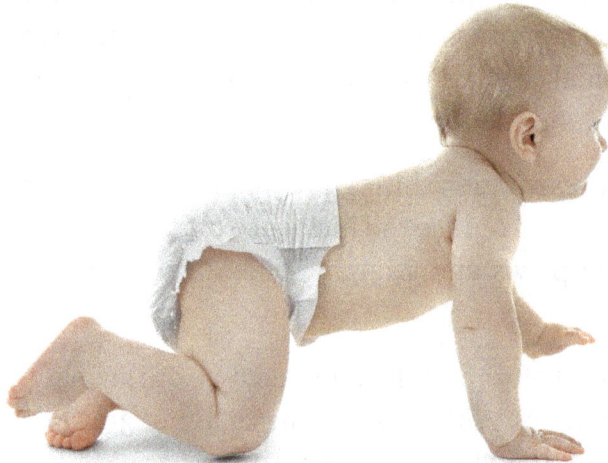

For developing babies, the ability to sit up, crawl, stand, and walk is dependent upon the development of their core strength. Core strength is gained by the child being face down and pushing up, commonly called "tummy time." Tummy time is very important for the development of infants. While on their stomach and pushing up, the baby is strengthening their upper body and mastering new motor skills such as reaching and pivoting, common precursors to crawling. They also develop the skills to support their head in an upright position, and learn to respond to stimuli from a new viewpoint. This new "view of the world" will stimulate the child to move their head around, learning to respond to stimuli while supporting the weight of the head (Shapiro, 2014).

A common mistake that parents make during tummy time is propping a baby up on a pillow. Propping the baby up diminishes the core activation, and can weaken the developmental skills necessary for initiating proper mobility patterns. Core strength and spinal curvature development are fundamental stages of pediatric development. Educating new parents of the importance of tummy time is essential to postural development. With each action parents do, they are either supporting the baby's natural development or preventing it.

New parents are often overwhelmed with suggestions of how to be "good parents", some of which may be confusing. Consider the "Back to Sleep" campaign, for example. This campaign to prevent Sudden Infant Death Syndrome (SIDS) educated parents not to lay babies on their stomachs. Although the intention of the campaign was to prevent SIDS, other side effects were noted from not laying babies on their stomach.

The increased presence of plagiocephaly, or having a flat spot on the baby's head from lying on their backs, was a notable effect. Lack of core strength and lagging head syndrome were also revealed. According to Porter (2006), 90% of children diagnosed with autism at age 3 or 4 showed evidence of head lag. Allowing adequate tummy time for infants plays a significant role in their physiologic and neurologic development.

When babies are given the environment to thrive, they are posture role models for adults. What seems to be a strange concept in reality makes complete sense. They are developing habits that support the natural framework of their bodies, whereas the majority of adults make lifestyle decisions that deteriorate their posture. Babies have flexible hips, allowing them to squat while keeping their backs straight and avoiding buckling forward at the waist. With a properly aligned spine, babies can perform foundational exercises of human movement.

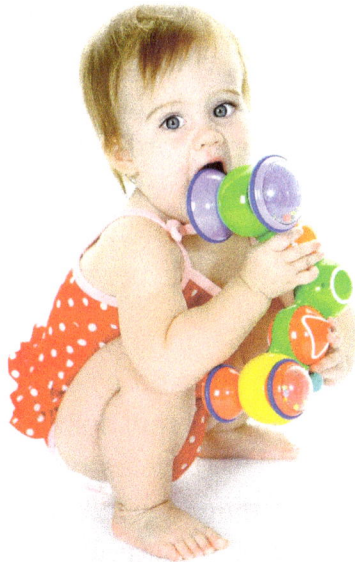

Babies also demonstrate efficient posture while seated. They have a well-anchored pelvis and straight, well-supported spine. When they bend forward while seated, they move with the whole pelvis and keep their spines straight. They don't buckle forward into a C-shaped curve like adults do. Babies truly are remarkable examples of proper posture. This is another concept supporting the fact that genetic predisposition supports proper posture; we were created to move properly. It is our lifestyle choices that prevent human beings from maintaining this postural presentation.

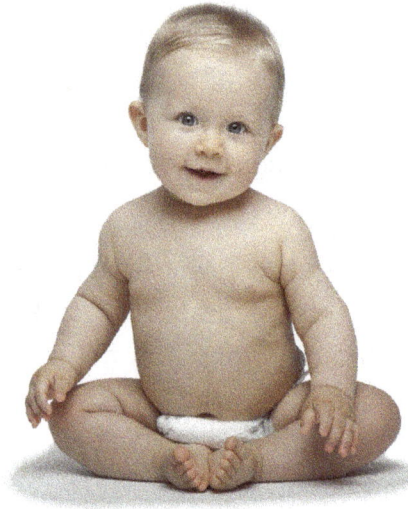

As babies develop into children, they begin experiencing events that shape their posture further. At approximately 6–7 years old, children develop good arch formation of the feet. With the development of strong arch formation, children's gait patterns change from a flat-footed walk to a much more coordinated, dynamic movement. Children who lack proper arch development will develop postural distortion patterns. Many young children also demonstrate hyperextension of their knees due to weak ligamentous development in younger years. Knee hyperextension generally autocorrects as ligaments strengthen.

There is a genetic predisposition in the far majority of people for left-brain dominance, or left cerebral lateralization. Common left-brain dominant characteristics include right hand and foot dominance. Between 8–10 years old, children develop handedness posture patterns. As children become more dependent on the utilization of their dominant hand at school and during hobbies, their posture begins to create compensatory patterns.

Between 10–15 years of age, children who present with abnormal lateral curvatures of their spine, or scoliosis, will start to show visible indications. Scoliosis affects 2–3%

of the population, or an estimated 6–9 million people in the United States. Scoliosis can develop in infancy or early childhood, idiopathic scoliosis being more common than congenital scoliosis. Females are eight times more likely to progress to a curve magnitude that requires treatment. Every year, scoliosis patients make more than 600,000 visits to private physician offices, an estimated 30,000 children are fitted with a brace, and 38,000 patients undergo spinal fusion surgery (National Scoliosis Foundation, 2007).

There are many contributing factors to the development of postural patterns, primarily: lifestyle choices, genetic predisposition, developmental influences, and structural asymmetries. The patterns that humans develop early in life affect their postural development for the rest of their lives. Smooth and fluid movements of the trunk and limbs characterize healthy posture, associated with positive health outcomes. Unhealthy posture is characterized as disconnected, labored, and less efficient movements due to unfavorable developmental conditions.

SECTION REVIEW

1. The development of strong *arch formation* changes children's gait patterns from a flat-footed walk to a much more coordinated, dynamic movement

2. Between 8–10 years old, children develop *handedness* posture patterns

3. Which population is more commonly affected by scoliosis during adolescence, females or males? *Females*

ANATOMY OF THE POSTURE SYSTEM

Human beings are extraordinarily complex functional organisms with a high level of intelligence. The human body is made up of many complex systems working together in synchronicity to keep the person within their normal range of homeostatic function. These auto-regulating systems include the neurologic system, respiratory system, digestive system, circulatory system, lymphatic system, and many more to produce life-sustaining actions. Each system works together, allowing the body to move, breath, digest food, produce energy, have clear thoughts, stay upright, and adapt to the world in which we live. In addition to these life-sustaining systems of the body is the posture system. Until this point, the posture system of the body has not been defined.

The posture system is equally as complex as the other physiologic systems of the body. The purpose of the posture system is to keep the body upright and erect against the ever-present force of gravity, stabilizing the core of the body while the limbs perform coordinated movements. The posture system integrates sensorimotor feedback from the brain to the body to adapt, balance, and stay upright in response to an ever-changing environment.

Anatomically, the posture system of the body includes an integrated system composed of osseous components, postural muscles, and neuroanatomical tissues. Principal osseous components of the posture system include the spine, in terms of the four essential curves (cervical, thoracic, lumbar, and sacral), the ribcage, the clavicles, the scapulae, the bony pelvis, the patellae, and the bones of the feet.

Principal postural muscles include: the rhomboids, the pectoral muscles, the diaphragm, the transverse abdominis, the external obliques, the multifidi, the pelvic floor, the iliopsoas, the hamstrings, the gluteus medius, and the tensor fascia latae. Principal neuroanatomical tissues include the cerebellum, the pontomedullary reticular formation, the vestibular system, and the reticulospinal tracts.

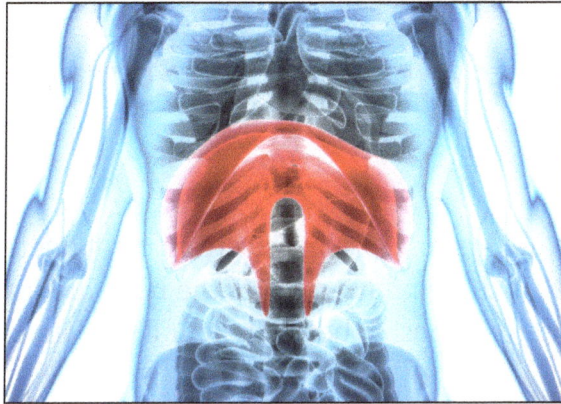

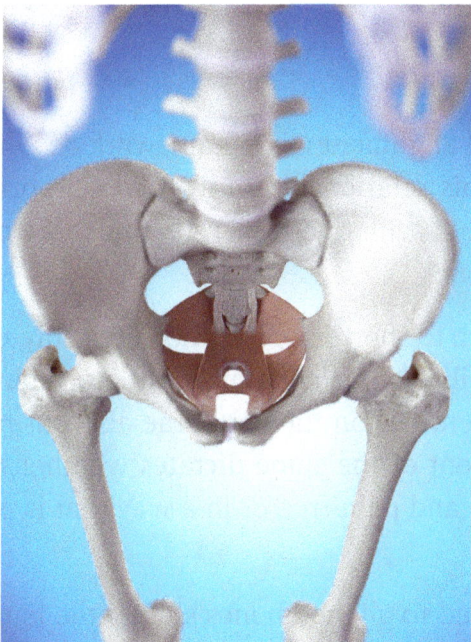

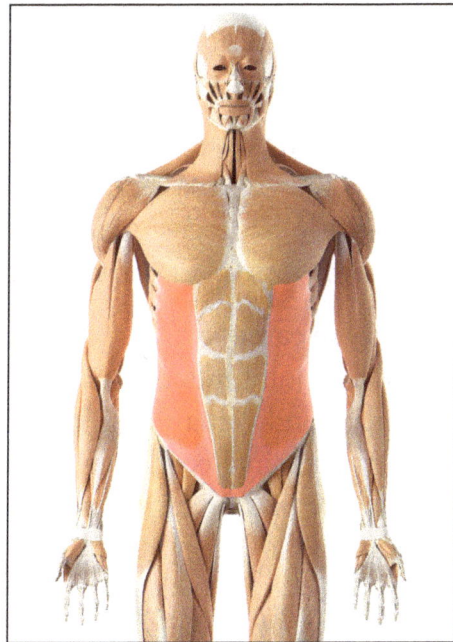

SECTION REVIEW

1. The purpose of the *posture system* is to keep the body upright and erect against the ever-present force of gravity

2. The posture system includes which three components? *Osseous, muscular,* and *neurologic*

PHYSIOLOGY OF THE POSTURE SYSTEM

Physiologically, the posture system combines certain components of the neuromusculoskeletal system. The structure and function of the body are interrelated at all levels. Human function is an interrelationship between neural, skeletal, and muscular function for postural control.

Skeletal physiology

The skeleton's role in posture is key. Skeletal alignment is the framework on which stability is constructed. By not recognizing this relationship of aligned support, many healthcare professionals focus solely on the muscular patterns, creating more postural distortion patterns instead of correcting them.

A misaligned spine causes muscles that attach to shorten or lengthen unevenly, creating chronic stress and joint immobility. Immobility of articulations will later manifest as arthritis for many individuals. Compressive forces on the vertebrae also put pressure on and distort the spinal cord. The alignment of the spine dictates whether muscles will work in a way that is natural, efficient, and pain-free or in a way that is prone to repetitive injury.

Muscles function best when they are attached to aligned bones so that the length and the configuration of the muscle fibers are elastic and balanced. Unbalanced actions eventually become tension, stiffness, and pain.

The bones of the skeletal system are dynamically alive; they are made up of nutrients and manufacture blood cells. They are able to withstand extraordinary compressive forces, but also malleable enough to undergo a continuous process of being remodeled and modified. Chronically distorted structural alignment can lead to spinal degeneration and malformation such as osteophyte formation.

Bones work as levers about the joints that are fulcrums for agile movement. Joints are bone-to-bone connections held together by fibrous, cartilaginous, or synovial tissue.

Joints vary greatly in their functions; some articulations allow full range of motion among diverse axes and other articulations limit motion to specific axes or are immovable. The more flexible a joint is, the less stability it has. The inverse is also true: the more stability the joint has, the less flexible it is. Dynamic movements occur at articulations, synchronously moving bones, muscles, and connective tissues.

Muscular physiology

As the muscular and skeletal systems interact within the posture system, they provide support, strength, stability, and flexibility while weight bearing. In addition, muscles contract and relax to perform movements of the skeletal system around articulations.

Muscles function best when they are attached to aligned bones so that the length and the configuration of the muscle fibers are elastic and balanced. A muscle should be long enough to permit normal mobility of the joints and short enough to contribute to joint stability. Muscle length is affected by postural distortion patterns; unbalanced muscular actions eventually become tension, stiffness, and pain.

There are vertical and horizontal muscular structures of the body, the majority being vertical. Vertical structures create movement. Consider powerful muscle groups of the lower extremity that contribute to ambulation, such as the quadriceps muscle group and the hamstring musculature. These vertical muscle groups are essential in producing powerful movements that contribute to human function.

Horizontal structures of the body serve another purpose. Their primary purpose is to stabilize the body upright while static or performing human movements. Principal horizontal muscles for postural stability include the diaphragm, the transverse abdominis, and the pelvic floor musculature.

Performing controlled movement requires an agonist and antagonist muscle. Agonist muscles are the main muscles utilized to perform motion. Antagonist muscles are the counterparts to dynamic motion. Antagonist muscles oppose the agonist muscle to stabilize the body and prevent hyperextension, but still allow full range of motion of the agonist muscle group.

Reciprocal inhibition is a process in which agonist and antagonist muscle groups work together to move and stabilize the body, supporting controlled motions.

Reciprocal inhibition is extremely important for postural correction, because as you strengthen one muscle, another one lengthens, and vice versa. It is important to recognize these relationships and to utilize reciprocal inhibition as a benefit for postural correction.

For long-term functional correction, it is not adequate to look at certain muscles individually. The Posture Expert must view the organism as a whole and correct all necessary components of coupled motion to improve overall postural fitness.

Skeletal muscle fibers are composed of two different types. Type 1 muscle fibers are red slow twitch fibers. These are predominately postural muscles to resist gravity. Type 2 muscle fibers are white fast twitch fibers. These are predominately the muscles of the limbs to carry out rapid and powerful movements.

Muscle fibers are arranged in three types of fasciculi arrangements. The arrangement of the fasciculi is correlated with the muscles' ability to exert power. Long fusiform muscles have greater range of motion, but less power. Muscles with pennate fasciculi arrangement have less flexibility but more strength. Fusiform muscular arrangement is when muscle fibers run parallel to the origin and insertion and attach to flat tendons at each end. Long fusiform muscles are most susceptible to stretch. In a pennate arrangement, muscle fibers run obliquely into the tendon that runs the length of the muscle. Pennate muscles are least vulnerable to stretch. Fan-shaped muscle fibers have their own origin with a common insertion.

Connective tissue physiology

Connective tissue joins anatomic structures to perform fluid movement patterns. Ligaments join bones together. They contain nerve endings that are important for reflexes and proprioception. Tendons attach muscles to bones. They are not highly vascularized, but they do have sensory nerve endings in the Golgi Tendon Organs. Tendons have great tensile strength but are inflexible.

Connective tissue is defined by Rolf (1990) as the "Organ of Posture" due to its intimate correlation with fluid bodily movements. Connective fascia is made up of ground substance that is a liquid crystalline matrix. Healthy fascia is composed of silky sheaths around muscles allowing them to glide easily as we move. Compression and stretching of connective tissue causes the matrix to become more fibrous. The greater the amount of fiber within the connective tissue, the more stiff the body becomes. Eventually fascial sheaths overlap and stick together, creating muscle adhesions.

Fascia is found in sheets or bands of fibroelastic connective tissue throughout the body. Comprised primarily of longitudinal fibers, fascia moves most freely during lateral bending and rotational movements. Deep fascia compartmentalizes organs, muscles, and nerves for protection.

Neurologic physiology

The neurological component of the posture system serves to stimulate and coordinate complex movements, to balance the body, and for purposes of training proper postural patterns.

Trying to change postural habits by commanding your posture with the cortical brain is inadequate. Posture programming requires activation of the subcortical centers, including the brainstem and limbic system, through sensations, perceptions, and emotions. Once the foundation for efficient posture is neurologically wired, the body becomes more adaptable because it is operating efficiently from a biological standpoint.

Postural control involves multisensory pathways, including visual, vestibular, and somatosensory data from proprioceptor and cutaneous receptors. The central nervous system uses this sensory information to create an internal frame of reference that regulates the center of gravity.

Somatosensory monitors include neck and lower limb proprioceptors and pressor receptors from the feet. Feedback from these receptors is used to initiate postural compensation resulting in the activation of muscle groups to maintain or restore equilibrium through body sway. The central nervous system can also prepare against or anticipate disturbance in the center of gravity or the center of mass through feed forward control from visual and vestibular input. The vestibular system is responsible for stabilizing the position of the body with the head and eyes in space.

Patterns of motion are controlled by three parts of the brain. The primitive brainstem organizes responsive motions such as digestion, heartbeat, reflexes, and monitors learned activities such as walking and riding a bike. The limbic brain monitors tactile, kinesthetic, and emotional connection of movement. The more developed cerebral cortex is activated while learning new movement patterns.

The upright posture and cognitive perceptions of the human being are neurologically the most developed system in nature. This postural presentation allows the neurology of the body to operate with optimal function. When the body is overwhelmed by stress, it causes neural connections of survival and physical breakdown, thus limiting the functional capability of the individual. Constant stress means the body is out of homeostasis, or out of balance. This is physically seen as "protective posture" or closed posture.

Proprioception is a neurologic experience that our bodies have with the environment to orient ourselves in time and space. Spinal mechanoreceptors provide continuous feedback of where our bodies are in space to keep us upright against gravity. Spinal mechanoreceptors are sensitive to the position of the body, bodily motion, vibration, pressure, and temperature. Depolarization of mechanoreceptors initiates cortical activity that is responsible for postural alterations (Kandel, Schwartz, and Jessell, 1991).

Mechanoreceptors are divided into four different types. Type IV mechanoreceptors are nociceptors, meaning that these mechanoreceptors provide the information to the brain that perceives pain. The stimulus of pain is transmitted along the spinothalamic tract to the sensory cortex where it is perceived and understood to be a painful stimulus. Nociceptors not only sense pain, but they initiate a sympathetic response. Sympathetic responses include conditions of sweating, vomiting, abdominal pain, and dyspnea.

Types I–III mechanoreceptors inhibit nociception. Thus to inhibit pain, the most effective way of doing so is by increasing the function of mechanoreceptors types I–III. Restricted joint motion causes an increased firing in nociceptive axons and a decrease in firing of large diameter mechanoreceptor axons (Hooshmand, 1993). Inhibition of nociceptive bombardment to the sensory cortex by types I–III mechanoreceptors occurs at the spinal column. When mechanoreceptors are activated, they shut down the nociceptive output via endorphins and enkephalins at that spinal level.

By inducing motion into a joint, mechanoreceptive feedback is processed in the cortex and midbrain, thus causing a change in the periaqueductal gray, the area that releases the neurotransmitter serotonin. The effect of serotonin is a feeling of wellness and happiness, initiating a down regulation of nociception. The more mechanoreception, or movement, a person has in their joints, the less pain they will experience. In addition, fluidity of movement among the spinal joints inhibits the central hyperactivity sympathetic state.

The cerebellum plays a significant role in postural control. The cerebellum has multiple functions such as coordination and fine-tuning of learned movements. One of the cerebellum's neurologic functions is to provide control over the timing of the body's movements. It accomplishes this by a loop circuit that connects the cerebellum and the motor cortex, modulating the signals that the motor cortex sends to the motor neurons.

The cerebellum consists of three regions. The vestibulocerebellum is connected to the vestibule of the inner ear and assists in balance control. The spinocerebellum is connected to the spinal cord and controls postural muscle activity by influencing muscle tonus. To play its role in maintaining body posture, a muscle must be tensed. The cerebellum therefore controls muscle tension at all times while releasing those muscles required to execute movements. The cerebrocerebellum contributes to controlled and coordinated voluntary movements.

Patients presenting with cerebellar syndrome have problems in coordinating balance, gait, and posture. These patients have an uncertain gait, spreading their feet more widely apart as they strike the ground. While standing in place, these patients have a wider base stance and they cannot tilt their trunks forward or backward without losing their balance.

The vestibular system also plays a significant role in postural control. The earliest indication of vestibular control is seen in the newborn with the labyrinthine reflex. This postural reflex depends upon stimuli from both vestibular organs and functions to automatically extend the head and hold it in an orthostatic posture. Each vestibular apparatus exerts control over the ipsilateral extensor or antigravity muscle on both sides of the body. The left vestibular apparatus primarily affects the left antigravity muscles while the right vestibular apparatus similarly affects the right side.

There is a congenital or genetic bias toward one-sided vestibular dominance called vestibular lateralization. Left vestibular dominance occurs in roughly two-thirds of the human population. Previc (1991) describes a possible prenatal mechanism for the origin of left vestibular dominance.

"Because the right side of the body faces outward in the left fetal position, the acceleratory component to the maternal walk would, from the standpoint of the fetus, be registered rightward. The more salient inertial force would consequently be leftward, providing for a more effective stimulation of the left utricle..."

Previc, 1991, p. 12

This promotes early growth and development of left vestibular neural and cortical control.

Antigravity extension is of utmost importance in achieving postural correction. Sick, degenerated posture is flexor dominant, while healthy posture is extensor dominant. Holding the body upright is maintained by monosynaptic stretch reflexes operating at the level of the spinal cord, excitatory ipsilateral input from the vestibular organs, and inhibitory input from the neck proprioceptors and the frontal cortex.

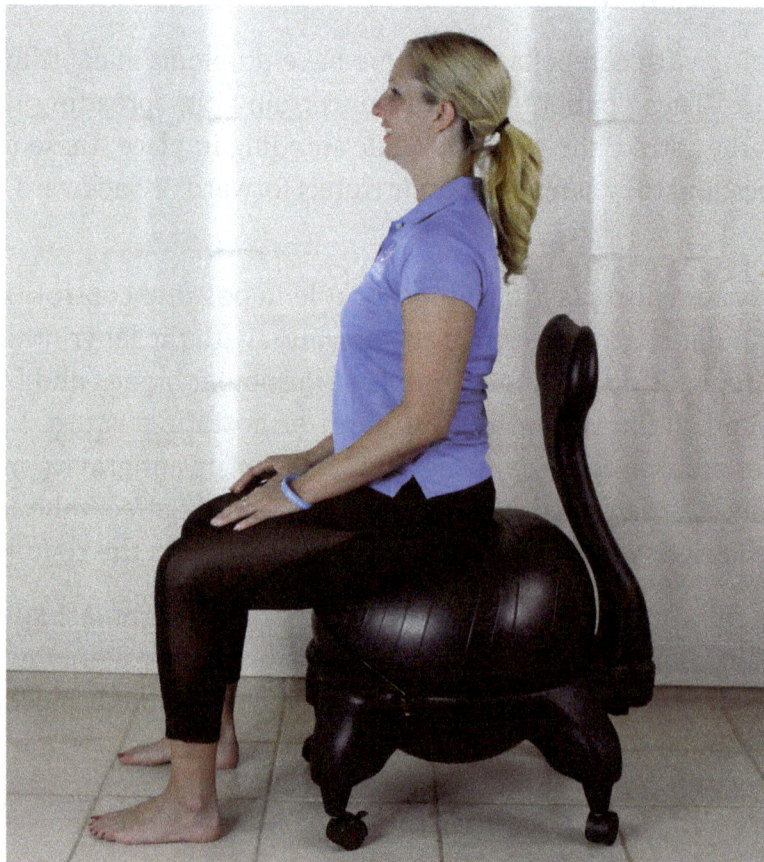

With general activities of daily living, one leg is primarily used for postural support (vestibular dominance) and the other for most voluntary activities (motor dominance). Kicking a ball is a very common example. Most people kick with the motor dominant right leg while simultaneously supporting themselves with the vestibular dominant left leg. In support for this premise it has been demonstrated that the majority of the adult population has greater size and muscle mass of the left leg (Pope, 2003).

There are multiple reflexes that affect patients' postural presentations. While we're standing or moving, our body tends to automatically assume particular postures based on the combination of these reflexive responses. The posture reflexes include the Tonic Neck Reflex, the Righting Reflex, and the Vestibulospinal Reflex.

The Tonic Neck Reflex describes the automatic positioning of the limbs in response to a movement of the head on the cervical spine. When the head is rotated in the yaw, there is an increase in the extensor tone on the two limbs on the side of the nose, or the side that the jaw is pointing to, and a decrease in extension and flexion on the opposite side.

When the position of the head or body changes, reflex movements occur that tend to return the head or body to the normal posture. This is called the Righting Reflex. The input to this reflex is a combination of vestibular, visual, and somatosensory.

The purpose of the vestibulospinal reflex is to stabilize the body. Extensor activity is induced on the side to which the head is inclined, and flexor activity is induced on the opposite side. Extensor tone changes according to the position of the head with respect to horizontal. Extensor tone is maximal when the angle of the head is 45 degrees with respect to the horizon.

SECTION REVIEW

1. Principal horizontal muscles for postural stability include: *diaphragm*, the *transverse abdominis*, and the *pelvic floor musculature*

2. Which type of musculature is for postural stabilization? *Type I?*

3. What do types I–III mechanoreceptors inhibit? *Nociception*

4. The purpose of the *vestibulospinal* reflex is to stabilize the body

NEUROLOGY OF THE POSTURE SYSTEM

Now we will take an even more in-depth look at the hierarchy of neurology that directly controls the posture system. There are multiple aspects of the neurologic system that contribute to proper posture. The main systems that work together for postural stability include the visual system, the vestibular system, and the somatosensory system.

The visual system contributes to postural control by delivering information from the retina to different areas in the brain that allow for object identification and movement control. Patients who present with visual impairments may have an impaired ability to control their posture and their balance, especially during movement.

The vestibular system, which consists of organs located in the inner ear, contributes by interpreting changes in movement, direction, and velocity or speed of movements. This information is sent to the brainstem, which then creates a response that allows your postural muscles to activate and increases your body awareness. The vestibular system can be affected in patients who present with balance disorders.

The somatosensory system is a complex system of nerve cells that responds to changes to the surface or internal state of the body. Somatic senses are those senses we feel with our bodies, including sensations of touch and pressure, pain and temperature, and muscle and joint position, also called proprioception. The somatosensory system contributes to the posture system by relaying information about body position to the brain, allowing it to activate the appropriate motor response or movement.

Specific receptors or gauges called proprioceptors are located in our muscles, tendons, and joints. These are the receptors that are able to tell our brain whether our knee is bent or straight, whether we are bearing weight or not, and which muscles are contracting and which are relaxing at any moment. Inadequate proprioception alters our body sense and causes faulty posture patterns.

The visual system

The visual system is very important to posture in order to keep our bodies vertical to the horizon and eyes parallel to the horizon. This is an evolved humanistic behavior.

Keeping our head upright with the eyes parallel to the horizon is literally one of the most important human characteristics that we possess. There are 3 Cranial Nerves—Cranial Nerve III, the Oculomotor Nerve; Cranial Nerve IV, the Trochlear Nerve; and Cranial Nerve VI, the Abducens Nerve—that are all dedicated to controlling the muscles that produce movements of the eyes throughout the cardinal fields of gaze.

Properly functioning eye muscles are vitally important to the posture and function of your patients. Consider each muscle and its actions. There are four recti muscles, all of which originate at the Annulus of Zinn.

- The Superior Rectus, innervated by the Oculomotor Nerve, performs in torsion and adduction from neutral

- The Inferior Rectus, innervated by the Oculomotor Nerve, performs extorsion and adduction from neutral

- The Medial Rectus, innervated by the Oculomotor Nerve, performs adduction from adduction

- The Lateral Rectus is innervated by the Cranial Nerve VI, the Abducens Nerve. It performs abduction from neutral

- The Superior Oblique, innervated by the Trochlear Nerve, Cranial Nerve IV, intorts, depresses, and abducts the eye from neutral

- The Inferior Oblique is innervated by the Oculomotor Nerve. It performs extorsion, elevation, and abduction from neutral

The function of the eye muscles can be tested by evaluating the fields of gaze of the patient. If they have double vision, nystagmus, inability to focus, or have a headache while performing this test, it is evident that they have visual dysfunction that needs to be improved.

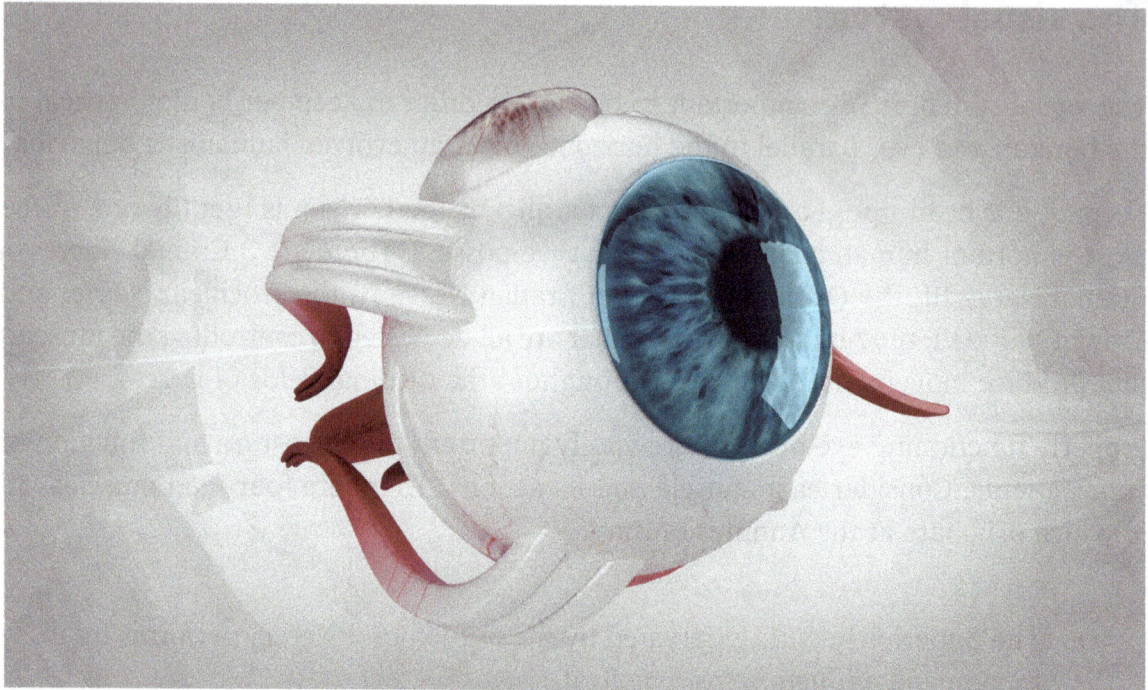

The movements of the eye, innervated by the Cranial Nerves, represent motor output. Let's consider also the sensory input that arrives from the eyes. The visual system is a primary sensation of human function.

The afferent motion perception consists of two visual systems: focal and ambient, or central and peripheral. Central vision is the focal system, specializing in object motion perception and object recognition.

The ambient or peripheral vision is sensitive to movement and is thought to dominate both perception of self-motion and postural control. Retinal slip, a part of the afferent motion perception, is related to a person's displacement by the central nervous system, and is used as feedback for compensatory postural sway (Guerraz and Bronstein, 2008).

The vestibular system is the primary sensory system used in postural balance. However, the visual system also plays an important role. Postural stability increases with the improvement of the visual environment. There are also other contributing parameters that affect visual control of posture such as object size and localization, binocular disparity, visual motion, visual acuity, depth of field, convergence, and spatial frequency (Gaerlan, 2010).

Peripheral vision plays an essential role in maintaining static posture. A study conducted by Berencsi, Ishihara, and Imanaka (2005) showed visual stimulation of the peripheral visual field decrease postural sway in the direction of the observed visual stimulus to the anteroposterior rather than medial-lateral. The authors concluded that peripheral vision operates in a viewer-centered frame of reference.

> "...peripheral vision used either for visual stabilization of spontaneous body sway or visually-induced body sway is more likely due to the size of stimulated field manipulated than to functional specialization of the peripheral vision for postural control."
>
> **Guerraz and Bronstein, 2008, p. 394**

In the absence of vision, proprioceptive information is primarily involved in postural control. This is most commonly seen during a Romberg's Test in which the patient is instructed to close their eyes and stand with their feet together. As the patient closes their eyes, they are reliant primarily on their proprioceptive system. In the majority of cases, the patient will demonstrate increased levels of postural sway with their eyes closed.

The vestibular system

The vestibular system is vitally important to posture for 2 primary reasons. The vestibular system controls balance and the reflexive extensor response. Regarding balance, the vestibular system answers two very important questions for the body: where is my body in relation to gravity, and which way is up? The vestibular system has intricate connections with the visual system to keep the eyes level with the horizon.

When stimulating the vestibular system, you are stimulating the extensors via the vestibulospinal tract. The vestibulospinal tract contributes to reflexive stabilization primarily through the lateral vestibular nuclei to the feet and medial vestibular nuclei to the neck and upper thoracic vestibular nuclei. These are stimulated by nerve projections from the otolith organs and the semicircular canals of the inner ear.

The vestibulospinal tract is a descending pathway that relays information from the vestibular nuclei to motor neurons. The vestibular nuclei receive information through the Vestibulocochlear Nerve about changes in the orientation of the head in relation to gravity. The nuclei relay motor commands through the vestibulospinal tract. The function of these motor commands are to alter muscle tone, extend, and change the position of the limbs and head with the goal of supporting posture and maintaining balance of the body and head.

The primary anatomy of the vestibular system includes the three semicircular canals, the otoliths, and Cranial Nerve VIII: the Vestibulocochlear Nerve. The semicircular canals measure rotational acceleration. The utricle and saccule are the otolith organs, which interpret linear acceleration. Vertical accelerations are perceived by the saccule and horizontal accelerations by the utricle.

The semicircular canals, the saccule, and utricle project to the central nervous system as well as visual and proprioceptive inputs. This intricate communication contributes to perceived orientation by the forebrain, postural control through communication with the cerebellum, and controlled eye movements of the oculomotor system.

Postural balance is maintained when there is good visual acuity and head movements are opposed by equal and opposite eye movements. For example, as the head turns right, the endolymph pushes the cupula to the left. The endolymph presses on the cupula. When it bends and the cilia is bent, it changes the frequency of firing of the Vestibulocochlear Nerve to the brain. When the cupula bends in one direction, it increases the frequency of firing; when it bends in the other direction, it decreases the frequency of firing. Movement then translates into neural signaling.

An enabled vestibulo-ocular reflex (VOR) also contributes to postural stability during movement. When the VOR is enabled, you can walk and move, but keep your eyes fixed on the horizon. A properly functioning VOR means that the patient can stabilize their gaze; their eyes don't move from parallel with the horizon when the head and the body move. This single reflex is vital to our functionality as human beings.

The VOR keeps your eyes on a target while moving. Consider 3 other reflexes controlled by the vestibular system. The vestibulocollic reflex keeps the head still in space while your body is moving beneath it, i.e. it keeps your head on a level plane while you're walking.

The vestibulospinal reflex adjusts posture for rapid changes in position, and the VOR Cancellation is exactly as it sounds. It cancels the VOR. This is important because sometimes we need to be able to turn our head and turn our eyes simultaneously to other directions to see different stimuli. You don't always want to keep your eyes fixated in daily life; you need to be able to move around and respond to stimuli in your environment.

For precise activation of a single semicircular canal, you must be able to activate 1 canal at a time via diagonal movements. For example, if the head goes "back," you are activating both posterior canals simultaneously.

The horizontal canals rotate in the horizontal plane in which they are paired. The left anterior and right posterior (easily remembered by the mnemonic LARP) have paired rotation in the vertical plane skewed 45 degrees anterior to the left. The right anterior canal goes with left posterior canal (or RALP).

The horizontal and posterior canals are easy to remember—they activate in the same direction. The canals are also connected to the eye muscles for synergistic movement with the VOR.

Somatosensory

The most basic understanding of the somatosensory system is this. The body perceives a stimulus, it sends the information of the stimulus to the brain for processing, and then the brain produces a motor response to the afferent input.

The CNS (central nervous system) processes a multimodal afferent input and integrates it at various levels in the spinal cord, brainstem, and cortex. Cortical processing of the somatosensory information results in efferent processing for coordinated firing of multi-alpha motor neurons and their corresponding muscle fibers (Shaffer and Harrison, 2007).

Proprioception is the ability to sense the body regarding position, motion, and equilibrium. Muscle spindles play an important role in proprioception.

It is mechanoreceptors that provide the nervous system with information about the muscle's length and velocity of contraction, thus contributing to the individual's ability to discern joint movement and position sense (Shaffer and Harrison, 2007). The muscle spindles also provide afferent feedback that translates to appropriate reflexive and voluntary movements.

Another organ that contributes to proprioceptive information is the Golgi Tendon Organ (GTO). The GTO located at the muscle tendon relays information about tensile forces, and is sensitive to very slight changes (Shaffer and Harrison, 2007). When the GTO of the muscles is activated, the afferent neuron synapses in the spinal cord. Interneurons inhibit the alpha motor neuron of the muscle, resulting in decreased tension within the muscle and the tendon.

Restricted spinal segments are a loop that creates less input to the brain. Restricted joints should be mobilized through exercise or manipulation or both to stimulate important feedback loops regarding body position and posture.

Pontomedullary reticular formation

The brainstem consists of the mesencephalon or the midbrain, the pons, and the medulla. The reticular formation is a set of interconnected nuclei that are located throughout the brainstem. The pontomedullary reticular formation (PMRF) is involved in posture and equilibrium as well as autonomic nervous system activity. It receives information from the hypothalamus.

The PMRF is located in the brainstem and is part of the descending brain pathways that cause primary motor commands to control posture. There are four primary functions of the PMRF that are important for our purposes.

First, the PMRF inhibits pain on the ipsilateral side of the body. It also inhibits the ipsilateral intermediolateral cell column (IML) of the sympathetic nervous system. This can cause an increase in blood pressure and heart rate ipsilaterally. Third, the PMRF inhibits the ipsilateral anterior muscles above T6 and the posterior muscles below T6. With a lack of inhibition, these muscles go into flexion and commonly result in chronic postural distortion patterns. The fourth role of the PMRF is the inhibition of inhibitory motor interneurons, or the Renshaw Cells, that work in conjunction with the ipsilateral cerebellum to create global tone ipsilaterally.

The nuclei of the cranial nerves that control eye movements (Cranial Nerves III, IV, and VI) and Cranial Nerve VIII, the Vestibulocochlear Nerve, are all located in the brainstem. Anytime your patient performs vestibular or eye exercises, they are activating the brainstem where the PMRF originates.

Why is this important for our purposes? The PMRF controls posture and autonomics, the vestibulospinal tract contracts the extensor musculature to stay upright, and the reticulospinal tract controls posture and blood flow.

The PMRF inhibits the ipsilateral anterior muscles above T6 and inhibits the posterior muscles below T6. The PMRF and the vestibulospinal tract are the preeminent designers of posture.

Postural distortion patterns are a reflexive flexor response to stress of the human physiology. This can be seen throughout the body. Consider the shoulders—they round forward in a primitive fetal position under stress.

The PMRF controls sympathetic tone and autonomic function ipsilaterally. If the patient presents with brainstem issues, they will have increased sympathetic output such as sweating on one side of the body. This can be evaluated clinically to locate PMRF dysfunction.

For long-term postural correction, you must do vision and vestibular training to target the neurology of the posture system. The neurologic system is hardwired to control simultaneous stabilization and movement, allowing humans to perform a vast variety of movements while maintaining proper posture.

Cerebellum

The cerebellum plays an important role in posture by supervising movement and making alterations to coordinate smooth gestures. The cerebellum creates flexor/extensor synergy for postural control. When this synergy is disrupted, we have overactive flexion or extension on either side of the joint, which creates jerkiness with intentional movements.

The cerebellum plays an important role in posture by supervising movement and making alterations to coordinate smooth gestures. The cerebellum creates flexor/extensor synergy for postural control. When this synergy is disrupted, we have overactive flexion or extension on either side of the joint, which creates jerkiness with intentional movements.

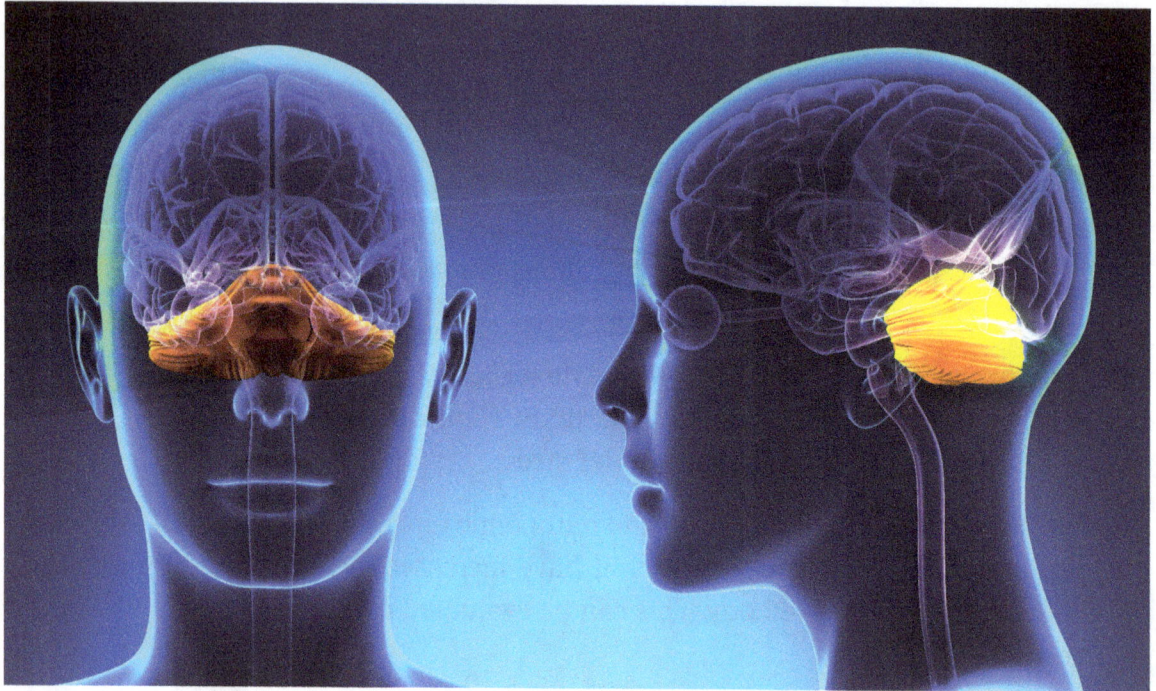

The cerebellum has four primary functions. It controls and coordinates complex movements ipsilaterally. It is in direct communication with the ipsilateral vestibular system. It directly stimulates the contralateral frontal lobe of the cerebral cortex. It also ensures accuracy and coordination with movement expression.

The midline aspect of the cerebellum is referred to as the vermis. The vermis coordinates movements of the eyes and spine, which is highly important for posture. The spinocerebellum, which includes the vermal and paravermal zones, is important in regulating muscle tone and in adapting the body to changing circumstances. This portion of the cerebellum receives extensive input from the spinal cord and has connections to the PMRF through the fastigial nuclei. The spinocerebellum can thus affect muscle tone and crude movements via the reticulospinal tracts.

The vestibulocerebellum, or flocculonodular lobe, is an important regulator of the vestibular system. Damage to this region will result in vertigo, nystagmus, and balance disorders.

The neocerebellum projects to the ventral lateral nucleus of the thalamus, which relays to the cerebral cortex. Therefore, the lateral hemispheres of the cerebellum are involved in regulating the cerebral cortical motor output through procedural learning. Learned activities such as riding a bike or knitting involve activity of the cerebellar hemispheres. Damage to the lateral hemispheres results in lack of coordination of limb movement, with overshoot and undershoot or intention tremors.

When a patient presents with a right cerebellar issue, we expect to see a compromise of the same side extensor tone, lack of coordination between flexors and extensors, lack of accuracy, and lack of balance all on the right side.

SECTION REVIEW

1. The *vestibular* system controls balance and the reflexive extensor response

2. *Proprioception* is the ability to sense the body regarding position, motion, and equilibrium

3. The *pontomedullary reticular formation* inhibits flexion of the posture system anteriorly above T6

4. The *cerebellum* creates flexor/extensor synergy for postural control

CLOSED LOOP SYSTEM

The posture system, like all other systems of the body, is a closed loop system. Consider the Control Theory of Closed Loop Systems. The Control Theory explains that dynamic physiologic systems behave based upon their inputs, and they respond via feedback. Your unique postural presentation is due to the sensory inputs received from your environment, particularly the repetitive inputs. These inputs are received and processed, and a response is produced. The response is sent to the appropriate anatomy via feedback, feeding the loop of adaptation.

The closed loop represents your posture in equilibrium. In postural equilibrium, stabilization and orientation is happening in perfect synchronicity to hold the body upright. When a disturbance disrupts the equilibrium, the Sensor evaluates the disruption. The Controller notes deviation from normal posture and computes an appropriate physiologic response. The Effector restores equilibrium in the system. This feedback-adaptation pattern is constant and continual to maintain equilibrium in the posture system. The Control Theory of Closed Loop Systems is an innate function of protection to maintain equilibrium within the body.

SECTION REVIEW

- The posture system is a *closed* loop system

ANATOMICAL POSTURE QUADRANTS

The posture system is a highly complex system that is broken down into four anatomic quadrants. Evaluating the structure and function of each posture quadrant provides a clear understanding of the health and integrity of the posture system.

Each posture quadrant has coordinated functions with the quadrants above or below it. Habitual stabilization occurring at each posture quadrant can either restrain or liberate the axis of that posture quadrant. Every action of the posture quadrants either promotes stable posture that supports efficiency of the body or promotes postural collapse.

- **Posture Quadrant 1**: cranium and cervical spine
- **Posture Quadrant 2**: shoulders, scapulae, thoracic spine, upper extremities, and the ribcage
- **Posture Quadrant 3**: core musculature, lumbar spine, and pelvis
- **Posture Quadrant 4**: lower extremity

Posture Quadrant 1 extends from the apex of the cranium to the seventh cervical vertebra. The orienting anatomy of Posture Quadrant 1 is the head and the stabilizing anatomy is the cervical spine.

Posture Quadrant 2 extends from the shoulder joint complex anteriorly to the base of the ribcage. Posteriorly, it extends from the first to the twelfth thoracic vertebrae. The orienting anatomy of Posture Quadrant 2 is the hands and the stabilizing anatomy is the shoulders, scapulae, ribcage, and the thoracic spine.

Posture Quadrant 3 extends from the top of the diaphragm to the femoral head of each leg anteriorly. Posteriorly, it extends from the first lumbar vertebra to the base of the ischial tuberosities bilaterally. Posture Quadrant 3 is the only quadrant that is primarily stabilizing.

Posture Quadrant 4 extends from the femoral head of each leg to the distal phalanges of each foot. The orienting anatomy of Posture Quadrant 4 is the feet and the stabilizing anatomy is the leg, lower leg, knee, and the ankle.

When you are performing posture analyses, it is recommended to perform the analysis from the head down to the feet. Visual analyses performed in this manner allow the Posture Expert to visualize each of the anatomical posture quadrants, and how they are in alignment with one another. The alignment of the posture quadrants provides a clear view of the overall postural alignment, from which Posture Experts can make assumptions of how the function of the organs or the physiology of the body will be affected.

SECTION REVIEW

1. Posture Quadrant 1 is the cranium and cervical spine

2. Posture Quadrant 2 is the shoulders, scapulae, thoracic spine, upper extremities, and the ribcage

3. Posture Quadrant 3 is the core musculature, lumbar spine, and pelvis

4. Posture Quadrant 4 is the lower extremity

POSTURE QUADRANT 1

Posture Quadrant 1 includes the head and the cervical spine. The head is utilized for orientation purposes and the cervical spine for stability and protection of the brainstem. The neck, with a natural anterior curve, supports the weight of the head in an upright position. The standard position of the head is to seek eye-level position with the horizon.

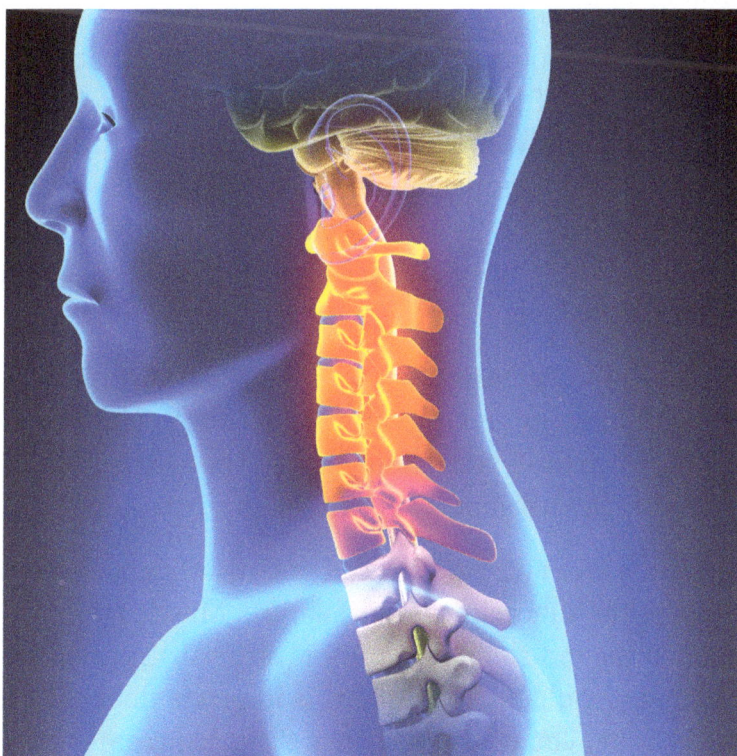

In typical faulty posture patterns, the head does not change position; the position of the cervical spine changes in response to the posture of the upper dorsal spine. If the upper back is straight, for example, the neck will straighten. If the upper back has an increased kyphotic curve, the neck will go further into extension to compensate.

Cervical extension among the sagittal plane occurs in the lower cervical area with the upper cervical vertebrae maintaining a level position to support the head. Lateral flexion of the cervical spine occurs in the coronal plane, and cervical rotation happens primarily in the transverse plane from C2–C7.

The occipital-atlantal area is an area of extensive mobility. This is the site of the tonic neck reflexes, which influence postural muscular tone throughout the trunk. Dysfunctional alignment of the occipital-atlantal transition area demonstrates disturbances in equilibrium, postural muscle tonus, and motor deficiencies.

The cervicothoracic junction is the most mobile section of the spine, where the supple cervical spine meets the rigid thoracic spine. There are insertions of important upper extremity and shoulder muscles in this transition zone and important neural pathways reside in the brachial plexus.

The suboccipital muscles are found at the base of the cranium and the upper cervical region, connecting the base of the skull with the upper two cervical vertebrae. The suboccipital musculature keeps your head aligned with your body as you move around in space. This small but highly significant muscle group contains more motion sensors than any other parts of the body. Inner ear sensorimotor feedback functions to help you keep your head upright; the suboccipital muscles help you keep your head in proper alignment with your body.

The upper cervical and suboccipital region is an important neurologic transition zone. The upper cervical vertebrae protect the integrity of the brainstem, and vital cranial nerves IX, X, and XI intersect this transitional zone. The rectus capitis posterior minor suboccipital muscle also directly meets with the dura mater here.

Fascial links between the face and the neck can greatly influence your posture; tension in the face immobilizes the suboccipital musculature. Muscles that open and close the jaw pull on the vertebrae and skull. Jaw muscle strain is transmitted to the cervical spine, down the throat, shoulders, diaphragm, and pelvic floor. Jaw tension can also transmit strain to the inner ear, causing balance disturbances.

Habitual cervical and head posture is directly linked with the position of the mandible at rest and during movement. "Good posture is important, yet many people don't realize how their posture affects their oral health," states Leibsohn, spokesperson of the Academy of General Dentistry.

Coordinated movement of the mandible is dependent upon coordination between the posterior cervical muscles and the muscles that lie anterior to the cervical spine. These muscles are used for mastication, respiration, deglutition, and speech. Darling et al. (1984) noted that postural imbalances of the head over the cervical spine caused positional imbalance of the mandible. Correcting cervical posture was thus associated with a more balanced position of the mandible.

Temporomandibular Joint Disorder (TMD) is described as pain and hypertonicity in the muscles of mastication, and in the muscles of the head, neck, and jaw complex. Goldstein and Makofsky (2005) have demonstrated the relationship between forward head posture and the painful effects of TMD.

When forward head posture is present, the supramandibular muscles pull the mandible toward the maxilla, causing a more retracted position. The suprahyoid and posterior cervical musculature shorten isometrically, and the infrahyoid muscles are stretched (Ayub et al., 1984). The effects of this postural distortion pattern may lead to an excessive amount of tension in the muscles of mastication and the supporting structures.

Munhoz et al. (2004) stated, "Patients suffering from TMJ disorder show a tendency toward increased morphologic and functional alterations of the cervical spine" after researching cervical radiographs of patients presenting with painful TMJ dysfunction. They discovered that patients with more severe TMJ symptoms exhibit cervical spine hyperlordosis.

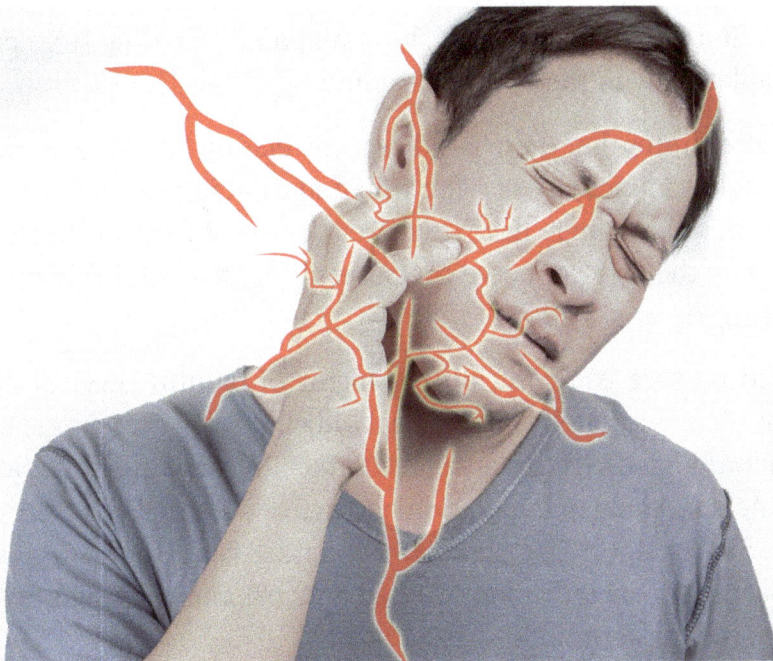

It was noted by Wright et al. (2000) that when patients are instructed to do posture training and TMD self-management, the results are significantly more effective than TMD self-management instructions alone, meaning that the patients with improved head posture had better results in managing TMD associated symptoms. Nikolakis et al. (2001) concluded similar findings. They concluded that a combination of exercise, manual therapy, correction of body posture, and relaxation techniques were significantly effective in alleviating jaw pain, restricted jaw movement, and orofacial impairment.

Goldstein and Makofsky (2005) concluded that correction of forward head posture resulted in decreased muscle tension in the neck, jaw, shoulders, and back; improved postural alignment that is efficient, functional, and aesthetic; diminished pain and stiffness of the head, neck, and jaw; decreased fatigue and improved mental state; and enhanced performance at work. The direct link between proper posture and TMJ function is an important consideration for how Posture Experts can best help their patients.

Harrison (2002) studied the stresses produced to the cervical spine by different cervical postures. It was discovered that stress in cervical kyphosis was 6–10 times greater than cervical lordosis. Extension of the cervical spine in forward head posture causes excessive pressure to the facets and the posterior bodies of the vertebrae, often resulting in cervical nerve root compression. Cervical nerve root compression of the lower cervical vertebrae is often felt by patients as "shooting pain," "tingling," or "pins and needles" sensations unilaterally in the upper extremity.

Research demonstrates that there is a direct correlation between reduction of the craniovertebral angle and increase of neck pain and disability. Patients who present with a smaller craniovertebral angle have a greater degree of forward head posture, causing more pressure to the cervical nerve roots, resulting in a greater level of neck pain disability (Ho Ting Yip et al., 2008).

Forward head posture is a contributing factor of painful cervical radiculopathy. To manage symptoms associated with cervical radiculopathy, non-surgical treatment plans to correct forward head posture are considered clinically effective. Non-surgical treatment plans include spinal manipulation and active and passive postural rehabilitation. According to Saal et al. (1996), patients who underwent a non-surgical treatment protocol for relief of cervical radiculopathy had a 92.6% clinically significant improvement from baseline to long-term follow-up.

Moustafa et al. (2012) stated that exercise programs to correct forward head posture are effective in reducing pain associated with cervical spine radiculopathy. Exercises that were found to be the most effective for pain management of cervical radiculopathy include neck retraction exercises. Neck retraction exercises contribute to correction of forward head posture and promote cervical root decompression (Lentrell et al., 2002).

Muscular associated cervical spine pain is generally associated with one of the two primary causes: muscle tightness due to gradual onset of symptoms, or muscle strain due to acute onset of symptoms. Neck pain and headaches associated with tightness in the posterior neck are often found in patients who present with forward head posture and an increased thoracic kyphosis. Unilateral muscle tightness is generally caused by environmental stressors, such as distorting the position of the neck unilaterally due to repeatedly holding a telephone on the same side of the head.

Faulty neck postures can have multiple different causes. However, one of the most common faulty neck postures, forward head posture, is generally caused as a compensation for a developed thoracic kyphosis. Hyperkyphotic presentations are often associated with postural distortion patterns of the lower back or pelvis. Postural correction of the cervical spine should include correction of the alignment and musculature of the rest of the spine and the pelvis.

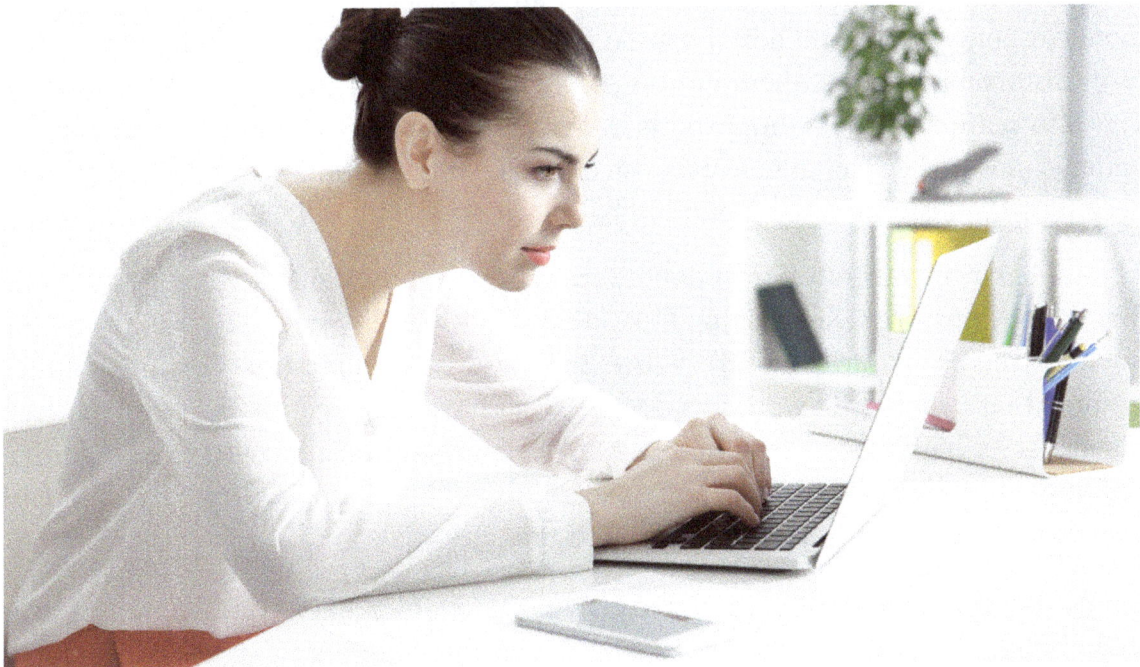

Consequences of faulty postural alignment in Posture Quadrant 1 range in levels of severity. Common symptoms include muscle strain, neck stiffness, pain and tingling in the arms, shoulder immobility, TMJ tension, and headaches. More severe consequences include migraines, cervical disc herniation, torticollis, trigeminal neuralgia, vertigo, balance disturbances, and high blood pressure.

There is a strong correlation between neck osteoarthritis and postural stability. Neck pain patients present with less postural control and less stability against gravity (Michaelson, 2003). As the trunk flexes forward and the head juts anteriorly into forward head posture, postural imbalance and impaired ability to regulate movement in the forward and backward directions are demonstrated (Jung-Ho Kang et al., 2012).

Neck pain patients have altered neck proprioception to brain communication, causing sensorimotor disturbances, that influences their ability to sustain sturdy balance. Due to instability, elderly patients who present with neck pain have an increased predisposition to suffering from falls (Uthaikhup, 2012). Posture and balance training for elderly patients can help prevent falls by up to 50% (Weiniger, 2008).

There is a relationship between neck alignment and the perception of the body during static and dynamic orientation. Pettorossi and Schieppati (2014) explain that tonic cervical proprioceptive input may induce persistent influences on the subject's mental representation of space, creating plastic changes associated with motion patterns, motor responsiveness, and head position. Thus, if a patient presents with cervical postural distortion patterns, their motion patterns and neural plasticity will be altered. This information helps Posture Experts understand how cervical cranial posture affects patients' position sense, motor responsiveness to stimuli, and how to correct chronic neck postural distortion patterns.

Beyond balance and body perception, there is also a connection between posture and high blood pressure (Deuchars and Edwards, 2007). Faulty neck posture affects the nucleus tractus solitarius (NTS), which regulates blood pressure. Edwards (2007) claimed that people who work at a desk job and have hunched forward neck posture are at risk of high blood pressure due to postural distortions. He also explained that patients who have damage to the musculature of their cervical spine, from car accidents for example, demonstrate changes in blood pressure.

Riddle and Purvis (2004) demonstrated how posture affects energy levels. Poor posture slowly decreases amounts of energy due to increased compression on the articulations throughout the body. They demonstrate that when you slouch, your muscles utilize more energy to hold the body upright. When the head is placed anteriorly in relation to the shoulders, it causes strain and fatigue on Posture Quadrant 2 to support the weight of the head.

> "[The] head in forward posture can add up to 30lb of abnormal leverage on the cervical spine. This can pull the entire spine out of alignment. Forward head posture may result in the loss of 30% of lung capacity."
>
> **Cailliet, 1987**

The patient will feel fatigued overall, have depressed lung function, degeneration of the spinal column, with imbalanced paravertebral muscle function.

Postural distortion patterns of the cervical spine are also associated with the presence of cervicogenic headaches, occipital headaches, and migraines. Goldstein and Makofsky (2005) state that approximately 50% of the population suffers from cervical spine pain or headaches, and that 70% of the population suffering from headaches demonstrate cervical dysfunction.

Watson and Trott (1993) performed a research study concluding that patients who present with cervicogenic headaches demonstrated a significantly more prevalent occurrence of forward head posture. In addition, it was noted that patients who present with forward head posture and have associated headaches also present with isometric weakness of the upper cervical neck flexor muscles. Postural correction of the cervical spine was thus indicated as a treatment method for cervicogenic headaches.

It is also important to consider postural correction in terms of frequency reduction. Research indicates a negative correlation between the craniovertebral angle and chronic tension type headache frequency, meaning that the amount of forward head posture the patient presents with is related to increased frequency of headaches (Fernández-de-las-Peñas, 2006).

With occipital headaches, misalignment of the occiput and C1 can cause increased tension to the occipital nerve, which innervates the splenius capitis, the semispinalis, and the scalp posteriorly. Patients will generally present with pain upon palpation in these areas with the exacerbation of an occipital headache.

The presence of trigger points in the sternocleidomastoid, temporalis, and the suboccipital muscles are associated with the initiation and perpetuation of migraines.

According to Fernández-de-las-Peñas et al. (2006), "Nociceptive inputs from trigger points in head and neck muscles may produce continuous afferent bombardment of the trigeminal nerve nucleus caudalis and, hence, activation of the trigeminovascular system." These researchers demonstrated that chronic migraine patients presented with trigger points of the cervical spinal musculature, an increased prevalence of forward head posture, and decreased cervical range of motion with flexion and extension.

A new age health condition that is also pertinent to the postural presentation of Posture Quadrant 1 is "tech neck." Tech neck has been coined as a medical condition due to the amount of time that modern day humans spend looking down at their cell phones and the dysfunction that this is causing to the health of the posture system.

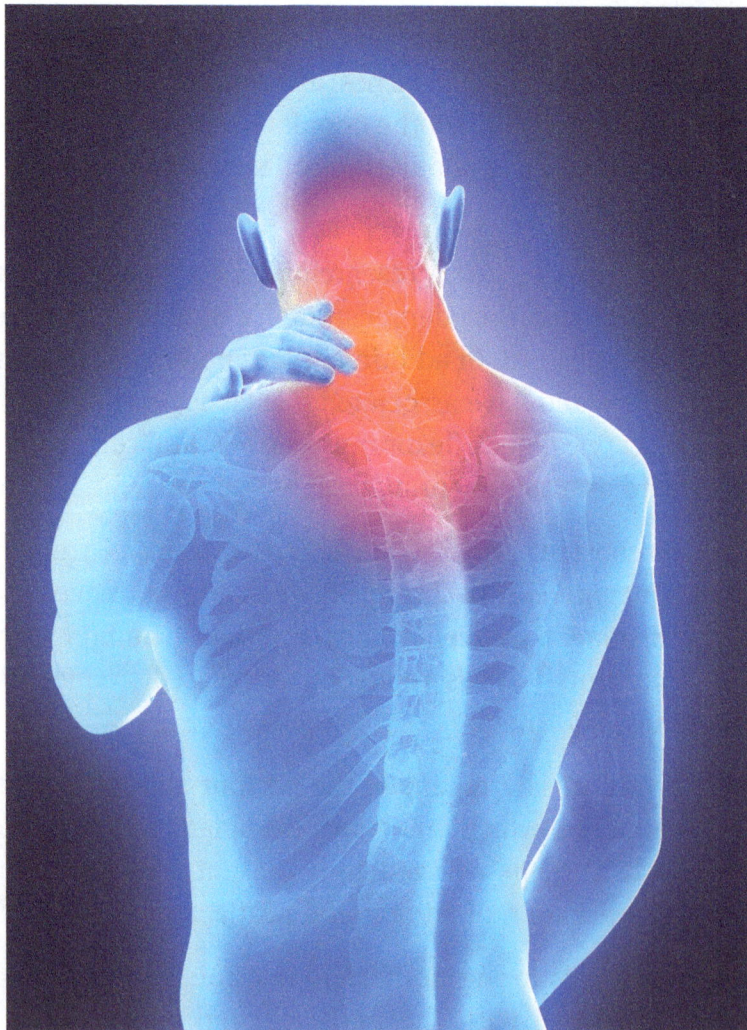

Hansraj (2015) evaluated the amount of pressure on the cervical spine when the neck is bent forward at varying degrees. He concluded that as the head tilts anteriorly (as it does while looking at a cell phone) by 15 degrees, the weight of the head increases from 10–12lb to 27lb. As the head tilts forward by 30 degrees, the head weight is increased to 40lb; at 45 degrees of tilt, the head weighs 49lb; and at a forward tilt of 60 degrees, the weight of the head is 60lb. This is a tremendous amount of unnecessary pressure to the posture system that has become the new societal norm. According to Hansraj (2015), people spend an average of 2–4 hours per day on their cell phone with significant anteriority of the cervical spine. Hansraj (2015) states, "In proper alignment, spinal stress is diminished" (p. 2).

Traumatic cervical spine injuries can occur in high impact sports. According to Proctor and Cantu (2000), sports-related injuries of the head and neck receive substantial public attention and are responsible for some of the most catastrophic athletic injuries seen. They explain that sports-related injuries of Posture Quadrant 1 cause 70% of traumatic deaths and 20% of permanent disabilities related to sports. Of all pediatric head injuries, 10% are estimated to be related to sports (Proctor and Cantu, 2000), and 10–15% of competitive football players suffer axial load injuries to the cervical spine (Thomas, McCullen, and Yuan, 1999).

Athletes who do not have correct posture may also experience functional health consequences in the future. According to McNeal (1992) changes in posture with age are of concern because of their association with impaired mobility and the possibility of falls. Traumatic injuries often lead to compensation patterns. If injuries, or their associated compensation patterns, are left uncorrected, it may lead to functional changes in the posture system.

SECTION REVIEW

1. Forward head posture is commonly caused by which postural distortion pattern of the thoracic spine? *Hyperkyphosis*

2. There is a correlation between reduction of the *craniovertebral* angle and increase of neck pain, disability, and forward head posture

3. *Tech neck* has been coined as a medical term due to the amount of time patients spend looking down at devices causing dysfunction of the posture system

POSTURE QUADRANT 2

The second posture quadrant includes the shoulders, scapulae, thoracic spine, upper extremities, and the ribcage. The second quadrant extends from the first thoracic to the twelfth thoracic vertebra posteriorly, and from the shoulders to the diaphragm anteriorly. The hands are utilized for orienting the person in space, and the shoulders, scapulae, and ribcage are important stabilizers. The primary functions of the second quadrant are to mobilize the upper extremity, to perform respiration, and for circulation.

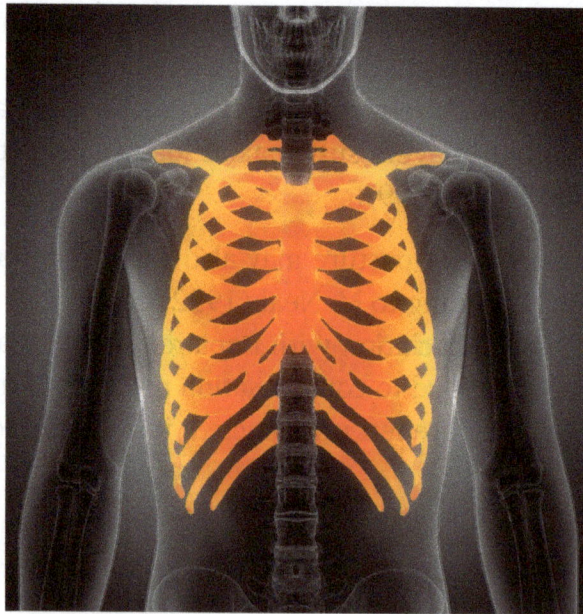

The brachial plexus is a prime connecter of Posture Quadrant 1 to Quadrant 2. Peripheral nerves of the nerve roots C4–T2 innervate many of the important muscles associated with function and mobility of Posture Quadrant 2. Postural distortions of Posture Quadrant 1 that affect the brachial plexus can cause debilitative function of Posture Quadrant 2.

The social dimensions of our bodies are expressed through the shoulders and arms. Our hands provide a primary interface with our surroundings. Sensory information from our hands tells us a lot about the environment that we are interacting with. This is why we instinctively put our hands out in front of us when we are in the dark or blindfolded. The interaction of our hands with our environment helps us orient ourselves to our surroundings.

As humans, we also instinctively tighten our grip when we want to maintain control of an object or situation. Humans have a natural tendency to favor the thumb side of the hands. For example, we don't reach for something with our pinky finger; this demonstrates weakness. A weak grip is without utilizing the fourth and fifth digits. When a grip is performed in this manner, the patient loses the connection between the hands, shoulder blades, and the spine. Tension in your hands communicates throughout your body, confusing your negotiation with gravity and distorting your posture. When gripping things tightly, you are then utilizing your hands as stabilizers, which can block their orientation capabilities.

How human beings hold their arms and hands demonstrates how they are feeling mentally and physically. Crossed arms and closed posture is associated with distress, concern, and anger, whereas open arms demonstrate love, caring, and nurturing. When people place their hands on their hips, it is a demonstration of confidence and sex appeal, but when they have their hands on their head, they are commonly expressing frustration. When you see someone fidgeting with their hands (such as tapping a pencil back and forth or drumming their hands), they are likely bored, impatient, or anxious. And of course, the strongest forms of social engagement, a handshake or a hug, are also performed with the arms and hands.

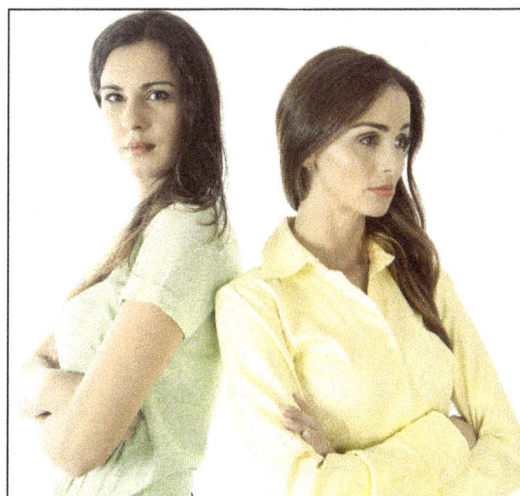

The structure and function of Posture Quadrant 2 are associated not only with our social behaviors, but also our response to stress. The upper extremity seeks stability with the trapezius muscles. Under high amounts of stress, the patient will experience a high level of trapezius muscle tension. Patients commonly complain that they "carry stress in their shoulders."

The upper trapezius muscles raise your shoulders toward your neck and the lower trapezius help secure your scapulae to the thoracic spine, providing a better foundation for arm movements. When people are stressed, or when they are cold, you will often find hyper-contraction of the trapezius muscles, resulting in decreased and rigid ranges of motion of the shoulder girdle and upper extremity.

Complaints of pain are associated with traction by the muscle on its bony attachments along the spine. Palpation generally elicits pain among the bony attachments to the spine or scapula. This results from habitual forward shoulders, or a round upper back, or both. In some cases, this is due to over-development of the anterior girdle muscles. Repetitive sports motions and occupationally related motions performed with the shoulders forward cause this.

In addition to heightened muscular tension, stress has a large impact on breathing patterns as well. As respiration rates increase, patients tend to recruit auxiliary muscles of respiration, all of which are located in Posture Quadrant 2. As the patient relaxes, their muscular tension lessens and their breathing patterns normalize.

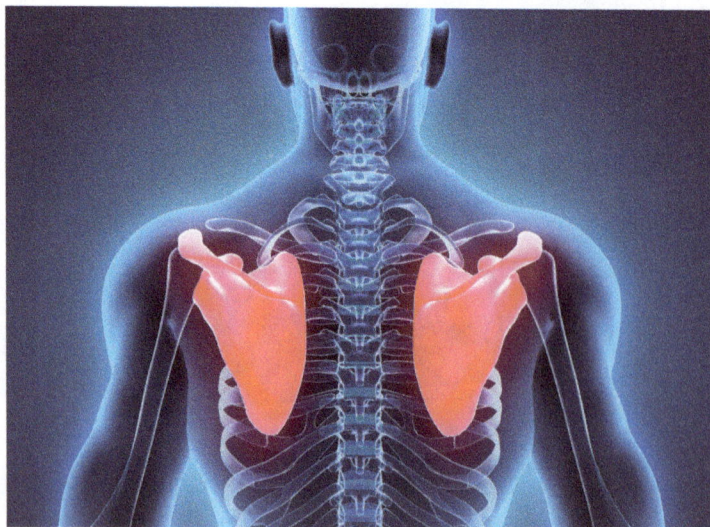

Important postural evaluation points of Posture Quadrant 2 are the scapulae. With the thoracic spine in good alignment, the scapulae lie against the thorax approximately between the second and eleventh ribs. The medial borders are essentially parallel and 4 inches apart. There is oblique orientation of the scapula muscles allowing for lateral and rotatory movements of the scapulae. Movements of the scapulae do not occur as individual movements; some degree of rotation or tilt accompanies lateral movements.

The serratus anterior muscles, located between the ribcage and the inside surface of the shoulder blades, draw the scapulae flat against your back ribs. Because the serratus anterior muscles wrap from back to front, they give the shoulders three-dimensional support. With dysfunction to the long thoracic nerve, which innervates the serratus anterior, marked winging of the scapulae is evident.

Movements of the wrist, elbow, and the shoulder girdle include a complex interaction of joints and muscles. Flexion and extension of the wrist occurs about the coronal axis, and abduction or radial deviation and adduction or ulnar deviation occurs about the sagittal axis. Wrist circumduction is the combination of flexion, extension, abduction, and adduction. The distal radioulnar joint allows supination and pronation of the forearm.

The elbow joint connects the upper arm via the humerus to the lower arm via the radius and ulna. Complex movements occur about the humeroulnar joint, which performs flexion and extension, the humeroradial joint, which is a ball and socket joint, and the superior radioulnar joint, allowing supination and pronation at the elbow.

The shoulder joint is of great complexity and importance to human anatomy. The shoulder girdle consists of three primary joints: the sternoclavicular (SC) joint, the acromioclavicular (AC) joint, and the glenohumeral joint. The SC joint is a synovial joint that connects the sternal end of the clavicle with the manubrium of the sternum, allowing mobility of the pectoral girdle. The AC joint is also a synovial joint formed from the articulation of the acromial end of the clavicle with the acromion of the scapula, allowing the scapula to rotate on the clavicle. The glenohumeral joint is the most mobile and least stable joint of the body. It is a ball and socket joint connecting the head of the humerus to the glenoid cavity. Movements of the glenohumeral joint include: flexion, extension, abduction, adduction, and circumduction.

Differential diagnoses of problems associated with the shoulder girdle require special attention be paid to the innervation of the muscles. The shoulder girdle and upper extremity contain muscles that are supplied by nerves that are motor only. As they have no sensory innervation, there can be a loss of function with no pain. The rhomboids and the serratus anterior are examples of this; they are supplied by nerves that have motor function only. The spinal accessory nerve to the trapezius contains some sensory and some motor fibers. Pain may occur both in and around joints as a result of faulty alignment, or where the muscle attaches to the bone. The loss of movement in one area may result in excessive movement of another area. Regardless of the cause of pain, the treatment is to correct the alignment and restore muscle balance by strengthening weak muscles and lengthening short muscles.

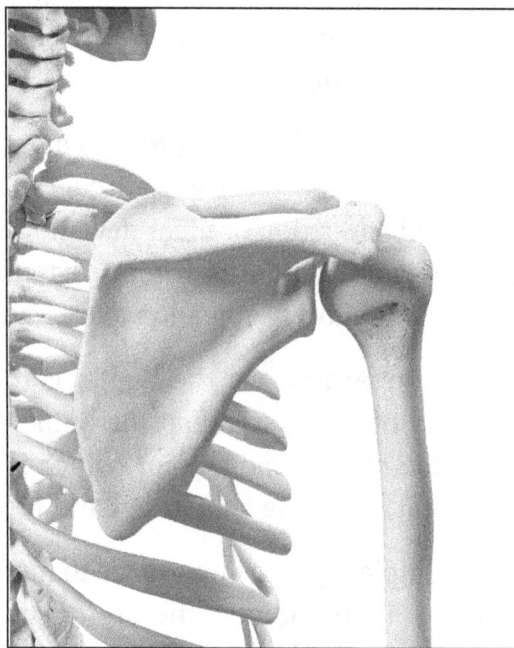

The shoulder complex is composed of the scapula, humerus, and the clavicle. The clavicle works like a yoke to evenly distribute weight among the shoulders while simultaneously stabilizing the shoulder. The clavicle draws its greatest strength from efficient, load-distributing Biotensegrity (not the surrounding muscles) unless the shoulder is misaligned.

Over-developed musculature of the shoulders restricts the range of motion of the upper extremity. An extreme example is bodybuilders. Bodybuilders with overly developed trapezius and deltoid muscles have minimal range of motion of their arms. They walk with their arms out, and some can barely touch their shoulders. Their upper bodies are very strong, but not very supple for performing activities of daily living. The joints and muscles of the upper extremity are highly vulnerable to overuse injuries caused by a person's occupation or recreational activities.

Painful conditions of the arm include many differential diagnoses. Localized or radiating pain in the arm is often the result of faulty alignment that causes tension or compression of the nerves or blood vessels of the cervical spine, upper back, or shoulder girdle. Oftentimes, all three components of misalignment are involved. This is an example of postural distortion compensation patterns. When one part of the kinetic chain is misaligned, the effects go far beyond that single misaligned segment.

Circulation is also affected by poor postural alignment of Posture Quadrant 2. Costoclavicular postural distortions affecting the subclavian vein can result in significant arm swelling and affect venous drainage. Misalignments of the cervical spine and muscular imbalances of the cervical and shoulder region can cause thoracic outlet syndrome (TOS).

TOS is compression of the subclavian artery or the brachial plexus within the space bordered by the scalenus anterior and middle muscles and the first rib. When compression of these important arteries supplying circulation to the arm occurs, the patient experiences the effects of poor circulation such as tingling, numbness, and diffuse pain in the arm. The condition is often aggravated by carrying, lifting, or activities performed with the arm over the head such as painting.

Overuse injuries are caused by repetitive motions performed for prolonged periods of time beyond the tolerance of the structures involved. Chronic overuse injuries result in irritation, inflammation, muscular imbalance patterns, postural distortions, and ligament and tendon tension. The joints and muscles of the upper extremity are highly vulnerable to overuse injuries caused by a person's occupation or recreational activities.

Common overuse injuries of the elbow include lateral and medial epicondylitis. Lateral epicondylitis is commonly referred to as tennis elbow, and is caused by inflammation of the extensor forearm muscle origins, causing lateral elbow and upper forearm pain and tenderness. It is caused by repetitive stress at the muscle-tendon junction and its origin at the lateral epicondyle.

Medial epicondylitis, or golfer's elbow, is caused from inflammation of flexor forearm muscles, causing medial elbow pain. Golfer's elbow is also caused by repetitive stress at the muscle-tendon junction, but its origin is at the medial epicondyle.

According to the National Institute of Neurological Disorders and Stroke (2014), carpal tunnel syndrome is the most common and widely known of the entrapment neuropathies in which the body's peripheral nerves are compressed or traumatized. Carpal tunnel syndrome occurs when the median nerve becomes compressed at the carpal tunnel, a narrow passageway of ligament and bones at the base of the hand. The median nerve controls sensations to the palm side of the thumb and fingers as well as impulses to some small muscles in the hand that allow the fingers and thumb to move. The result may be pain, weakness, or numbness in the hand and wrist, radiating up the arm.

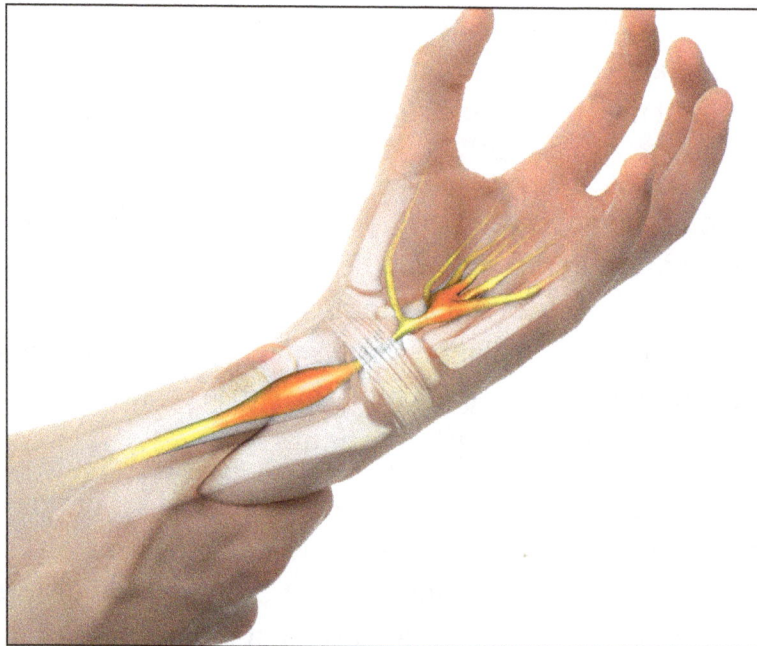

Contributing factors to carpal tunnel syndrome include a congenital predisposition, trauma to the wrist that causes swelling, hyperactivity of the pituitary gland, hypothyroidism, rheumatoid arthritis, mechanical problems in the wrist joint, work stress, repeated use of vibrating hand tools, fluid retention during pregnancy or menopause, or the development of a cyst or tumor in the canal.

Coracoid pressure syndrome is a condition of arm pain that involves compression of the brachial plexus. It is associated with muscle imbalances and posture distortions. Where the pectoralis minor attaches to the coracoid process of the scapula, the three cords of the brachial plexus and the axillary artery and vein pass through these structures and the ribcage. Postural distortions causing the coracoid process to tilt downward narrow this space. The pectoralis minor depresses the coracoid process anteriorly, thus tight pectoralis minor musculature contributes to coracoid pressure syndrome. Tightness of latissimus dorsi indirectly contributes, and weakness of the lower trapezius muscle contributes to a faulty position of the shoulder. Patients often complain of loss of grip strength, and carrying a backpack or heavy bag on the associated side exacerbates pain.

Teres syndrome occurs when the quadrilateral space of the axilla is bounded by the teres major, teres minor, humerus, and the long head of the triceps, causing compression to the axillary nerve which emerges through this space. Pain in the shoulder is prevalent, with restricted shoulder range of motion. The teres major is a medial rotator. When it is shortened, it holds the humerus in internal rotation. This appears as internal rotation when the patient is evaluating the posture from a standing position.

A cervical rib is a rare congenital bone anomaly that may or may not cause nerve irritation. Symptoms are generally based upon the presence of a faulty postural alignment. Forward head posture, rounded shoulders, and an increased kyphosis in addition to a cervical rib will likely exacerbate nervous system symptoms. Treatment is based upon correcting the alignment of the cervical and thoracic spine and the shoulder girdle. Asymptomatic patients likely don't know they have a cervical rib. It is discovered on X-ray.

Other neural and arterial impingements that may occur in Posture Quadrant 2 include the teres major with the axillary nerve, supination with the radial nerve, pronation with the median nerve, the flexor carpi ulnaris with the ulnar nerve, the lateral head of the triceps with the radial nerve, the trapezius with the greater occipital nerve, the scalenus medius with C5, C6, and the long thoracic nerve, and the coracobrachialis with the musculocutaneous nerve.

The most common traumatic injuries to occur in Posture Quadrant 2 include wrist fractures such as distal radius fractures, ulnar fractures, and scaphoid fractures, and shoulder problems. The most common shoulder problems are a dislocation of the glenohumeral joint, a separation of the acromioclavicular joint, rotator cuff injuries, frozen shoulder, or arthritis.

In the case of traumatic injuries to the upper extremity, it is important to note that immobility patterns will develop on the side of the injury. Contralateral muscles and joints will commonly be used more to compensate for the injury. After rehabilitation of a traumatic injury, the patient may have developed new movement and postural patterns that will be important for the Posture Expert to identify.

Beyond the upper extremities in Posture Quadrant 2 is the thorax. The thorax is the ribcage, with ribs connecting from the sternum to the spine surrounding and providing protection to the vital organs, the heart and lungs. Lifting the chest upright elevates the thorax and straightens the upper back. The thorax is depressed when a person is sitting or standing in a slumped position. When the thorax is depressed due to poor posture, there are functional respiratory and circulatory effects.

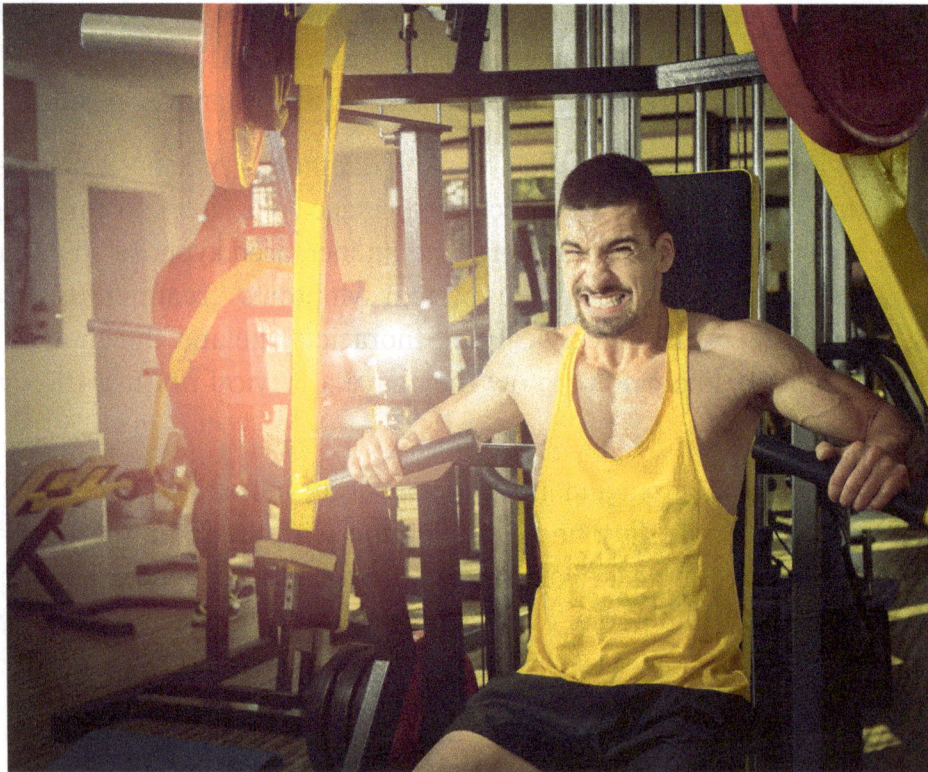

A primary metabolic process of Posture Quadrant 2 is the vital function of respiration. Respiration is the exchange of gases between the cells of an organism and the external environment. Oxygen is transported to the tissues of the body and carbon dioxide is excreted. Respiration consists of ventilation and circulation; ventilation is the movement of gases into and out of the lungs, and circulation is the transport of gases to the tissues. Muscular effort is required to enlarge the thoracic cavity and lower the intrathoracic pressure.

The principal muscle of respiration, the diaphragm, is found in Posture Quadrant 3. However, the accessory muscles of respiration are found in Posture Quadrant 2. The intercostal muscles, located between the ribs, cause the ribs to pivot where they meet the spine. Your whole ribcage expands and contracts when you're breathing. Due to the connection of the ribs and the spine, postural alignment directly affects efficiency of breathing patterns.

The anterior, medial, and posterior scaleni are accessory muscles of inspiration and function together as a unit. By elevating and firmly fixing the first and second ribs, they aid in deep inspiration. They are also active in quiet breathing. The expiratory function is to fix the ribs against contraction of the abdominal muscles and to prevent herniation of the apex of the lung during coughing. Some texts refer to the scalene muscles as primary respiratory muscles as they are highly active in respiration.

Other muscles associated with respiration include the sternocleidomastoid, the latissimus dorsi, the serratus anterior, the pectoralis major, the pectoralis minor, the trapezius, and the thoracic erector spinae musculature.

The diaphragm is the principal respiratory muscle, separating the thoracic and abdominal cavities. It attaches to the bottom of the ribs, the spine in the back, and the breastbone in the front. It connects to the pleura of the lungs. When the diaphragm is relaxed, it pushes air out, called expiration. With expiration, intrathoracic pressure increases due to decreased volume in the thoracic cavity. Simultaneously, the volume of the abdominal cavity is increased, which decreases pressure. The opposite of expiration is inspiration, which occurs when the diaphragm is contracted and pushes air in. With inspiration, the volume of the thoracic cavity increases which lowers the pressure. The volume of the abdominal cavity decreases, which increases abdominal pressure. Limited or excessive excursion of the diaphragm reduces its effectiveness in inspiration and expiration.

Normal respiration is 10–14 breaths per minute. Exhalation should be longer than inhalation. Exhalation is generally 3 seconds and inhalation is 2 seconds with a 1 second pause. Breathing can be altered by positional changes, emotional state, activity level, disease, wearing tight garments, etc. When breathing is altered, the ventilatory muscles work harder, and additional muscles are recruited to meet the demands of breathing.

Deep breathing techniques do not refer to the amount of oxygen taken in; rather, they refer to the amount permeated by the cells of the body. In diaphragmatic breathing (also commonly called "belly breathing"), oxygen is drawn to the lowest and widest part of the lungs. When the bones of the skeleton are organized symmetrically along the vertical axis, the diaphragm is free to rise and fall with full efficiency.

Nose breathing engages the diaphragm and lower ribs, also drawing air deep into the lungs, where oxygen absorption is most efficient. Nose breathing is related to parasympathetic function, as it is slow with increased efficiency of oxygen exchange, a slower heart rate, and relaxed muscles. Mouth breathing activates the upper chest, and draws air into the upper lungs for quicker and shallower breaths. Mouth breathing is related to sympathetic nervous system function and is vital in stressful fight or flight situations. Hyperventilation may also occur in stressful situations. In hyperventilation, the blood becomes more alkaline, called respiratory alkalosis. The blood cells release less oxygen to the tissues, reducing oxygen delivery to the brain by up to 40%. Carbon dioxide levels decrease, and in severe cases the body feels like it is suffocating.

The combination of nose and diaphragmatic breathing improves posture. Breathing through the nose expands the lower ribcage, elongates the trunk, and decompresses the spine. According to Kendall et al. (2005) "Optimal breathing capability derives from a posture of optimal muscle balance" (p. 234).

Muscle balance causes efficient energy expenditure. Muscular imbalance due to postural distortion patterns may affect the volume of pressure that can be attained or maintained. Very weak protruding abdominal muscles are not able to generate maximum expiratory pressures to meet the needs of exertion. Weakness of the erector spinae and the middle and lower trapezius muscles interferes with the ability to straighten the upper back, limiting the ability to raise and expand the chest, thus limiting lung capacity. Postural problems associated with kyphosis, kyphoscoliosis, and pectus excavatum restrict breathing and decrease chest wall compliance.

According to Saha et al. (2007), when patients present with a trunk flexed posture, their level of oxygen consumption is greater, and the change in muscle activation leads to greater energy expenditure. An interesting study evaluated the kinematics of running for triathletes and marathon runners. The study found that triathletes tend to have less energy at the end of a race because they have a more flexed forward posture after biking than marathon runners do from just running. Upright posture supports efficiency in energy expenditure (Hausswirth, 1997).

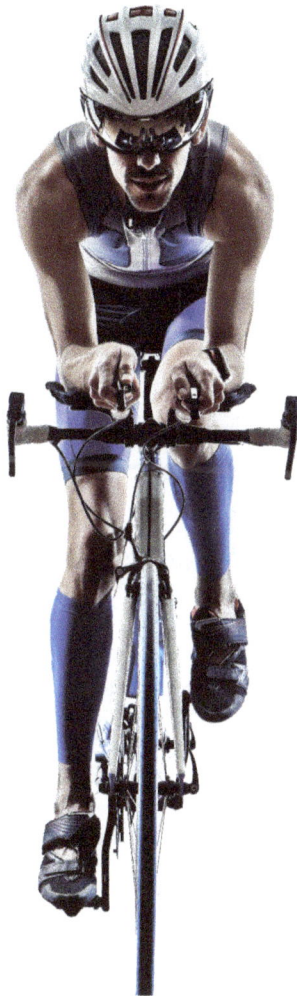

When patients present with postural collapse, the posture system utilizes more metabolic energy to stay upright, leading to lethargy. The use of more energy in this case has a negative health impact. Postural collapse is associated with greater stress to the body with a higher release of cortisol.

The neuroendocrine effect of proper posture is the opposite of postural collapse. Carney et al. (2010) demonstrated that patients who present with proper posture have lower levels of cortisol. Levine et al. (2013) determined the connection between proper posture and decreased obesity, stating that individuals with intentional changes of posture during activities of daily living burn 350 calories more per day on average in comparison to patients who present with sedentary postural presentations.

Patients with persistent asthma have been shown to have postural distortion patterns that increase airway resistance, making it more difficult to breath. Abnormal postural adaptations of asthmatic patients also showed muscle shortening of respiratory musculature (Lopes et al., 2006). Proper posture for asthmatic patients is a fundamental way of reducing the severity of asthma related symptoms.

Due to the amount of accessory muscles assisting in respiration, it is evident how increased stress to Posture Quadrant 2 can affect the function of the rest of the body. Postural imbalances of the thoracic spine and ribs with associated muscular compensation patterns can be detrimental to the respiratory system.

Try this at home in front of a mirror: round your shoulders forward in a position of collapsed, faulty posture. Really slump your shoulders forward. Try taking a deep breath in. Does it feel heavy? Does your breath feel limited? Do you notice how you utilized additional muscles to take a breath in? Now roll your shoulders back and straighten your spine in good posture. Take another deep breath in. Do you feel a difference? Do you feel how much easier it is to breathe in good posture? Now imagine the effect unresolved postural distortion patterns will have long-term on the efficiency of the respiratory system.

Another reported compromise of chest flexion of Posture Quadrant 2 is gastroesophageal reflux disease (GERD). Approximately 7 million people in the United States have symptoms of GERD, with more than 20% of them reporting weekly occurrence (Amos, 2012). The symptoms of GERD occur when the digestion process is disrupted such as when the stomach acid used in the breakdown of the food flows backwards into the esophagus, causing a burning sensation in the chest.

It has been shown the postural position your patients maintain while eating and after digesting their food has an effect on the symptomatic presentation of GERD. Upright posture with a reduction in forward flexion has been shown to reduce the symptoms of GERD. Patients with a hunched posture during meals and after eating may suffer from a more intensified burning presentation associated with GERD (Spiegel et al., 2000).

Discussion of Posture Quadrant 2 would be incomplete without discussing the thoracic spine. The thoracic spine has a natural kyphotic curve. Hyperkyphotic curves are an extremely significant postural distortion affecting the function of Posture Quadrant 2, as well as the alignment and function of Posture Quadrants 1 and 3.

The thoracic spine is unique in that the spinal nerves associated with it go directly to organs innervating their vital functions. In the cervical and lumbosacral areas of the spine we have important plexuses that branch into peripheral nerves innervating the upper and lower extremities.

The thoracic spine plays a major role in trunk stability and protection of the spinal cord. Due to uncorrected postural distortion patterns, a large majority of the population presents with postural faults of their thoracic spine. Up to 40% of the elderly population presents with hyperkyphosis (Kado et al., 2007). Abnormal lateral curvatures of the thoracic spine are less common, but affect 6–9 million Americans per year (National Scoliosis Foundation, 2007).

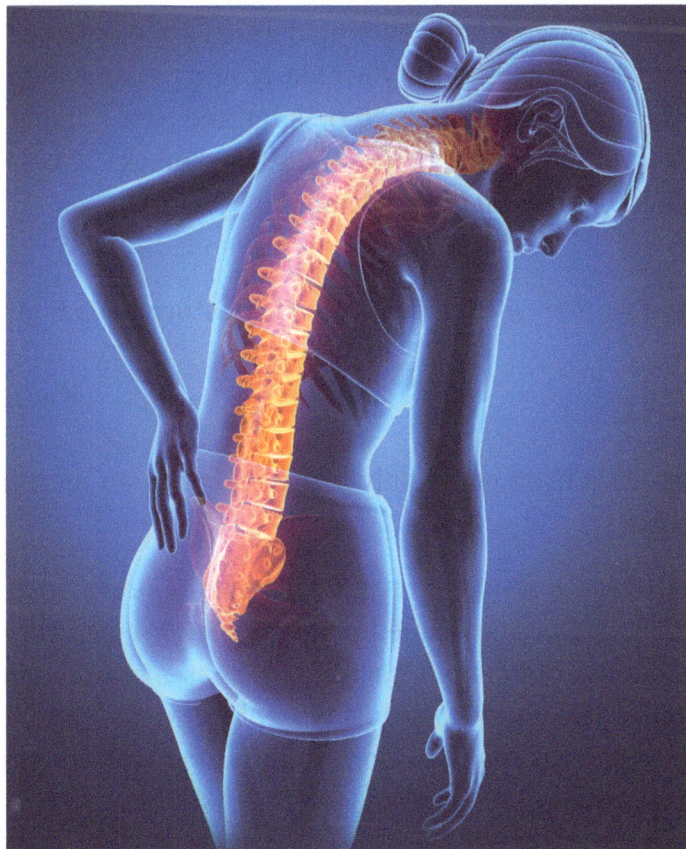

Hyperkyphosis of the upper thoracic spine can be severely debilitating. Studies of birds with hyperkyphosis demonstrate spinal cord flattening and severe demyelination of the anterior funiculus. The anterior funiculus contains the vestibular tracts that control posture and muscle tone (Shimizu et al., 2005). Kyphotic spinal cord compression interferes with blood flow to the anterior spinal cord and mechanical compression of blood vessels (Murphy, 2005).

Patients who present with a hyperkyphotic spine demonstrate an increased risk to many health disorders.

> "Hyperkyphosis may be independently associated with an increased risk for adverse health outcomes, including impaired pulmonary function, decreased physical function capabilities, and future fractures."
>
> **Kado et al., 2007, p. 330**

It has also been demonstrated that even a moderate kyphosis of the thoracic spine is associated with increased risk of falls in the elderly, and patients with high trunk angle of inclination are 3.5 times more likely to be admitted to a nursing home or require assistance at home than patients with good posture (Speck, 2013). The most severe consequence of hyperkyphosis is early mortality.

> "Older men and women with hyperkyphotic posture have higher mortality rates."
>
> **Kado et al, 2009**

Hyperkyphotic posture is most commonly associated with an increased rate of death due to atherosclerosis.

Katzman et al. (2010) did a research review to show the prevalence and implications of hyperkyphosis. The authors concluded that this postural distortion pattern impairs mobility, increases the risk of falls and fractures, increases mortality in the elderly, and is associated with impaired physical performance, health, and quality of life. They determined that hyperkyphosis may develop from muscle weakness and degenerative disc disease, or from vertebral fractures.

Complications associated with scoliosis, or an abnormal lateral curvature of the spine, are variable. Scoliosis patients experience back pain to varying degrees and varying frequencies. Rare cases of scoliosis restrict space in the ribcage needed for optimal heart and lung function (O'Brien and Newman, 2008).

SECTION REVIEW

1. What is the prime neurologic connector between the first and second posture quadrants? *The brachial plexus*

2. The social dimensions of our bodies are expressed through the *shoulders* and *arms*

3. *Carpal tunnel syndrome* is the most common and widely known of the entrapment neuropathies

4. The *hyperkyphosis* postural distortion pattern is associated with increased risk of falls in the elderly

POSTURE QUADRANT 3

Posture Quadrant 3 is of primary importance for postural anatomy. Posture Quadrant 3 is the principal stability quadrant from which you stabilize your internal environment. This is the only quadrant of the body that does not play a role in orientation; the purpose of Posture Quadrant 3 is solely for stabilization. The majority of postural distortion patterns are initiated in Posture Quadrant 3, causing alignment compensations and muscular inefficiencies in other parts of the kinetic chain. Complex anatomic structures and physiologic functions occur in Posture Quadrant 3. The primary functions include respiration, mobility, stability, digestion, reproduction, and detoxification.

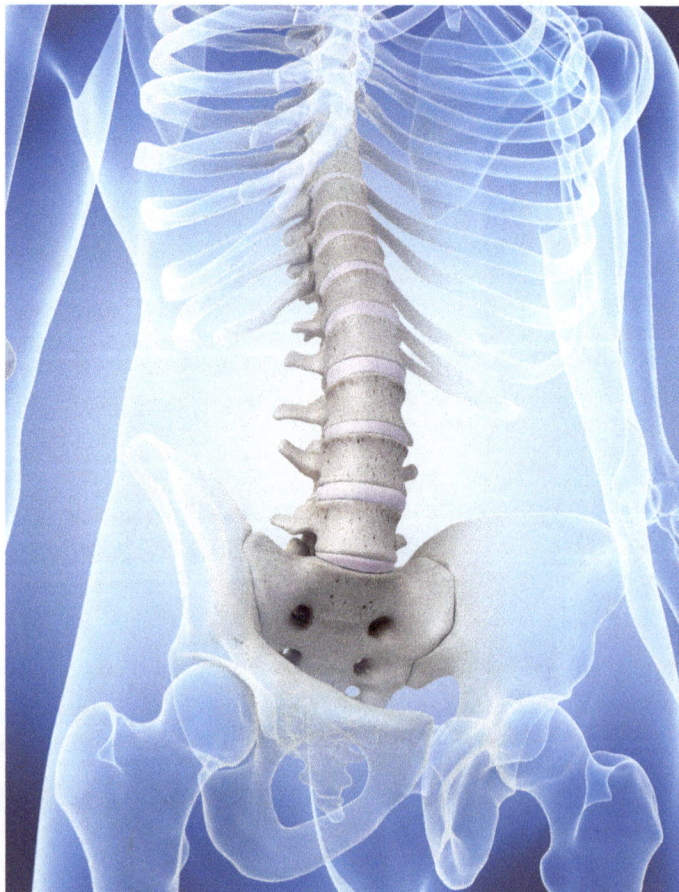

Physiologic discrepancies in this posture quadrant can significantly debilitate the quality of life of your patients. For example, faulty posture affects the ability of the body to properly digest food. A misaligned body means a misaligned digestive tract. This affects the ability of the food to move comfortably and fluidly through the digestive tract.

A body with poor postural presentation is a body under stress. As digestion is a parasympathetic process, the digestive system is able to process food with more efficiency when it is in a parasympathetic state. Sympathetic overdrive can be caused by many factors, including postural distortion patterns. When the body is in a chronic state of stress, the ability of the body to digest and process food for energy is limited. Interestingly, one of the most common factors among patients who seek professional medical attention for low back pain is the presence of associated digestive dysfunction or gastrointestinal discomfort (Coté, 1998).

The anatomic components associated with Posture Quadrant 3 include the core musculature, made up of the diaphragm, the rectus abdominis, the internal and external obliques, the transverse abdominis, the multifidi, the pelvic floor, and the iliopsoas. Also in Posture Quadrant 3 reside the lumbar spine, with its associated paravertebral musculature, and the complex pelvic girdle. These structures are prime stabilizers, keeping the body in an erect position countering the force of gravity.

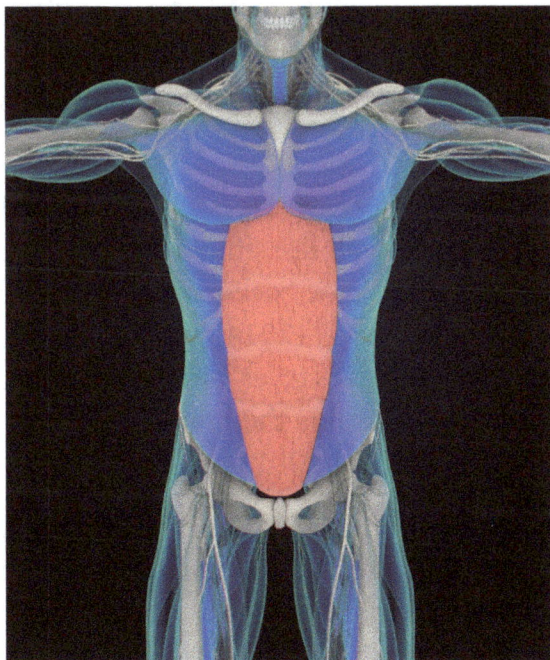

The lumbopelvic transition zone forms the base of the spinal column. When misalignments are found in this area of the spine, compensation patterns arise in other posture quadrants. For many patients, lumbopelvic misalignments and weak core muscle activation are the primary causes of faulty posture patterns. Postural distortions of Posture Quadrant 3 often result in postural collapse of Posture Quadrant 2 and decreased efficiency in movement patterns of Posture Quadrant 4.

Transition zones of the spine are where function changes. Movement from the legs is transmitted to the rest of the spine via the lumbopelvic transition zone. Transition zones are of utmost importance in synchronizing dynamic movements between posture quadrants. Spinal transition zones are often weak areas due to increased compressive forces. For example, patients commonly present with pain and postural instabilities at the cervicothoracic and lumbopelvic junctions. Chronic postural distortion patterns of Posture Quadrant 3 cause lumbosacral strain, sacroiliac strain, facet slipping, and/or disc herniations.

Low back pain is the most common musculoskeletal dysfunction affecting millions of people each year. The Global Burden of Disease Study (2010) is the largest study to describe the global distribution and causes of a wide array of major disease, injuries, and health risk factors. Musculoskeletal conditions were shown to be the second greatest cause of disability globally. They affect over 1.7 billion people worldwide and have the fourth greatest impact on the overall health of the world population, considering both death and disability. The Global Burden of Disease Study showed that low back pain is the leading cause of disability and that osteoarthritis is one of the fastest growing conditions.

The consequences of low back pain reach far beyond localized pain and discomfort. Patients with low back pain move with less efficiency, less controlled motion of their extremities, and decreased balance. Low back pain affects the movement patterns of the rest of the body. According to Haavik (2014), when a spinal segment doesn't move properly, it influences how the brain perceives and responds to all other sensory information. Dysfunction of the spine disrupts the brain's ability to sense accurately what is going on in the rest of the body (Holt, 2013).

In addition, balance and equilibrium suffer. Patients who present with postural dysfunction of their lower back stabilize themselves differently against gravity, because they perceive their bodies less accurately. A lack of bodily awareness disrupts coordinated balance. Low back pain patients are less sturdy on their feet, demonstrating that patients who present with low back pain have poor overall postural control (Sohn, 2013).

Jones, S. et al. (2011) demonstrate that people with low back pain have different postural stabilization patterns and move differently. Neuromotor alterations to pain were noted which represent either movement patterns that have developed in response to pain or underlying impairments that may contribute to recurrent episodes of low back pain. Understanding the relationship between pain and how postural distortion patterns disrupt dynamic movements helps the Posture Expert make predictions of kinetic chain dysfunction.

Decreased postural control affects the movement patterns of the limbs. In the presence of pain, the body naturally stabilizes the injured area (in this case, the lumbar spine), and recruits other muscles and joints to move in its place. The change in muscle activation patterns due to low back pain results in abnormal recruitment, sequencing, and muscle control during dynamic movements (Suter et al., 1999).

The global effects of low back pain are demonstrated through faults of the central nervous system. Chronic low back pain has been shown to cause premature brain aging. Patients presenting with chronic low back pain demonstrated 10–20 times more loss of gray matter on MRI than the control group (Apkarian, 2004). This renowned research study demonstrates a direct link between spinal function and central nervous system function. When the central nervous system is compromised, the patient may suffer from a myriad of negative health consequences.

O'Sullivan et al. (2002) demonstrated the relationship between passive postures and low back pain. They evaluated pain levels and electromyographic activation of lumbopelvic musculature in pain free adults during different seated and standing postures. They concluded that low back pain may be exacerbated when a patient assumes a passive posture such as a slumped posture or a swayback. In addition, the lumbopelvic stabilization musculature demonstrates weaker activation during passive postures.

Types of low back pain

Lumbosacral strain is one of the most common types of back pain. There are two associated causes: faulty alignment and undue compression on bony structures. The spine may have good alignment in weight bearing, but if the low back muscles are tight, they will undergo sudden stress and acute muscle tension with forward bending. Or, the spine may have very faulty alignment such as a lordosis, swayback, or a scoliosis with associated tightness of the low back muscles. For those with faulty alignment and muscle tightness, both stationary positions and movements may give rise to pain. Compressive stress of the spine is often caused by weak core musculature. The pain is usually a gradual onset.

Movement of the spine is critical. The movement of the spine compresses and opens the discs, providing nutritional needs to them. Without motion, the spine will deteriorate at a faster rate, accelerating postural aging.

Most sacroiliac (SI) strains are the result of undue tension on the ligaments with pelvic displacement. The SI joints are supported by strong ligaments; no muscles cross directly over them to support them as there is very little movement from these joints. Muscle tightness in adjacent areas, such as the low back and hips, however, causes a further restriction of motion during forward bending. Men are more likely than women to have SI joint strain with flat back posture, whereas women are more likely to experience SI joint pain with an increased lordosis. SI joint strain may be bilateral, but is more commonly unilateral. Pain is generally exacerbated from sitting in unsupported flexion of the lumbosacral region

Facet slipping occurs when the facet joints that connect one vertebra with another show abnormal deviations of alignment. Facet slipping may occur at the limit of range in flexion or hyperextension. Patients often describe acute facet slipping as "hearing a click" or feeling "out of place". Facet slipping most often occurs in flexion.

Intervertebral foramina (IVF) protrusion is another common cause of low back pain. Vertebral discs bulge anteriorly during flexion, posteriorly during extension, and toward the direction of the concavity on lateral bend. Acute radiating nerve pain is often caused by a sudden twist and extension of the spine from a forward bent position, such as twisting the trunk while lifting a weight.

Sciatica occurs from neuritis of the long sciatic nerve. Pain patterns associated with sciatica include radiation down the posterior thigh and lower leg to the sole of the foot and along the lateral aspect of the lower leg to the dorsum of the foot. The sciatic nerve runs a significantly long course from the spine and is susceptible to irritation at multiple different sites. Irritation may occur to the nerve root at the level that the spinal nerves exit the spinal canal, or at the sacroiliac region where the nerve exits from the sacral foramen, causing strain on the sacral plexus. Sciatic irritation may also occur from a lesion along the course of the nerve of peripheral extensions.

Another common cause of sciatica is Piriformis Syndrome. The piriformis has multiple standing functions. It externally rotates the femur and pulls the sacrum down, tilting the pelvis posteriorly. Faulty alignment of the piriformis occurs when the leg is in adduction and internal rotation in relation to an anteriorly tilted pelvis. This position causes marked stretching of the piriformis and irritation of the sciatic nerve.

Residing below the lumbar spine is the pelvic girdle. The pelvic girdle has many muscular attachments, including the following:

- The erector spinae and the quadratus lumborum attach to the posterosuperior aspect of the pelvis, exerting an upward force posteriorly

- The anterior abdominals, especially the rectus abdominis, attach to the pubic symphysis, and the external obliques attach to the anterior iliac crest, exerting an upward pull anteriorly

- The gluteus maximus, gluteus medius, and the hamstrings attach to the posterior ilium, sacrum, and ischium, exerting a downward pull posteriorly

- The rectus femoris, tensor fascia latae (TFL), and the sartorius attach to the anterior superior and anterior inferior spines of the ilium and the iliopsoas, with attachment on the lumbar spine and inner surface of the ilium, exerting a downward pull anteriorly

- Lateral opposition occurs when the hip abductors on one side and lateral trunk muscles on the other side combine in action to tilt the pelvis laterally
  - Right abductors pull downward on the right side of the pelvis as left lateral trunk muscles pull upward on the left side
  - Leg abductors, mainly the gluteus medius and minimus, which arise from the lateral side of the pelvis pull downward on the pelvis when the leg is fixed in standing
  - The lateral trunk muscles, attached to the lateral side of the ilium, pull upward laterally on the pelvis

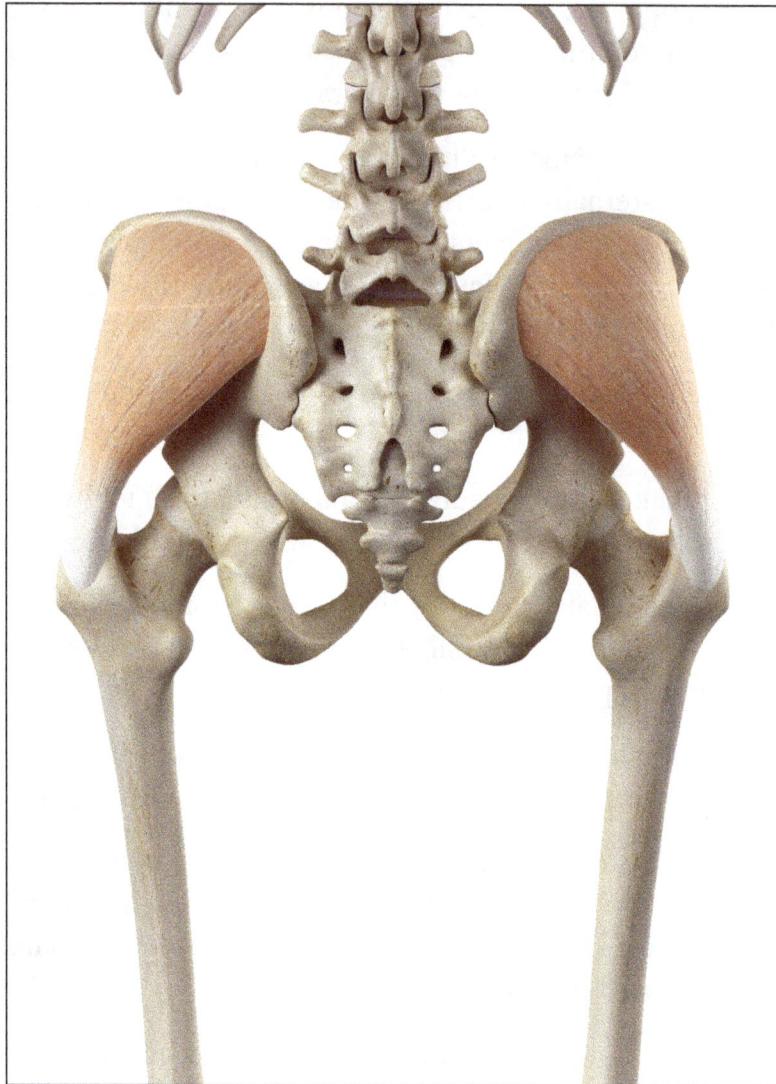

Many of the muscles of the hips and the pelvis perform similar movements, thus it is important to evaluate for accommodation in cases of muscle shortness and substitution in cases of muscle weakness. If muscle length is excessive, avoid stretching exercises and postural positions that maintain elongation of the muscle. These conditions indicate the need for strengthening exercises. When muscles are short and stretching is indicated, attention should be paid to stretching the appropriate muscle group.

A common differential diagnosis in muscle weakness is among the abdominal muscles and the hip flexors. Abdominal muscles receive their innervation from the thoracic branches of the ventral division of the spinal nerves. Trunk raising movement is utilized as an analytical test combining two parts for differential diagnosis: spinal flexion and hip flexion. When the patient is supine, spinal flexion occurs as the abdominal muscles curl the trunk forward. The spine is completely flexed and the feet are on the ground. Hip flexion occurs as the hip flexors contract, lifting the trunk and pelvis off the table anteriorly. The crucial point of the test is the moment in which hip flexion is initiated. If the feet rise as the hips flex forward, this indicates hip flexor weakness.

The spine may have good alignment in weight bearing, but if the low back muscles are tight, they will undergo sudden stress and acute muscle tension with forward bending. The spine may have very faulty alignment such as a lordosis without tightness of the low back muscles. In this case, the back feels fine with movement, but prolonged positions such as sitting or standing cause pain. For those with faulty alignment and muscle tightness, both stationary positions and movements may give rise to pain.

Core musculature

The musculature of Posture Quadrant 3 makes up the core musculature. The core is the center of gravity for the body, the primary area of stabilization. The core of an object is its most central and essential part. The key to authentic core strength is the relationship between an anchored pelvis in proper alignment and a freely moving ribcage.

Core training has gained a tremendous amount of attention in the literature from exercise enthusiasts and trendy exercise programs promising to improve core strength. Although the "popularity" of core training for athletes and professionals alike is a positive thing, often these core training programs equate core stability with abdominal strength. A strong core requires much more than doing crunches to strengthen the rectus abdominis. All core muscles need to be activated to improve strength. Injury prevention and optimal human performance lie much deeper than simple abdominal strength. A combination of mobility, stability, and strength is essential among each core muscle for optimal function of the body.

Restrictions of core movement are most commonly due to tension of the pelvic floor musculature, shortened outer corset musculature, restricted diaphragmatic breathing, or misalignments of the pelvic girdle. Effective rehabilitation plans focus on all muscles of the core, not just the recuts abdominis. Unnatural strength arises from over strengthening the abdominals by doing too many crunches and sit-ups. This shortens the distance between the sternum and pubic symphysis, causing the pelvis to tuck, hamstrings to shorten, the psoas to clench, the diaphragm to be constricted, and contraction and compression of the spine. Although these muscles look good when contracted on the beach, they can be counterproductive to maintaining good posture.

Abdominal muscles have three primary layers. The outer layer, running vertically from the ribcage to the pelvis, is the rectus abdominis. The rectus abdominis muscles are easily seen; these are the muscles associated with having "6 pack abs". The second layer is made up of the external and internal obliques, which run diagonally from the lower ribcage to the pelvis. The deepest layer contains the transverse abdominis, which runs horizontally beneath the other layers. As the muscle fibers of the transverse abdominis are horizontal in nature, they are not affected by torso crunches or flexion exercises. To locate the transverse abdominis, place your fingertips medial to the ASIS (anterior superior iliac spine) bilaterally, keep your spine straight, and lightly cough. You will feel muscular contraction of the transverse abdominis.

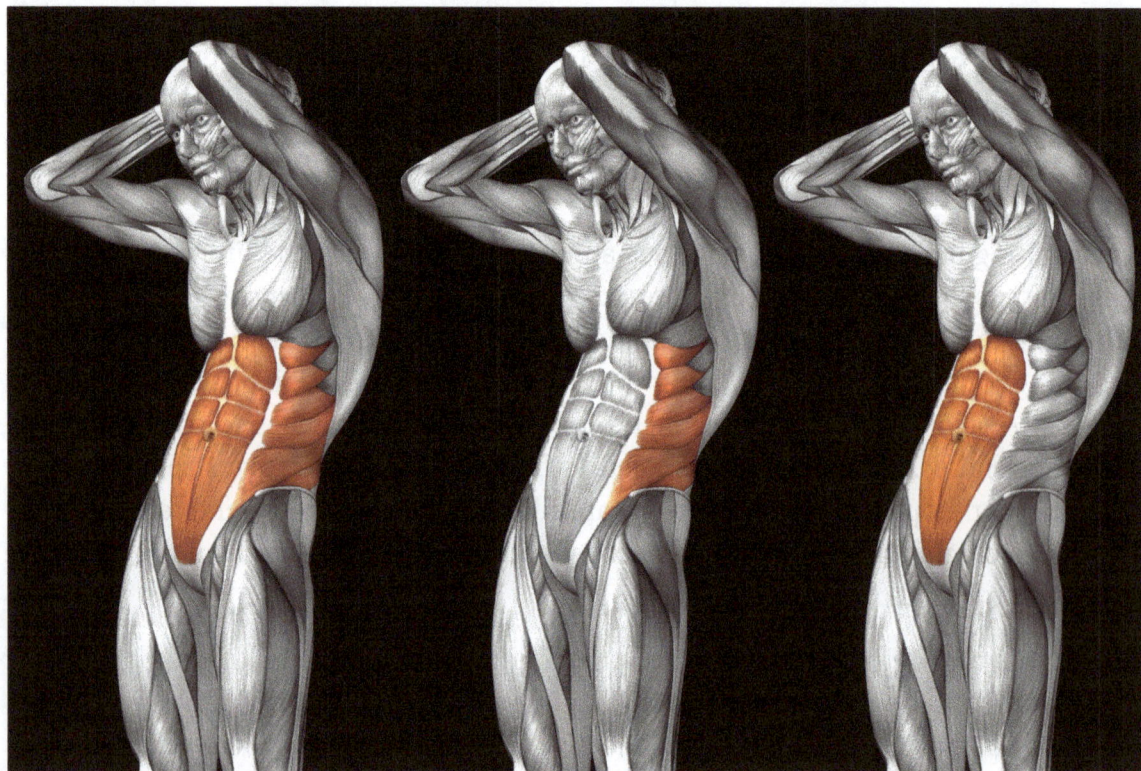

In typical activities of adults, few movements require strenuous use of the core muscles, but most activities tend to activate the low back. Low back pain patients with postural distortion patterns tend not to stabilize or engage the core muscles properly while performing daily activities. This is easily seen with a flaccid belly. When people bend forward and their stomach sticks out instead of contracting, this is an example of flaccid belly. The person is able to perform the movement of bending by activating their lumbar paraspinal muscles and hip flexors instead of their core musculature.

The core musculature is divided into the inner corset, which has direct connection with the spine, and the outer corset, which bends and twists the trunk. The primary muscle of the inner corset is the transverse abdominis, a broad sheath that wraps around the visceral core. The transverse abdominis is the natural corset of support for the upright body, harnessing the vital organs in place. This muscle is equally underdeveloped in fitness professionals who do crunches religiously as it is in sedentary individuals. Contraction of the transverse abdominis compresses the abdomen and tightens the lumbar fascia. The transverse abdominis squeezes, but does not bend, twist, or tilt the trunk. This makes it different from outer corset muscles.

The transverse abdominis has connections between the pubic bone and the navel, which is crucial for lower back stability. When the transverse abdominis activates the lumbar fascia, the multifidi are stimulated to control the lumbar segments. The transverse abdominis stabilizes the lumbar spine during fundamental movements of limbs. In fact, in healthy individuals the transverse abdominis contracts to stabilize your body before activating the muscles of the extremities to move your arms or legs. The transverse abdominis also supports the rotary motion of the lumbar spine as you are walking.

Studies show that the transverse abdominis is only active prior to movement of the limbs in patients who haven't experienced low back pain. Hodges and Richardson (1998) determined that healthy patients activate their core musculature (the transverse abdominis and the internal obliques) to stabilize their trunk before moving their extremities. Patients with low back pain, however, do not activate their core muscles for stabilization. Thus these individuals are more susceptible to future injuries.

"The secret to prevention and elimination of low back pain is sustained contraction of the transverse abdominis."

Bond, 2007, p. 95

Even a contraction of 10–25% of maximal effort is adequate to support and prevent low back pain (Bond, 2007).

The multifidii muscles also protect the spine from injury. Multifidii are deep back muscles that oppose the rectus abdominis. They perform back extension as well as stabilize the lumbar spine. When the transverse abdominis and the multifidii are engaged, they act as an inner corset for the lumbar spine, protecting the body from injury. MRIs of patients with postural distortion patterns of the lumbar spine demonstrate multifidus muscular atrophy, making patients more susceptible to acute injury (Cholewicki, 2005).

The muscles of the outer corset are highly active in trunk mobility and stability. They act to bend your trunk forward and twist it. They are not attached to the spine, therefore do not give direct support to the spine. Outer corset muscles are mainly fast twitch fibers, whereas the inner corset muscles are slow twitch endurance muscles.

When the muscles of the outer corset become shortened, they draw the chest and pelvis together, flattening the curve of the lumbar spine, resulting in excessive pressure on the lumbar intervertebral discs. Rigidity of the outer corset musculature also restricts range of motion of the diaphragm, leading to less efficient upper chest breathing.

Shortened outer corset muscles cause postural collapse, but strong outer corset muscles help support proper alignment of the spine. Where is the happy medium between strength and excessive pull? Balanced posture and proper spinal support are maintained through two techniques of core stabilization: abdominal hollowing and abdominal bracing.

Abdominal hollowing, developed by Hodges (1996), is a method of activating the deep core musculature. This method of core stabilization occurs when the navel is pulled posteriorly toward the spine, activating the transverse abdominis. This method has been adopted by many fitness programs, including yoga and Pilates courses, and has been demonstrated to be efficient for postural correction.

Abdominal bracing, developed by McGill, is a form of global core stabilization. If you were to be punched in the stomach, the natural reaction would be to brace all abdominal muscles simultaneously. In abdominal bracing, the entire abdominal wall is activated from all angles, sides, and directions, causing the layers of muscles to physically bind together. This binding enhances the stability of the core to a much greater degree. According to McGill (2007), abdominal bracing provides 360 degrees of spinal stability, making patients injury resilient.

In a research study performed by Vera-Garcia et al. (2007), they compared the effectiveness of abdominal hollowing and bracing in response to sudden, unanticipated perturbations. They concluded that under these circumstances, abdominal hollowing was ineffective for spinal stabilization, but that abdominal bracing was highly effective. However, spinal bracing caused more compression of the lumbar spine.

The diaphragm is the principal respiratory muscle and is highly significant in postural correction. It attaches to the bottom of the ribs, the spine in the back, and the breastbone in the front. The diaphragm connects to the pleura of the lungs and separates the chest cavity from the internal abdominal organs. When the diaphragm is relaxed, it pushes air out of the lungs, or expiration. When the diaphragm is contracted, it pushes air into the lungs, or inspiration. Contraction and relaxation of the diaphragm control respiration and intra thoracic abdominal pressure gradients, providing the pumping mechanism for venous and lymphatic circulation.

Deep breath

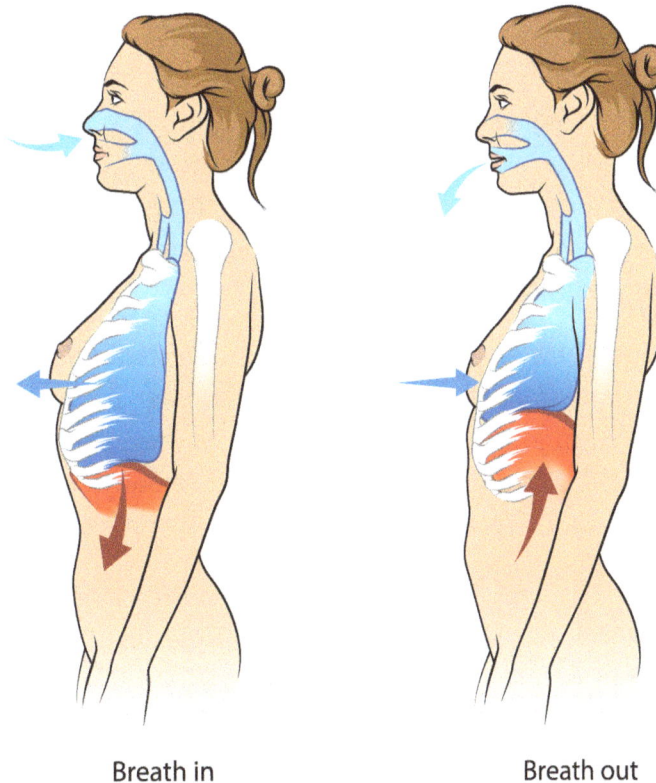

Breath in   Breath out

The psoas major is another major muscle of the core posture zone. This muscle is complex, and highly important for postural correction as it is the only muscle attaching the spine and leg. The psoas major passes along the front of the pelvis and the hip joint and attaches to the inside of the femur. Located deep within the torso, behind the abdominal organs, it merges with the iliacus muscle at the pelvic rim to form the iliopsoas. The actions of the iliopsoas are to bend the hip forward, swing the hip forward when taking a step, and to stabilize the pelvis. The iliopsoas has a symbiotic relationship with the hamstrings.

The iliopsoas muscle is of utmost importance to postural correction. A properly functioning iliopsoas promotes efficiency in movements at the level of the spine, the hip, and the leg. Chronic iliopsoas tightness may be a primary reason for postural asymmetry; or postural asymmetry may be the reason for a tight iliopsoas. Long-term correction of pelvic unleveling is difficult to achieve with iliopsoas tightness. Asymmetric psoas strain can increase pelvic unleveling and lumbar strain. As the pelvis is the base of the spine, chronic asymmetric postural patterns of the pelvis will lead to sustained compensation patterns, including scoliosis in more severe and prolonged cases.

When the pelvis tucks under in a posterior tilt, it causes the psoas and hamstrings to ipsilaterally shorten on the side of the high hip. Similarly, if the trunk prevents the spine and pelvis from rotating with full range of motion, it causes chronic shortening and tension of the iliopsoas. Tightening of these muscles is commonly felt as back or hip pain to patients. Actively stretching the muscles brings only short-term relief if the underlying pelvic misalignment is not corrected.

You can see iliopsoas tightness in your patient as the patient is lying supine on the table. When the pelvis is in a neutral position, the lower back should have a normal anterior curve and the hip joint is in a zero position. When the patient presents with a tight iliopsoas, a lordotic position of the lower back remains and they may find it difficult to flatten their lumbar spine against the table.

Another muscle that plays an important role in posture is the gluteus medius. The gluteus medius performs hip extension, lateral hip rotation, and abduction. In paralysis or marked weakness of the gluteus medius, displacement of the trunk occurs laterally toward the side of gluteus medius weakness, shifting the center of gravity over the weak side. With gluteus medius weakness on one side, the pelvis will ride higher on the side of the weakness. Weakness of the right gluteus medius, for example, allows the pelvis to deviate toward the right and elevate on that side, appearing like a longer leg. Habitual standing with the weight shifted to one side will weaken the hip abductors. Slight gluteus medius weakness is often found in handedness posture patterns.

The pelvic floor is another important component of the Core Posture Quadrant. Stretching across the floor of the pelvis, the pelvic floor musculature serves as a hammock supporting the internal organs. Dysfunction of the pelvic musculature can lead to accidents in controlling the release of urine. This dysfunction is particularly prevalent among women, especially women who have given birth one or multiple times.

Pelvic floor muscle control is directly related to postural symmetry and core activation. In fact, research demonstrates that electromyographic activity of the pelvic floor musculature increases significantly when patients go from a slumped posture to an upright posture. The activity increases even further as patients extend their posture to tall, erect sitting positions (Sapsford et al., 2007). Therefore, proper posture stimulates activation of the pelvic floor to prevent urinary leakage.

Efficient muscle activation of the pelvic floor restores proper load transfer through the lumbopelvic region, while strengthening the transverse abdominis (Critchley, 2002). The transverse abdominis, a deep core muscle, plays a crucial role in supporting proper postural alignment of the lumbar spine. The majority of patients who present with dysfunction of Posture Quadrant 3 demonstrate weakness of the transverse abdominis.

Also consider the relationship between the alignment of the pelvis and sacrum, and how this affects urinary incontinence. Weakness of pelvic floor musculature can generate a backward rotation of the sacrum, as seen in both males and females. In females, there has also been noted stiffening of the sacroiliac joints with pelvic floor alteration (Pool-Goudzwaard et al., 2004).

The lumbar curvature should also be considered. Asymptomatic women tend to have a greater depth of lumbar lordotic curvature, in particular while seated, than women with urinary incontinence. Women who present with urinary incontinence tend to demonstrate anterior pelvic translation while seated with related slumped spinal posture.

According to Norton and Baker (1994), "Postural changes are an effective means of reducing urine leakage in women with stress urinary incontinence and should be an integral part of the management of this condition." For improved pelvic floor control, postural coordination is necessary. As the lower back goes into extension, it causes weakness of the pelvic floor and susceptibility to urine release. Strengthening occurs through specific Kegel exercises in which the pelvic floor is contracted. Sustained contraction results in greater strength.

SECTION REVIEW

1. The other posture quadrants are for stabilization and for orientation. Posture Quadrant 3 is different because it solely does *stabilization*

2. The *core* is the center of gravity for the body, the primary area of stabilization

3. The *inner corset* of the core has connection to the spine

4. The *diaphragm* is the principal respiratory muscle and is highly significant in postural correction

POSTURE QUADRANT 4

Posture Quadrant 4 extends from the femoral head of each leg to the distal phalanges of each foot, including the thigh, knee, lower leg, and the foot. The primary function of this posture quadrant is to perform coordinated ambulatory movements. Posture Quadrants 3 and 4 are connected via the pelvic girdle and the nerve supply of the lower extremity via the lumbar and the sacral plexuses.

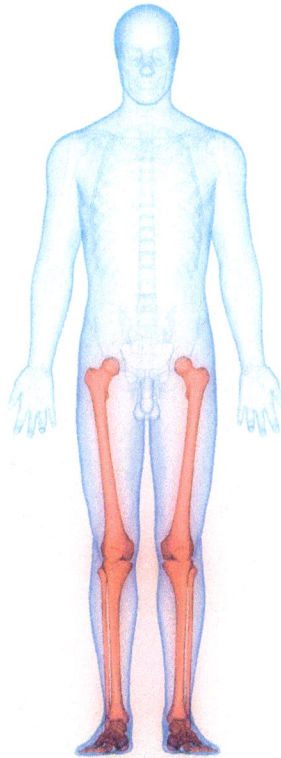

Coordination of the lower extremities is fundamental for performing common human movements including walking, running, and bending. While the majority of postural muscles in Posture Quadrant 3 are Type 1 slow twitch muscles to stabilize the body upright against gravity, the muscles of the limbs are predominately Type 2 fast twitch muscles to perform rapid and powerful movements.

Proper function of Posture Quadrant 4 is necessary to perform common daily movements, as well as to protect the body in instances of survival. The ability to run away from a harmful stimulus quickly without injuring the joints or pulling a muscle is a life-sustaining function.

The orienting anatomy of Posture Quadrant 4 is the feet and the stabilizing anatomy is the leg, lower leg, knee, and ankle. The feet are the foundation of the body, and are highly active in orientation. Unlike the foundation of a building that is static, our feet are dynamic and are designed to support a moving body. Sensation of the feet is transmitted throughout the posture system for stabilization, even activating the musculature of the inner corset.

The feet are perceptual organs; they interact directly with the external environment, keeping us "grounded" in space. The perception of the feet tells the body where "down" is within our external environment. The sole of each foot has more than 7,000 nerve endings that work together with the ankle joints for balance and proprioception. The feet are highly durable and resilient and are designed for complex movements. On a daily basis, the feet respond to uneven surfaces, repetitive shocks, and uneven impacts. The feet absorb 3 million tons of pressure per day (Porter, 2006).

Each foot has 26 bones, 32 joints, 56 ligaments, and 38 muscles. One fourth of the bones of the body are found in the feet. There are three arches to the foot: the outside and inside longitudinal arches run vertically from the heel to the ball of the foot and the mid arch runs horizontally across the foot. The outside arch, or the lateral longitudinal arch, is for "stance" as it contacts the ground first during a gait cycle. The inside arch, or the medial longitudinal arch, is more prominent in weight bearing and for walking as it propels the body in forward momentum. The foot acts as a spring, absorbing energy with each step and distributing it through the fasciae to contribute to the body's forward movement.

The way patients balance on their feet has tremendous effects on their posture. By putting more weight on the heels, for example, they cause the muscles on the front of the body to tighten to avoid falling forward. Standing on the heels is also an associated cause of upper chest breathing due to a restriction in the pattern of movement of the chest.

Having the feet too close together also causes postural instability for many people as it creates a small base of support for the weight of the rest of the body. With an instable base of support, the body feels like it is falling; this causes more tension on the postural muscles and increased postural sway.

The lower extremity is made up of primary muscle groups and important joint complexes for ambulation and locomotion. The primary muscle groups of the upper leg are the divisions of the quadriceps and the hamstrings. The quadriceps and the hamstrings act as agonists and antagonists to one another during movement. Primary muscle groups of the lower leg are the gastrocnemius and soleus and the tibialis anterior.

The tensor fascia latae (TFL) muscle also plays a significant role in posture. The TFL abducts, flexes, and internally rotates the hip joint and assists in knee extension. Tightness of the TFL is not only painful for patients, but it can contribute to rotational posture distortions of the pelvis. As the dermatome distribution is similar, a tight TFL is commonly misdiagnosed as sciatica. Pain is present at the lateral thigh, and can extend superiorly to the buttocks. If the TFL is weak, there is strain on the high side of the pelvis.

The hip joint is a ball-and-socket joint formed by the articulation of the acetabulum of the pelvis with the head of the femur. Movements about this joint include the hip and the leg and how they interact with one another. Flexion and extension occur around the coronal plane, and abduction and adduction occur around the sagittal axis. Lateral and medial rotation occurs around the longitudinal axis.

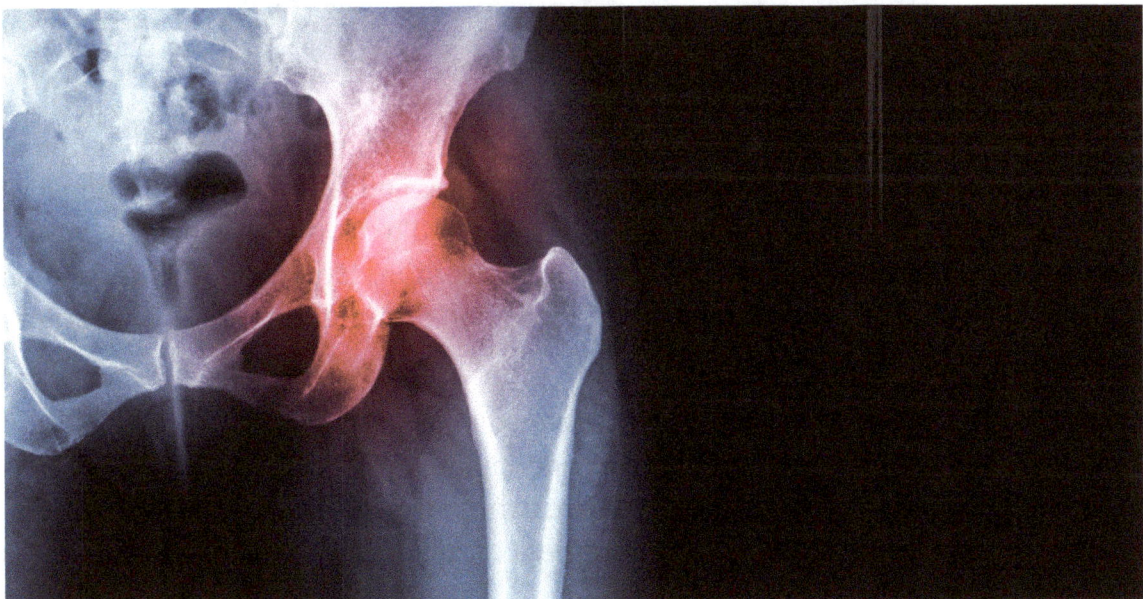

The knee joint is a hinge joint that includes articulation of the condyles of the femur with the condyles of the tibia, and the patella articulating with the patellar surface of the femur. Flexion and extension occur around the coronal axis. Lateral rotation and medial rotation are movements about a longitudinal axis. Rotation does not occur with the knee in extension, but medial and lateral rotation is possible with flexion.

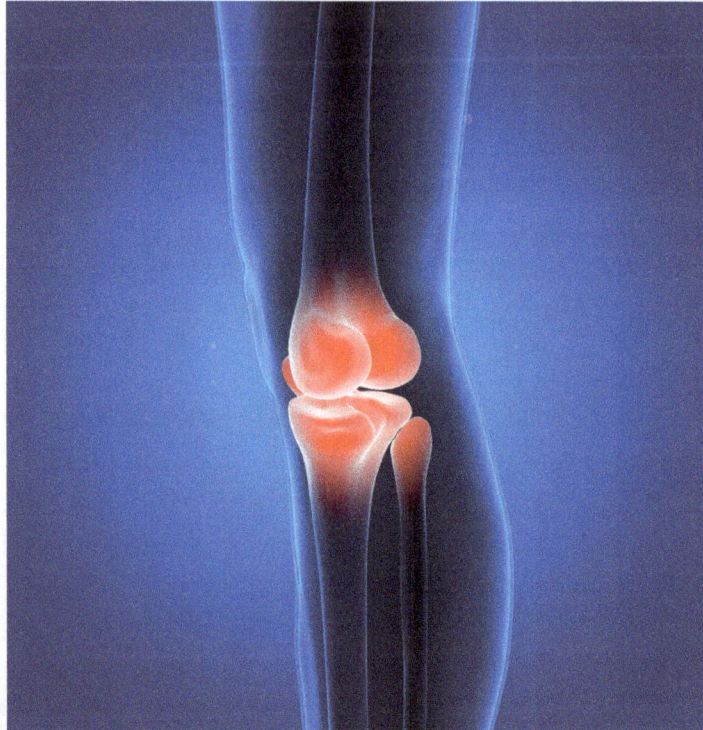

The orientation of the knees is often due to the rotation of the thighs, which is due to the hips. If the pelvis is tilted back, the thighs, knees, and feet tend to turn outward when the patient is standing or walking. If the pelvis is tilted forward, with an increased lumbar curve, the thighs, knees, and feet tend to turn in. Hyperextension, extension of the knee joint past the zero position, is a common postural distortion. This is more common in children than adults.

Knee hyperextension causes undue compression on the anterior aspect of the knee and undue tension for the posterior ligaments and muscles. Pain in the popliteal space is common. If the popliteal muscle becomes weak from hyperextension, it causes lateral rotation of the knee. Knee flexion is much less common than hyperextension, but is present in the elderly population.

Muscle tightness of musculature in Posture Quadrant 2 and 3 can affect the position of the knees and feet. Muscles that insert on the anterior aspect of the femur are medial rotators, and muscles that insert on the posterior aspect are lateral rotators. The medial rotators include the TFL, gluteus minimus, and gluteus medius. Weakness of these muscles results in lateral rotation of the lower extremity, whereas shortened musculature will cause medial rotation of the hip, in-toeing, or knocked knees. Lateral rotators of the femur are the piriformis, quadratus femoris, obturator internus, obturator externus, gemellus superior, and the gemellus inferior. Weakness of the lateral rotators causes medial rotation of the femur, knocked knees, and pronation of the foot. Shortness of the lateral rotators causes lateral rotation of the thigh, and associated out-toeing.

The ankle joint is a complex joint made up of three bones: the tibia, fibula, and the talus. It is a hinged synovial joint. The primary joint movements are plantar flexion and dorsiflexion about the oblique axis. The subtalar joint is a gliding joint located directly below the ankle joint; combined range of motion of the ankle and subtalar joints results in universal joint movement. Numerous ligaments surround the ankle and subtalar joints, including the anterior and posterior ankle capsular ligaments and the medial and lateral ankle ligaments, which bind the bones of the leg to each other and to those of the foot.

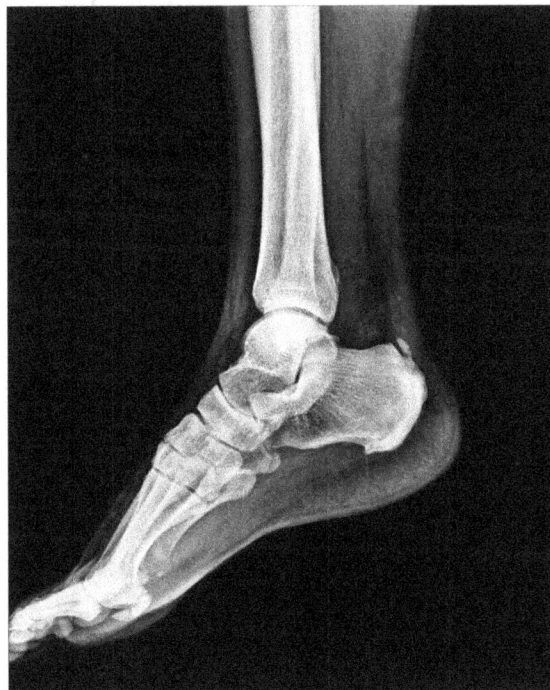

The primary function of Posture Quadrant 4 is ambulation, or movement from one place to another. Walking, a seemingly easy task for healthy humans, is actually a complex movement pattern. Walking involves three motions: front to back where the heel contacts first, from side to side, and rotation around the center of gravity. The ball and socket joint of the hip allows these motions to occur simultaneously. Walking occurs most efficiently when all three motions move with proper coordination.

In a healthy walking pattern, your back leg is the active one, not the front. The downward pressure of your push off foot activates the kinetic chain of the ipsilateral leg and hip up to the opposite shoulder, as seen in the cross crawl pattern. The pelvis should move freely to be centered over the stepping foot to ensure balance. Heel strike occurs from use of the whole heel, not just the back edge.

The gait cycle is a complex movement pattern consisting of 6 steps: heel strike, foot-flat, midstance, heel off, toe off, and mid-swing. The stance phase includes heel strike to heel off. As the stance phase ends, the swing phase begins. This phase is the phase between the toe off and the next heel strike. The gait cycle is a repetitive pattern involving steps and strides. A step is one single step; step time is the time from one foot hitting the floor to the other foot hitting the floor; a stride is a whole gait cycle.

When you are walking, your heel strikes first and orients you into space. In midstance, the mid foot and arches are responsible for resilience and adaptability. The majority of people actually have poor awareness of the mid foot. This can cause a disturbance in the transfer of weight from the heel to the toes during a gait cycle. A sprained ankle, for example, is often the result of poor awareness of the mid foot. The forefoot to the toes is where the power of the foot is found. The forefoot pushes off the ground to propel the leg forward in the final phase of gait. People who lack push off from the toes tend to over utilize the knee joint, which over time causes repetitive motion injury.

Physical consequences of poor structural alignment of the fourth posture quadrant are commonly associated with acute traumas or altered movement patterns associated with unresolved chronic injuries. Imbalances of the feet can be caused as compensation for postural distortion patterns of the spine, or postural distortion patterns of the spine can be compensating for unbalanced feet. In older people, their feet may become painful because of the loss of normal padding on the soles. Insoles that cushion the foot can improve comfort of elderly patients.

Ankle sprains are common fourth quadrant injuries, referring to tearing of the ligaments of the ankle. Two ligaments are most commonly sprained, including the anterior talofibular ligament and the calcaneal fibular ligament. Although ankle sprains can occur on the lateral or medial aspect of the joint complex, more commonly injuries occur on the lateral aspect of the ankle joint. Patients with weakness of the peroneal muscles are more susceptible to inversion ankle sprains.

Chronic ankle instability (CAI), present in up to 70% of individuals who suffer an initial lateral ankle sprain, is the occurrence of repetitive ankle instability, often resulting in subsequent ankle sprains (Waterman et al., 2010). Research suggests that individuals with chronic ankle instability use different movement strategies to maintain postural control than individuals with healthy ankles. These changes may be related to alterations in movement variability associated with ankle instability.

McKeon and Hertel (2008) stated that postural control appears to be adversely affected in patients with CAI compared with healthy patients. As a result of ankle instability, patients with CAI position their center of pressure more anteriorly and laterally on their base of support. Pope et al. (2011) determined that the plantar aspect of the foot, where CAI patients distribute their weight, is the most unstable data point for postural control.

The most common foot misalignment is over pronation. Approximately 92% of the population has pronated feet. Of this 90%, about 60% present with excessive pronation (Griffith, 2014). Indications of pronation include out-toeing, a dropped navicular, posterior lateral heel wear and tear of the shoes, patellar approximation and inward rotation of the tibia, superior lateral tracking of the patella, decreased muscle tone of the hip abductors (TFL, ITB), inward bending of the Achilles tendon, and callus formation under the 2–4 metatarsals.

There is almost always no symptomology with pronation, but it affects the postural presentation of the patient. With pronation, the patient walks and stabilizes on the inner arch of the foot. This leads to flattening of the inner arch as it was supposed to be utilized for movement, not stabilizing. The tendons of several calf muscles run underneath the feet to support the arches. If the foot is over pronated or supinated, it prevents normal rotation of the tendons.

Pronation without flatness of the longitudinal arch is often found among women who wear high heels. This pronation pattern causes more strain medially at the knee. In the actual foot, the anterior arch is subject to more strain than the longitudinal arch.

Pronation with flatness of the longitudinal arch occurs when the foot is in dorsiflexion and eversion with out-toeing of the forefoot. Excessive tension is present on the muscles and ligaments of the inner side of the foot, supporting the longitudinal arch. Compression is placed on the outside of the foot at the talocalcaneonavicular joint. The tibialis posterior and abductor hallucis are usually weak and the peroneal muscles tend to be tight.

Pronation misalignments of the foot and lower leg include the talus being misaligned anteriorly and laterally. The calcaneus is everted and plantar flexed, and changes in the soft tissue components of calcaneus lead to misalignment of the fibular head. The fibular head misaligns posteriorly and laterally. Stretching of the anterior talofibular ligament in inversion sprains of the ankle leads to fibular misalignment.

Out-toeing of the foot may be caused by multiple different postural distortion patterns. External rotation that occurs at the hip level is also associated with strain on the longitudinal arch as weight is transferred from heel to toe. Lateral rotation of the tibia is often accompanied with tightness of the Achilles tendon. Abduction may also occur in the foot itself as a result of the breakdown of the longitudinal arch.

The supination pattern of the foot is the opposite of pronation; it is characterized by in-toeing, a high arch, and weight distribution on the outside of the foot. Supinated feet present with a pigeon toed appearance. Postural fault may occur at various anatomic levels. If the legs are internally rotated at the hips, the patellae will face inward. With in-toeing due to medial rotation of the tibia, the patellae face forward but the feet point inward. Problems of the feet show the hips and knees in good alignment, but anterior foot varus is present (foot adduction).

Collapsed arches occur from medial rotation of the knees, causing the ankle to roll in and the leg bones to be misaligned with the ankle. Arches of the feet have minimal muscular support; they are primarily ligamentous in nature. For correction purposes, then, it is important to correct the alignment of the foot. For plastic deformation of the feet, low intensity forces for prolonged periods of time can create permanent plastic changes. Developing young children should spend as little time as possible in shoes (and wear soft, flexible shoes), allowing for full movement of the toes and arches.

A common knee injury is the "unhappy triad" or tears of the anterior cruciate ligament (ACL), the medial cruciate ligament (MCL), and the medial meniscus. This injury occurs from lateral force applied to the knee while the foot is fixed on the ground. It is common in contact sports such as football, rugby, soccer, etc. With the exception of direct knee trauma, the majority of knee problems are due to poorly supported feet or restricted hip motion. In the case of the unhappy triad, prolonged pronation of the foot and ankle complex produces excessive internal tibial rotation, which produces a pre-loading effect on the ACL.

Bowed legs can be actual (structural) or apparent (postural). Actual bowed legs are caused from Rickets and correction requires bracing. Apparent bowed legs are caused from faulty posture: medial hip rotation, medial thigh rotation, hyperextended knees, and pronated feet. Correction of postural bow legs includes alignment of the hips, strengthening lateral rotators, correct shoe support for pronated feet, and attention of the patient not to hyperextend their knees.

The knocked knee presentation is the opposite of bowed legs, in which the knees are shifted medially. It is characterized by tension on the medial ligaments and compression on the lateral surfaces of the knee with a tight TFL and ITB. Treatment of mild knocked knees in-cludes stretching the TFL and ITB, proper shoes with an inner border wedge, and strengthening of the medial rotators. Severe knocked knees may require surgery or bracing.

To prevent common painful foot and leg conditions, proper shoe choice is of utmost importance. Shoes should support the natural arches of the feet and provide ankle sta-bility. They should be the right size and should be tight enough to support the foot, but not so tight it disrupts the circulation to the foot.

Shoes that do not support the feet appropriately cause postural changes throughout the body. Slip on shoes, for example, cause you to lean back, scuff your feet, and con-tract your feet muscles to keep them on. Shoes with heels or high wedges decrease the interaction of your foot with the ground, making you susceptible to ankle injury. Women who wear high heels have adaptive shortening of the soleus and are susceptible to metatarsalgia, hammer toes, and tightness of the Achilles tendon. Clinical trials con-ducted by Cronin et al. (1985) demonstrated that long-term high heel use compromises muscle efficiency in walking and often causes muscle fatigue.

The use of orthotics and lifts in shoes can be highly beneficial for the patient when uti-lized correctly. However, if postural distortion patterns can be corrected and the correction maintained without the use of orthotics or shoe inserts, this will render long-term benefits for the patient. Rigid orthotics can actually weaken foot muscles, making it more difficult to maintain proper posture.

SECTION REVIEW

1. The muscles of the limbs are predominately *Type 2 fast twitch* muscles to perform rapid and powerful movements

2. A tight *TFL* muscle is commonly misdiagnosed as sciatica

3. The primary function of Posture Quadrant 4 is *ambulation,* or movement from one place to another

4. The most common postural distortion pattern of Posture Quadrant 4 is *pronation*

PHYSIOLOGY OF A SPINAL MISALIGNMENT COMPLEX

After examining the structural anatomy and physiologic functions associated with the posture system, we will now look at the physiology of a spinal misalignment complex. As previously mentioned, postural distortions of the spine may be the primary postural distortion pattern, causing weakness in the related kinetic chain. Or, the opposite may be true. Spinal distortions may be caused as a secondary compensation from postural distortions elsewhere in the body.

The Posture Expert should pay special attention to this concept and be certain to correct the primary and ancillary causes of postural asymmetry in the body. Without the Posture Expert correcting the whole postural pattern, the postural distortions will continue to present when the body is stressed.

We begin with a properly aligned spinal joint complex. The principle functions of the vertebral column are to keep the body upright against gravity (posture) and to protect the spinal cord, which is vital to life function. The multifaceted joints give the spine its ability to be fluid and mobile, not rigid.

There are three normal curves of the spine: the cervical curve which has a forward convexity or slight extension of the neck, the thoracic curve which has posterior convexity or slight flexion of the upper back, and the lumbar spine which has forward convexity or slight extension of the lower back.

The spine supports the head and torso, providing support for multidimensional movements. The vertebral bodies give the spinal column the power to absorb and distribute compressive forces, the facet joints enable hydraulic lift, and the intervertebral discs have shock-absorbing qualities. With proper spinal alignment, the body moves with muscular efficiency and proprioceptive control.

There are 31 pairs of spinal nerves. The ventral root of the spinal nerve is motor, and the dorsal root is sensory. The dorsal and ventral nerve roots meet at the IVF of the spinal segment. This is where the spinal nerve is created, containing motor and sensory fibers. After the spinal nerve exits from the foramen, it divides into a dorsal and ventral primary ramus. The dorsal rami are directed posteriorly to innervate skin and extensor muscles of the neck, trunk, and the facet joints. The ventral rami contain nerve fibers that innervate the arms, legs, and intervertebral discs.

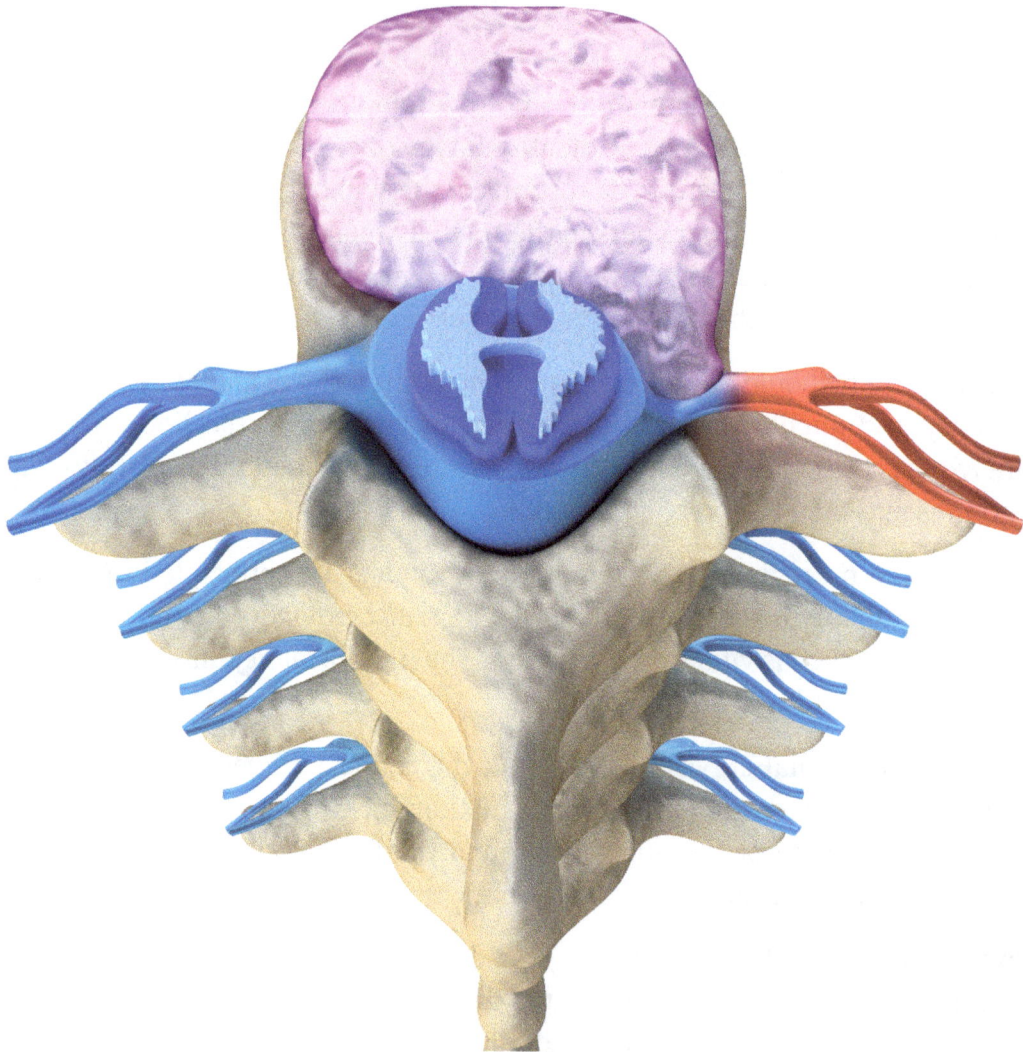

Disturbed kinematics of the spinal joint complex lead to unequal movements of the spinal joints and compromised neurologic function. The complexity of physiologic compromise expands much further than the spinal joint complex, but has the ability to affect the function of the vital organs of the body. Consider each of the physiologic disruptions listed below that occur when a spinal joint complex is misaligned.

Physiologic compromise of a spinal misalignment complex

1. Unequal load sharing, with higher load on one of the facets

2. Elastic deformation of the muscles and tendons
   a. Muscles are the first to weaken and the first to heal. It takes 6 hours for atrophy to begin. Once atrophy begins, you lose 1.5% of muscle mass per day of non-use
   b. Tendons break down based upon the load of the muscle-tendon junction, causing tendonitis

3. Plastic deformation of the ligaments (which is more likely to become permanent)
   a. Ligaments change according to the load applied. Loss of muscle tone decreases joint tension and increases the load to the ligaments

4. Cartilage is where the most severe damage can occur; it heals the slowest and the least. Nutrition is critical for repair of cartilage

5. Vertebral discs degenerate causing decreased rotational torque. The spine may suffer from 25% less rotational ability at the affected joint complex

6. Spinal nerves demonstrate a lower threshold, meaning they fire easier

7. Nerve pathways become de-facilitated with restriction, and the associated body part becomes weak and clumsy
   a. The weight of a dime is the amount of pressure needed to a nerve to cause damage. The longer the nerve is not functioning, the more likely the effects will become permanent. There is an approximate 2 year period of time to regain function of the nerve before it becomes permanently affected

8. Vasculature becomes compromised causing hypoxia in certain tissues, and decreased circulation

9. Adhesions and bony degeneration such as osteophyte formation occur
   a. Wolff's Law states that any abnormal stress to the bone creates bony abnormalities

10. Osteoarthritis or DJD is caused by improper biomechanics and mechanical stress of joints due to weight bearing forces or repetitive activities

11. Joints with abnormal movement result in abnormal stimulation to the brain by the surrounding muscle spindles.

    a. The central nervous system is not controlling the movement of that spinal segment properly. Motor control and stability are different at this level

Postural distortion patterns with spinal misalignments can be very debilitating to the structure and the function of the body. Distortions of the pelvic girdle also contribute to the presence of postural distortion patterns. The pelvic girdle is located at the base of the spine. Postural distortions of the pelvis can also cause spinal misalignments. The neutral position of the pelvis is one in which the anterior superior iliac spines (ASIS) are in the same transverse plane and the ASISs and the pubic symphysis are in the same plane. Any deviation from neutral is considered a postural distortion.

With an anterior pelvic tilt, the vertical plane of the ASIS is anterior to the vertical plane through the symphysis pubis. In standing, an anterior pelvic tilt causes hyperextension of the lumbar spine (increased lordosis) and flexion of the hip joints. Posterior pelvic tilt occurs when the vertical plane through the ASIS is posterior to the vertical plane of the pubic symphysis. While a patient is standing, a posterior pelvic tilt causes flexion of the lumbar spine and extension of the hip joints.

Pelvic unleveling may also occur in the presence of a lateral pelvic tilt. Lateral pelvic tilt means that one ASIS is higher than the other. While the patient is standing, lateral pelvic tilt is associated with lateral flexion of the lumbar spine and with adduction and abduction of the hip joints. If the right iliac crest is higher than the left iliac crest there is lumbar lateral flexion to the right, with the convexity of the curve to the left.

SECTION REVIEW

1. What are the three curves of the spine? *Cervical, thoracic,* and *lumbar*

2. *Cartilage* is where the most severe damage can occur; it heals the slowest and the least

3. With an *anterior pelvic tilt,* the vertical plane of the ASIS is anterior to the vertical plane through the symphysis pubis

PHYSIOLOGY OF THE DISEASE PROCESS IN RELATION TO POSTURAL DISTORTION PATTERNS

With the majority of patients living in a hyper-stressed state of life within their environment, a global postural pattern has emerged that is contributing to structural and functional human breakdown.

In a state of stress, the posture of the body reverts to its most primitive posture, flexor or adductor dominance. Patients in a hyper-stressed state present with anterior tightness above the T6 spinal level: the shoulders and neck are forward with internal rotation of the arms. They also present with posterior tightness below the T6 spinal level including the lumbar paraspinals, the gluts, and hamstrings. External rotation occurs at the hip, causing toe-out foot flare and pronation of the foot.

Flexor dominance above T6 causes hypertonic scaleni and SCM musculature. SCM hypertonicity leads to first rib elevation, and compression of the brachial plexus at C8/T1 primarily. Compression of the neural tissue leads to peripheral neuropathies, and compression of important vasculature leads to conditions such as thoracic outlet syndrome (TOS) and Raynaud's syndrome. Anterior rolling of the shoulders with upper back extensor weakness also causes elbow flexion, which stretches the ulnar nerve and can cause neuritis, or a hypertonic pronator teres, which can lead to pronator teres syndrome. Associated wrist flexion may lead to carpal tunnel syndrome.

Stretched and weakened erector spinae below T6 lead to hypotonic multifidii, spinal misalignments, vertebral disc herniations, peripheral neuropathies, psoas flexion, sciatica, and piriformis syndrome. As the pelvis misaligns, the high hip tends to be on the side of cortical dominance, with ipsilateral psoas tightness. Internal rotation of the femur and tibia occurs on the opposite side of the weak cortex with pronation and gastrocnemius and soleus tightness that can lead to Achilles tendonitis.

There is decreased chest expansion, leading to decreased lung expansion by 12–15%. With decreased lung capacity, hypoxia, or lack of oxygen for certain tissues, occurs. Hypoxia increases the acidity, making the tissues more infectious, and decreases afferent input to the brainstem. The cerebellum receives information from the muscles and tendons of the peripheral limbs and communicates this information to the cortex to stimulate tone. Inhibition of mechanoreceptor flow to the cerebellum will cause a disruption of controlled movement.

A continued sympathetic nervous system response leads to anaerobic glycolysis, causing lactic acid and diffuse pain such as in fibromyalgia or myofascial pain syndrome. Anaerobic glycolysis also leads to inefficient ATP production, associated with chronic fatigue and depression of the immune function. In response to stress, cortisol levels are higher, leading to sugar cravings, and eventually obesity and type 2 diabetes if prolonged.

SECTION REVIEW

1. What is the most primitive posture pattern? *Flexor dominance*

2. *Hypoxia* increases the acidity, making the tissues more infectious, and decreases afferent input to the brainstem

3. A continued *sympathetic* state leads to anaerobic glycolysis, causing lactic acid and diffuse pain

BIOMECHANICS OF THE POSTURE SYSTEM

After understanding the anatomy of the postural system and the posture quadrants, we now transition into postural biomechanics. Postural biomechanics is how the structures and functions of the postural system interact with one another for human performance. Regarding postural biomechanics, alignment and muscle balance are inseparable.

Irvin (2000) explained the concept of postural boundaries. This means that each anatomical structure functions optimally within the boundaries of that structure's biomechanics. This function is inversely proportional to trauma, somatic dysfunction, and disease.

Poor posture is synonymous with an overstretched rubber band. Once the rubber band is stretched it becomes lax and less efficient. Motion collapses in a kinetic chain at the level of the weak muscle. Due to the all-or-none firing patterns of muscles, other areas of muscles with similar functions absorb the responsibility of producing the movement.

From a mechanical standpoint, two types of faults relate to alignment and mobility: increased compression on articulating surfaces of bone or increased tension on bones, ligaments, or muscles. Lack of mobility is associated with persistent faulty alignment. When mobility is lost, stiffness occurs, and a certain alignment remains constant. This can be due to the restriction of motion by tight muscles, which is more common, or the inability of weak muscles to perform their full range of motion.

Muscles do not succeed in functioning for both movement and support. They perform one or the other, but not both simultaneously. When muscular symptoms occur, such as muscle tightness or soreness, the patient will experience muscle fatigue first, then pain.

Muscle weakness allows separation of the origin and insertion of the muscle. Stretch weakness is weakness that results from muscles remaining in an elongated condition, beyond the physiological rest position, but not overstretched (which means past the normal range of the muscle).

One-joint muscles, such as the gluteus medius and minimus, iliopsoas, hip external rotators, abdominal muscles, and middle and low trapezius, are most commonly affected. Treatment for stretch weakness is *not* to do stretches. Proper treatment protocols include realignment of the part causing it to be past neutral, and stabilizing this structure in this position while weak muscles gain strength.

The weak musculature should not be overworked while it is recovering from stretch weakness. Once the muscle gains strength, however, the patient utilizes the muscle to maintain proper muscle balance and good alignment. Also consider ergonomic improvements to support stability of weak muscles once realigned.

Muscle shortness is the opposite of muscle weakness. Muscles shortness is characterized by holding the origin and insertion closer together. Adaptive muscle shortening is tightness due to chronically shortened muscles. Unless the opposing muscle can pull the shortened muscle to neutral, it remains shortened. Several weeks of stretching is generally needed to restore full range of motion of the muscle. Common examples of muscle shortness include sedentary individuals who generally present with adaptive shortening of the iliopsoas, and women who wear high heels, who have adaptive shortening of the soleus.

Muscle guarding occurs to stabilize injured tissue. Just as with an injured neck, shoulder, or ankle, if the spine is injured, the surrounding muscles will naturally contract to stabilize the injured area. The body creates muscle spasms as a protective method. Although stabilizing an injured area is good for acute injuries, the transition from acute injury to recovery requires moving from immobilization to the restoration of fluid movement. Continuing to stabilize an area in recovery will perpetuate the problem.

Tensegrity is the balance of tension and compression resulting in maximum efficiency. Maintaining this balance is an important biomechanical consideration for postural correction. Postural asymmetry leads to unbalanced forces of tension and compression with usually too much reliance on the tensile (muscular) aspect of the design. With a properly aligned spinal column, the tensegrity is better balanced, and the muscles work with increased efficiency.

Elastic creep occurs from loss of rebound of muscles, tendons, and ligaments due to prolonged stress. For example, while a patient is sitting, certain ligaments of the spine shorten. Even after the patient changes postures, the ligaments remain shortened and stiff for a longer period of time.

When treating abnormal conditions of joints and muscles, you must first determine the treatment-based objective of increasing stability or mobility. This differentiation will be essential when evaluating the postural system. We will analyze the parts of the postural system and determine if muscles need to be strengthened or lengthened and if joints need to be mobilized or stabilized. Joints with greater mobility are less stable, and more stable joints have less mobility.

SECTION REVIEW

1. *Stretch weakness* is weakness that results from muscles remaining in an elongated condition, beyond the physiological rest position

2. Adaptive *muscle shortening* is tightness due to chronically shortened muscles

3. *Tensegrity* is the balance of tension and compression resulting in maximum efficiency

ARTICULATION AND SPATIAL ORIENTATION TO BALANCE THE POSTURE SYSTEM

We have already discussed in depth the role that the neurological system plays in balancing the postural framework of the body. To conclude this module, we will now discuss postural balance through articulation.

Articulation is a term used to describe the way in which the parts of a joint work together. API's postural correction system is designed to increase the "articulate capacity" of how the body moves. Energetic articulation is the synchronization of dynamic movement based upon the alignment of the joints, efficiency of the muscles, and fluidity of the fascia. Human bodies move with optimal efficiency when the body is upright in a manner allowing for complete distance between the feet and the top of the head, and when it is balanced equally from side to side.

To improve articulation, Posture Experts should help their patients overcome any habits that close the posture quadrants of the body, restore fluidity to parts of the body that are not moving freely, and improve spatial orientation.

It is easy to stay "grounded" due to gravity. However, it requires spatial orientation to stay upright. Spatial orientation is our relationship with our environment. There are two components of movement: spatial orientation and weight distribution. Our sense of ourselves in space allows us to have goals of how or where to move our bodies. Our weight rebounds off the earth, allowing movement to happen. When the posture quadrants are chronically closed, it draws your dynamic axis closer to the ground, restricting fluid motion.

Healthy posture has articulation and dual orientation. Dual orientation is the ability to interact efficiently with your surroundings and with the ground, to be grounded, and to resist gravity in an efficient manner that does not strain the joints and muscles. When you are dually oriented to the ground and your spatial environment, the postural muscles have optimal length and efficiency. This lengthening prevents chronic shortening and tightness, and prepares the body for more fluid and graceful dynamic movements.

We have already discussed in detail the interacting mechanisms for balance: vestibular, muscle and joint position sensors, and cerebellar control. When there is even distribution of weight bilaterally, the brain perceives the body as being in balance. We have not considered in detail, however, the role that vision plays.

The eyes relate us to our surroundings. For many people, eye orientation is the primary mechanism for balance. Peripheral vision is linked to the subcortical brain, the part of the brain that organizes movements. When your eyes focus tightly, you use the cortical brain, which causes you to use your analytical brain and interferes with coordination. If you expand your vision before doing balance exercises, it is easier to maintain postural balance.

You can find your center of gravity while standing or seated. The center of gravity point while you're standing is two finger widths below the navel and between the spine and the intestines, in front of the third lumbar vertebra. While you're seated, the center of gravity is the point between the shoulder blades.

SECTION REVIEW

1. *Articulation* describes the way in which the parts of a joint work together

2. *Dual orientation* is the ability to interact efficiently with your surroundings and with the ground

Module 3
STRUCTURAL, FUNCTIONAL, AND NEUROLOGICAL POSTURE EVALUATION

INTRODUCTION

Module 1 provided a strong theoretical basis of the posture principle and why proper posture is a key component in achieving optimal human performance. A symmetric and balanced bodily framework is a vital factor for having a healthy lifestyle.

In Module 2 we took a much closer look at the scientific principles of posture and how postural patterns affect the structure and the function of the body. Module 2 provided an in-depth analysis of the posture system and the principal anatomic posture quadrants with their associated physiologic functions. By understanding the structure and the function of the posture system, and the most commonly associated pathologic consequences when postural distortion patterns are present in the posture quadrants, Posture Experts are equipped to make important clinical decisions to optimize the human performance of their patients.

Module 3 will begin by identifying the most common postural distortion patterns, including spinal and bodily joint misalignment patterns and compensatory muscular dysfunction. Once you are able to identify the primary postural distortion patterns, you will then learn how to perform an accurate structural, biomechanical, and functional posture evaluation. Module 3 provides a clear understanding of how to perform an efficient and accurate postural evaluation on any patient.

At the American Posture Institute, we believe in systems and patterns. A systematic approach to clinical evaluation of postural patterns is key to performing a thorough evaluation and immediately interpreting the results. You will learn what tools are necessary to perform the evaluation, and what principle posture patterns to be looking for.

In addition, you will learn the importance of not skipping steps, but analyzing patients' postures from start to finish in a specific sequence. Once you understand how to perform a thorough initial evaluation, you will then learn how to perform a posture scan that can be completed in about 1 minute each time the patient presents to your practice after the initial postural examination. This will provide you as the Posture Expert with the information you need for every patient visit.

Prepare to get up out of your seat while reading the information presented in this module, and try these clinical application tips immediately while they are fresh in your mind. Module 3 and Module 4 are full of practical applications that you can implement into your practice instantly.

In addition to reading the information provided in this textbook, you are highly recommended to participate in the Certified Posture Expert course produced by the American Posture Institute (AmericanPostureInstitute.com). The course will provide you with videos and real life case examples to analyze and learn from. This course ensures mastery of posture to improve clinical accuracy and efficiency.

Examples will also be provided in this section that you can look at and analyze. This will help you become comfortable with the most common postural distortion patterns that patients present with. While you are analyzing the examples, think about your current patients and how the information learned in this module can be utilized to improve your patient care strategies immediately.

IDEAL POSTURE PRESENTATION

Before we analyze postural distortion patterns, it is pertinent to understand what an ideal postural presentation is. Notice the choice of heading for this section; we are not talking about "normal" postural presentations, rather "ideal" posture. The far majority of the population presents with postural distortion patterns, thus "normal" posture will be insignificant information at this time.

Ideal posture is symmetrically balanced bilaterally, and from the anterior to the posterior aspect in relation to the patient's center of gravity. The patient has strong core musculature that supports the proper alignment of the spine and the pelvis. The postural muscles and the joints among the kinetic chain of movement have accurate recruitment patterns and full range of motion. Agonist and antagonist muscle groups fire and stabilize together in synchrony. The connective tissue is fluid, not tightly bound into contracture. The patient has strong postural muscles and mobile joints, so that when they perform dynamic movements, they don't have postural collapse. The brain, cerebellum, and the body produce coordinated and controlled movements. The patient's body is in proper alignment and they have developed postural fitness to maintain this.

More specifically, ideal posture has the following structural components. Consider ideal posture patterns from the anterior, lateral, and posterior aspect of the patient.

Anterior view of the patient:

- Head: neutral position (no lateral flexion or rotation)

- Eyes: parallel to the horizon

- Ears: level with one another bilaterally

- Chin: centered (not rotated to one side)

- Shoulders: level bilaterally (not elevated or depressed), even muscular development, and pulled back (not rotated forward)

- Arms: neutral position, at even lengths, palms toward the lateral aspect of the body with the thumbs pointed forward

- Pelvis: level, both anterior superior iliac spines and pelvic crests are in the same transverse plane

- Hip joints: neutral position (no abduction or adduction, or flexion or extension)

- Patellae: level bilaterally, pointed forward

- Feet: parallel with slight out-toeing. The medial malleoli are in the same vertical plane (no pronation or supination is present)

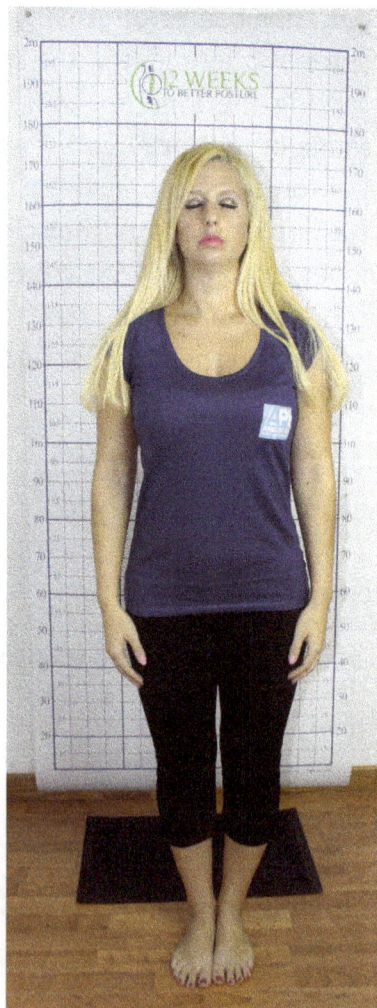

Lateral view of the patient:

- Head: neutral position (no flexion or extension)

- Eyes: parallel to the horizon

- Ear: aligned over the shoulder

- Cervical spine: normal curve with slight anterior convexity

- Thoracic spine: normal curve with slight posterior convexity

- Shoulders: back (not rotated forward), aligned over the hips

- Arms: neutral position, at even lengths, palms toward the lateral aspect of the body with the thumbs pointed forward

- Lumbar spine: normal curve with slight anterior convexity

- Pelvis: neutral position, the anterior superior iliac spine is in the same vertical plane as the pubic symphysis

- Hip joint: neutral position, neither extended nor flexed

- Knee: neutral position, neither extended nor flexed

- Ankle: neutral position, leg is vertical and at a right angle to the sole of the foot

- Feet: pointed forward

Posterior view of the patient:

- Head: neutral position (no lateral flexion or rotation)

- Ears: level with one another bilaterally

- Shoulders: level bilaterally (not elevated or depressed), even muscular development, and pulled back (not rotated forward)

- Scapulae: medial borders are parallel and about 4 inches apart

- Arms: neutral position, at even lengths, palms toward the lateral aspect of the body

- Thoracic spine: no lateral deviation

- Pelvis: level, both posterior superior iliac spines and pelvic crests are in the same transverse plane

- Hip joints: neutral position (no abduction or adduction, or flexion or extension)

- Achilles tendons: parallel bilaterally (no supination or pronation)

- Feet: parallel with slight out-toeing. The medial malleoli are in the same vertical plane (no pronation or supination is present)

The position of the pelvis is a key factor to having symmetric posture. In a neutral position, the anterior superior iliac spines are in the same vertical plane as the pubic symphysis, and opposing muscle groups have equal mechanical advantage. Imbalance between opposing muscles, anteroposteriorly and laterally, changes the alignment of the pelvis and adversely affects the alignment of the posture quadrants above and below.

Patients with ideal postural presentation also demonstrate symmetry among the central axis. The central axis divides the body evenly, weight-bearing joints are in alignment along the central axis, and muscles throughout the body are symmetrically balanced and flexible. With symmetric postural design, the internal organs are positioned naturally and not compressed, allowing ease of natural organic function.

SECTION REVIEW

1. Ideal posture is symmetrically balanced bilaterally, and from the *anterior* to the *posterior* aspect in relation to the patient's center of gravity

2. Which anatomical views should you view the patient's posture from? *Anterior, posterior,* and *lateral*

PRIMARY POSTURAL DISTORTION PATTERNS WHILE STANDING

When you are considering the primary postural distortion patterns that patients present with, it is important to realize that the most common postural distortion patterns while they are seated and standing are different. When a patient presents to your office, don't just consider their standing posture. During the patient history, ask them if they spend more time seated than they do standing during their activities on a normal day (at work or school generally). This will help you as the Posture Expert make more appropriate recommendations for their plan of care.

Primary Postural Distortion Patterns While Standing:

- Forward head posture
- Kyphotic-lordotic spine
- Anterior pelvic tilt
- Pelvic unleveling
- Foot pronation

FORWARD HEAD POSTURE

It has been estimated that 66–90% of the population presents with forward head posture (Chiropractor's Association of Australia, 2010). Forward head posture is defined by Sylva et al. (2009) as "the protrusion of the head in the sagittal plane so that the head is placed anterior to the trunk." Raine and Twomey (1997) suggest that forward head posture is the result of an extended cervical spine, protracted shoulder girdles, and a hyperkyphotic thoracic spine.

When a patient presents with forward head posture, their eyes seek eye level with the horizon causing the cervical spine to go into extension. When the cervical spine is extended, there is approximation of the occiput and C7. The neck extensor musculature is shortened and strong, leading to adaptive shortening, and the neck flexors anteriorly present with stretch weakness. Forward head posture can be evaluated by looking at the position of the head in relation to the shoulders, by measuring the craniovertebral angle on X-ray, or by evaluating the Burns Cervical Angle on a posture image.

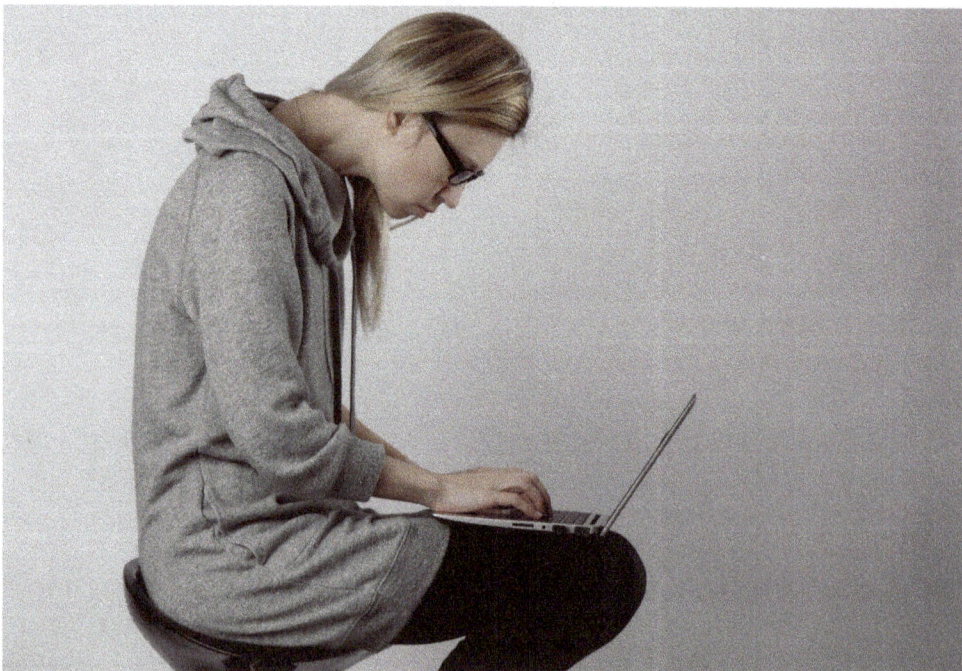

There is an association between forward head posture and pain presentation. Fejer et al. (2006) conducted a study comparing patients with neck pain of non-traumatic origin to patients without neck pain. The results of their study showed that patients with neck pain typically have more forward head posture in standing.

There are three ways in which the cervical spine presents as "forward head posture" as there are multiple ways in which forward head posture occurs.

The first is due to neck flexion. This is the classic "tech neck" presentation in which the person is looking down for a prolonged period of time and the eyes are fixed at a target below—such as a cell phone when sending a text message.

Let's consider what that would look like on the spine. The cervical vertebrae, starting from C7, will bend forward anteriorly. The majority of flexion will take place at lower cervical vertebrae. The eyes stay fixed downward. There is no extension of the cervical spine; the coupled motion of the individual vertebrae is flexion. The neck flexors will be activated, whereas the neck extensors will be elongated.

According to new research by Hansraj (2015), at a neutral position, the force to the cervical spine is approximately 10–12 lbs. As the cervical spine flexes to 15 degrees, the weight increases to 27lbs; at 30 degrees, the weight is 40lbs; at 45 degrees it's 49lbs; and at 60 degrees of flexion, the force to the cervical spine increases to 60 lbs.

What do these patients look like when they come into your office? You may have some sitting in the waiting room right now. They are checking their cell phones or reading, and staring downward for a prolonged period of time.

Now consider the second case presentation of forward head posture. You likely will see a lot of these people in your office too. Now, the first group we mentioned is looking downward with forward head flexion. As it is necessary to interact with our environment, the eyes are more commonly seeking to be upright and parallel with the horizon than they are to be looking down at a fixed object. This is associated with the righting reflex where the head seeks to be upright.

A common chronic presentation of forward head posture is when the head protrudes forward in the sagittal plane so that the head is placed anterior to the trunk (Sylva et al.). As the eyes seek to be level with the horizon, this results in an extended upper cervical spinal posture.

The lower cervical vertebrae protrude forward, causing an anterior vertebral stacking, commonly referred to as a "decreased spinal curve" or a "straight spine appearance". The upper cervical vertebrae are in extension, meaning the spinous processes, or the posterior tubercle in the case of the atlas, are drawn together posteriorly and the interspinales muscles are shortened.

Anterior translation and extension in the coronal plane occur at the facet joints. As the facets are surrounded by articular cartilage, chronic irritation of the articular cartilage can be debilitating to the joint complex.

Extension of the cervical spine in forward head posture causes excessive pressure to the facets and the posterior bodies of the vertebrae, which can often result in cervical nerve root compression.

When we consider the influence that forward head posture has on the cervical musculature, it is evident that certain muscles are stretched and weak, and others are contracted and often hypertonic.

Muscles that tend to be weak include the lower cervical extensors and the upper cervical flexors. More specifically, the splenius, longissimus, and semispinalis cervicis for the lower cervical extensors, and the suprahyoid muscles, the rectus capitis anterior, and the longus capitis upper cervical flexors are all considered weak.

The neck muscles that cause anterior protrusion will be contracted, including the lower cervical flexors such as the SCM and the anterior and medial scaleni, and the upper cervical extensors such as the suboccipitals and the splenius, longissimus, and semispinalis cervicis.

There is also a strong correlation between forward head posture and backward lower jawbone posture. Patients who suffer from TMJ disorder typically have both forward head posture and backward lower jawbone posture. How does this occur? The bite, or how your teeth line up, determines the position of your lower jaw. If the posture of the rest of the body causes mechanical strain to the lower jaw, the lower jawbone is shifted back and the head is shifted forward.

The muscles of the jaw complex are small, and perform precise functions to open and close the mouth. They are not intended to support additional weight of the head caused by forward head posture. As the head goes forward, the jaw goes back, and the muscles become restricted.

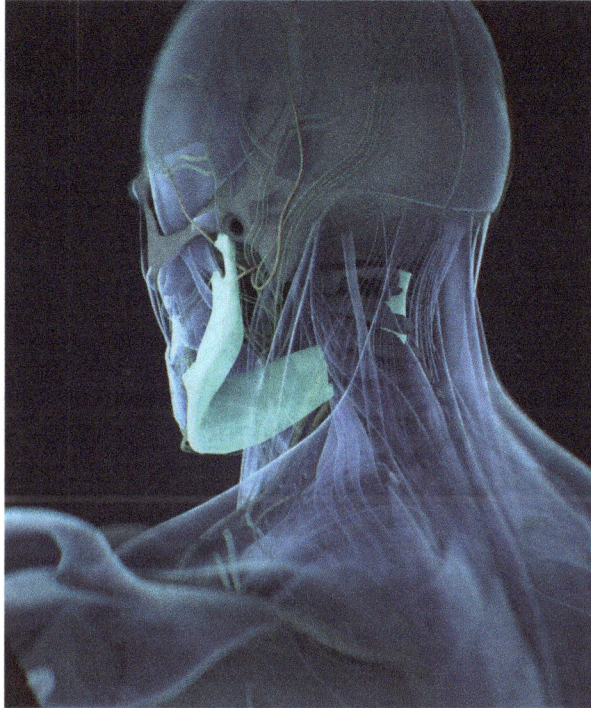

The musculature that closes the jaw includes the masseter, temporalis, and the internal and external pterygoids. The muscles to open the jaw are the hyoid muscles, including the anterior belly of the digastric, the geniohyoid, and the mylohyoid.

Muscular stress results in an inability to move the jaw smoothly and freely, resulting in clicking and cracking of the jaw, tension, stiffness, and often pain. These patients will present to your office with different complaints, most commonly tension and occipital headaches, neck pain and stiffness, and TMJ dysfunction.

Now consider the third presentation of forward head posture, which is very common. Forward head posture may also arise as a postural compensation in response to hyperkyphosis of the thoracic spine.

With an exaggerated kyphotic curve of the thoracic spine, the compensation is an exaggerated lordotic curve of the cervical spine. This will look different on X-ray and posture imaging than the other types of forward head posture just previously mentioned.

The patient will present with an evident hyperkyphosis. If the patient didn't seek to have their eyes level with the horizon, the head would fall more and more forward over the years in an extremely compromised position for the patient.

The lordotic curve occurs because our eyes seek to be level with the horizon in order to interact with the world around us. With hyperkyphosis, the upper thoracic vertebrae are anterior. When patients have a gibbus formation, you can actually see a "hunchback" presentation at the level of the upper thoracic vertebrae.

There will be a similar presentation of symptoms to those explained above. In addition, the patient will present with symptoms associated with the hyperkyphotic thoracic presentation and anterior chest flexion such as restrictions of circulation, digestive dysfunction, and a decreased respiratory capacity, along with neck and back pain.

With an increased lordotic cervical curve, the posterior aspects of the spinous processes will be drawn together. The facet orientation of the C2–C7 vertebrae is approximately 45 degrees (ranging from 35–65 degrees). With an increased cervical lordosis, there appears to be "jamming of the facets".

Three Types of Forward Head Posture:

- Forward head flexion

- Anterior head carriage with upper cervical extension

- Thoracic hyperkyphosis with cervical hyperlordosis

SECTION REVIEW

1. Which type of forward head posture is Tech Neck classified as? *Forward head flexion*

2. There is a correlation between forward head posture and *backward* lower jawbone posture, which may result in symptoms of TMD.

3. When the patient presents with hyperkyphosis, which type of forward head posture is this classified as? *Thoracic hyperkyphosis with cervical hyperlordosis*

KYPHOTIC-LORDOTIC POSTURE

Kyphotic-lordotic spinal presentation is an increased posterior curve of the thoracic spine with an increased anterior curve of the lumbar spine. With this common postural distortion pattern, patients present with the shoulders elevated and medial rotation of the shoulder joints. Patients with medially rotated shoulders, or shoulder anteriority, have shortened pectoral muscles and weak rhomboids; they present with their hands facing posteriorly in the anatomic position instead of anteriorly with the palms of their hands at the lateral side of the body.

The thoracic spine demonstrates increased flexion, or kyphosis. Muscle imbalances of the thoracic region demonstrate weak upper back erector spinae, external obliques, anterior abdominal muscles, and hip extensor muscles.

With an increased lordosis, or hyperextension of the lumbar spine, the pelvis tilts anteriorly and the hip joints are flexed. An increased lumbar curve results in shortened hip flexors.

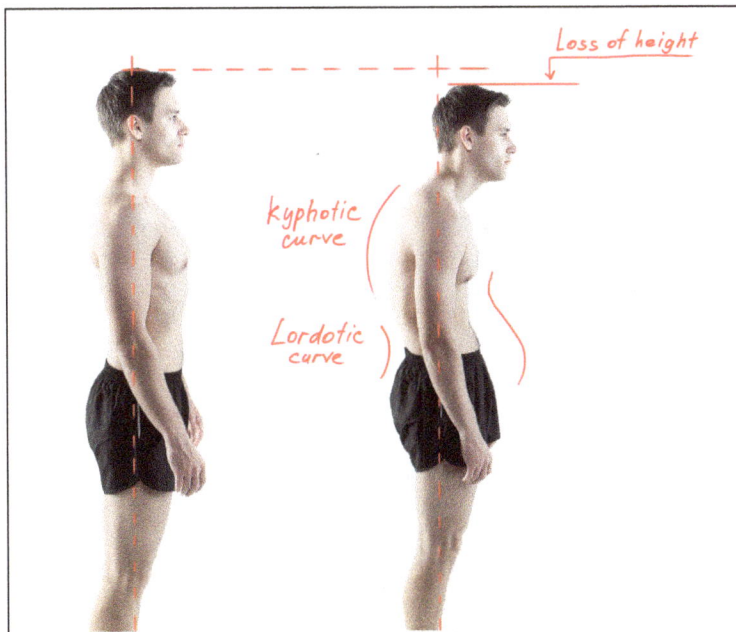

HYPERKYPHOSIS OF THE THORACIC SPINE

The sagittal kyphotic thoracic curve is the first curve to develop from an early fetal position. A normal thoracic curve ranges between 20–40 degrees in adults. Hyperkyphosis, which is an exaggerated kyphotic curve, is classified as a curve that is 45–50 degrees or more (some resources say 45 degrees whereas others say 50 degrees) and is associated with anterior flexion. Hyperkyphosis of the thoracic spine is a highly debilitating postural presentation.

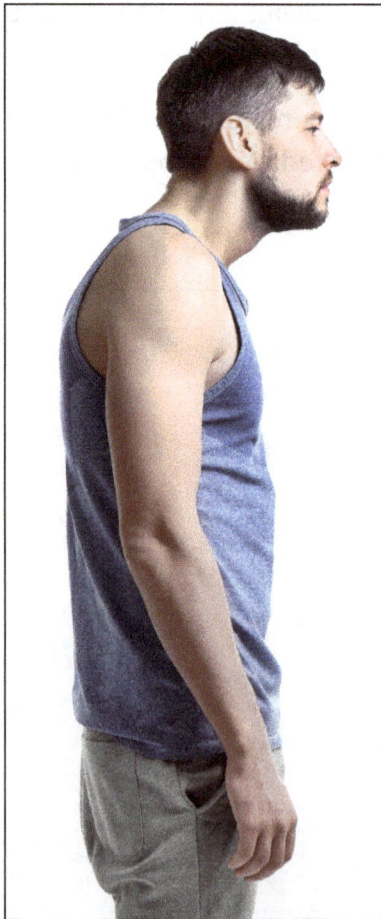

Hyperkyphosis is classified as either postural or structural. Postural means the kyphosis is attributed to poor posture, usually presenting a smooth curve, which can be corrected with conscious attention of postural changes. Postural hyperkyphosis is usually associated with slouching. The patient sits in a slouched position, but they have the ability of straightening their spine when prompted to do so.

Structural hyperkyphosis is caused by an abnormality affecting the bones, intervertebral discs, nerves, ligaments, or muscles. Common causes of structural hyperkyphosis include Scheuermann's disease, Vitamin D deficiency which softens the bony skeleton, vertebral fractures, trauma, gibbus deformity, and a small population even presents with congenital hyperkyphosis.

Due to the connections of the thoracic spine to the ribcage, the thoracic spine is less mobile than its cervical and lumbar counterparts. The thoracic spine plays an important role in protecting vital anatomy including the spinal cord in the foramen magnum posteriorly and the heart and the lungs anteriorly due to the costovertebral connection of the thoracic spine to the ribs making up the bony thorax.

Normal thoracic posture viewed from the lateral aspect of the patient demonstrates an "S" shaped curvature. When a hyperkyphosis is present, there is a visible "C" shape of the thoracic spine from the lateral aspect of the patient.

Biomechanically, thoracic hyperkyphosis can be associated with higher spinal loads and trunk muscle force in upright stance. This may accelerate degenerative process and contribute to dysfunction and pain. As the thoracic kyphosis curves posteriorly, trunk flexion occurs anteriorly and the anterior aspect of the vertebral bodies and the anterior anatomy of the thorax become compressed.

In the thoracic spine the facet joints are orientated in the coronal plane, which means the primary movements of the thoracic spine are axial rotation and lateral flexion. Toward the lower thoracic spine, the facet joints progressively orientate more into the sagittal plane, allowing for greater flexion and extension movement.

Thoracic vertebrae also have facets on either side of their bodies, which form joints with the heads of the corresponding ribs, which we know as the costovertebral joints. The transverse processes, with the exception of the eleventh and twelfth thoracic vertebrae, articulate with the corresponding ribs via the costotransverse joints. Together, the costovertebral and costotransverse joints allow rotational movement of the ribs, which assists ventilation of the lungs.

With anterior flexion of the thorax associated with hyperkyphosis, these joints are less mobile and the chest cavity space decreases, compressing the respiratory capacity of the lungs and associated respiratory organs.

The musculature of the thoracic spine is highly complex, including the deep intrinsic musculature and the superficial extrinsic musculature. The extrinsic muscles include large muscle groups such as the trapezius, latissimus dorsi, levator scapulae, serratus anterior and posterior, and the rhomboids. The intrinsic muscles include the iliocostalis, the longissiumus, and the spinalis.

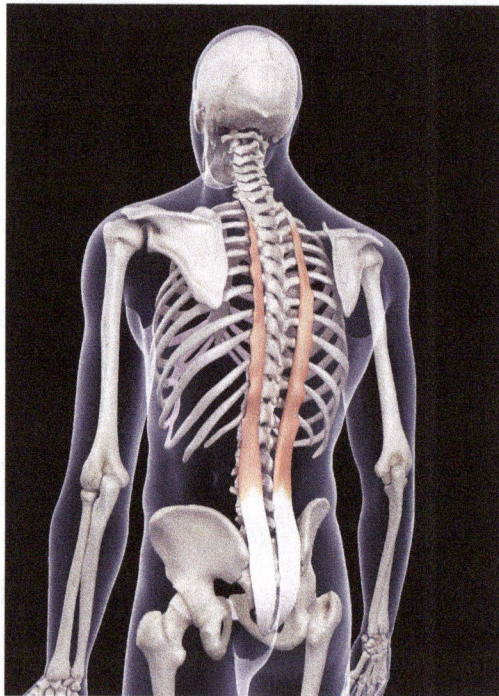

Primary spinal extensors will be elongated and weak with a hyperkyphosis postural presentation. These muscles include the intrinsic muscles, the rhomboids, and the lower trapezius. The contracted or tonic muscles include the pectoral muscles, the upper trapezius, and the levator scapulae. This will be the classic upper crossed syndrome position.

Although there are no anterior muscle attachments to the thoracic spine, the abdominals act as a spinal stabilizer and the rectus femoris are highly active in anterior thoracic flexion.

The posterior ligaments, such as the supraspinal, the posterior longitudinal ligament, and the ligamenta flava will have more stretch, whereas the anterior longitudinal ligaments will be shortened.

An important connection between the thoracic spine and the shoulder girdle is the scapulothoracic joint. The scapulothoracic joint is unique in that it actually doesn't follow the rules of a normal joint because there is no ligamentous attachment, just musculature attachments of the serratus anterior and the subscapularis. The movement of the scapulothoracic joint is dependent on the motion of the acromioclavicular joint and the sternoclavicular joint, as well as the tonicity of the muscle attachments.

When the pectoralis muscles become tightened, as with upper crossed syndrome associated with hyperkyphosis, the pectoral muscles protract anteriorly. This is the anterior shoulder displacement that is commonly seen in association with hyperkyphosis.

Two Types of Hyperkyphosis:

- Postural hyperkyphosis: an increased thoracic curve that can be instantaneously corrected with conscious attention. This postural presentation is associated with slouching

- Structural hyperkyphosis: due to structural deformation of the thoracic spine

SECTION REVIEW

1. Hyperkyphosis is classified as an increased thoracic curve of *45–50* degrees

2. Which type of kyphosis is attributed to poor posture, usually presenting a smooth curve, which can be corrected with conscious attention to postural changes? *Postural hyperkyphosis*

3. Normal thoracic posture viewed from the lateral aspect of the patient demonstrates an "S" shaped curvature. When a hyperkyphosis is present, there is a visible *"C"* shape of the thoracic spine

HYPERLORDOSIS OF THE LUMBAR SPINE

Lumbar hyperlordosis is a condition that occurs when the lumbar region of the lower back experiences stress or extra weight and arches anteriorly. Lordosis of the lumbar spine is normal. An accentuation of that normal curve is considered to be a "hyperlordosis".

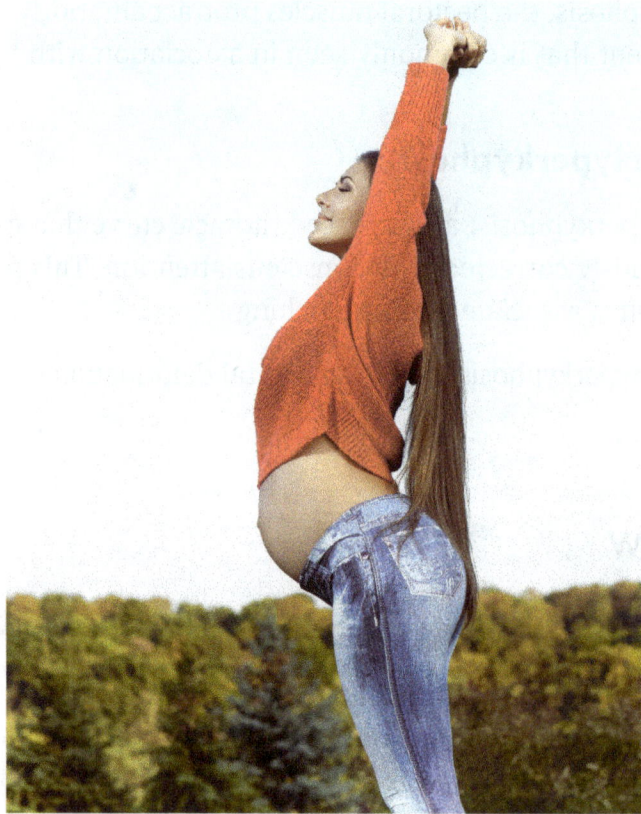

Hyperlordosis is classified by a bilateral anterior pelvic tilt greater than 10 degrees from horizontal in females and greater than five degrees for males (although different sources will quote slightly different angles). For our purposes, we will say 10 degrees for females and 5 degrees for males.

The hip joints are held in flexion with the pelvic rim flexed anteriorly. The posterior aspect of the vertebrae, or the spinous processes, are drawn together. There is an approximation of L1 toward S1 with posterior "jamming" of the joints and anterior lengthening. In the anterior aspect, the intervertebral discs have space and minimized pressure, whereas in the posterior aspect of the disc, the IVF space is compromised.

Lumbar hyperlordosis is a classic lower crossed syndrome presentation where the hips tilt anteriorly and there is a muscular imbalance of the lower back and pelvis. The postural muscles of the lower back and pelvis shorten in responses to stress, and they in turn inhibit their antagonists on the other side of the joint due to reciprocal inhibition.

With lower crossed syndrome, the major muscle groups that are compromised include the iliopsoas, rectus femoris, and the lumbar erector spinae. Other muscle groups that are involved are the tensor fascia latae (TFL), pectineus, adductors, and the quadratus lumborum. The abdominal muscles and the gluteus maximus are weak.

- **Muscles that are tight and require stretching**: trunk extensors called the erector spinae, the quadratus lumborum, and the hip flexors, in particular the iliopsoas muscle.

- **Muscles that are weak and require strengthening**: abdominal muscles called the rectus abdominis, internal oblique, external oblique, the hip extensors, hamstrings, and gluteus maximus

The iliopsoas is the pivotal muscle in hyperlordosis. A shortened iliopsoas tilts the pelvis anteriorly, increasing the natural lordotic lumbar arch. It simultaneously inhibits the gluteus maximus through reciprocal inhibition. In this case, the gluteus maximus cannot help tilt the pelvis posteriorly to correct the hyperlordosis because it is switched off by the iliopsoas. Implications of weak gluteus maximus muscles are evident in gait. You can see the hamstrings and the latissimus dorsi compensate for weak gluts.

Obesity and pregnancy are potential causes of hyperlordosis. The increased weight on the anterior aspect of the abdomen pulls the lumbar arch forward. If a patient is overweight and has weak abdominals, it will be even more difficult to correct the posture of the spine.

Another common cause of hyperlordosis is wearing high-heeled shoes. The weight of the female is shifted to the anterior aspect of the foot; 4-inch high heels shift a woman's weight forward at a 45 degree angle. To prevent the woman falling anteriorly, the lumbar spine compensates by tilting the pelvis forward and arching the lumbar spine. The woman appears to have curves when she wears high heels. In this case, though, it is not desirable to have an increased curve of the lumbar spine.

Anterior pelvic tilt can be viewed from the lateral aspect of the patient. Anterior pelvic tilt is characterized by tight hip flexors and lumbar paraspinal musculature, and weakened hip extensors such as the gluteus maximus and the hamstrings as well as weak rectus abdominis muscles. Weakness of these muscles is seldom the primary cause of anterior pelvic tilt, but when they are weak in conjunction with other factors causing anterior pelvic tilt, it worsens the lordosis.

Patients who present with anterior pelvic tilt can sit for extended periods of time, but experience pain when shifting from seated to standing. Lying on the abdomen is not recommended as the tight hip flexors hold the lumbar spine into lordosis.

Lower Crossed Syndrome:

- Anterior pelvic tilt

- Tight musculature: hip flexors and lumbar paraspinal muscles

- Weak musculature: hip extensors and gluteus maximus

SECTION REVIEW

1. Hyperlordosis is classified by a bilateral *anterior* pelvic tilt

2. A shortened *iliopsoas* muscle tilts the pelvis anteriorly, increasing the natural lordotic lumbar arch and inhibiting the gluteal muscles

3. Which muscles are weak in lower crossed syndrome? *Hip extensors and the gluteus maximus*

PELVIC UNLEVELING

With pelvic unleveling, there is a visible high hip with an ipsilateral visible leg length discrepancy (this can be seen when the patient is lying prone or supine). Pelvic unleveling is viewed from the anterior and the posterior view of the patient. From the anterior perspective, pelvic unleveling is evaluated by comparing the level of the iliac spines and the pelvic crests. From the posterior aspect, evaluate the level of the pelvic crests, the iliac spines, and the sacroiliac joints.

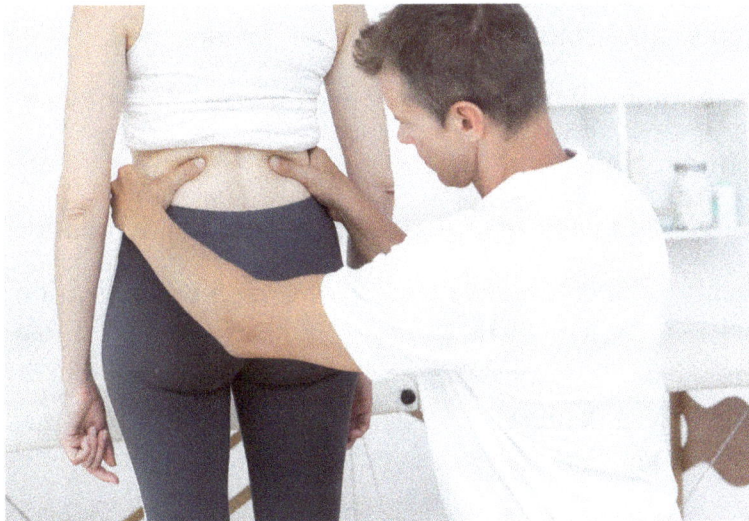

With pelvic unleveling, there is also commonly an increased sacral base angle with flexion, increased lumbar lordosis, normal flexion range of motion, but decreased extension. Pelvic unleveling contributes to whole body postural distortion patterns.

Common compensatory postural patterns include shoulder and scapula unleveling contralateral to the high hip side. Lateral flexion, or slight rotation of the head, is also commonly noted.

There are three primary regions of anatomic or postural asymmetry in relation to pelvic unleveling. At the lumbosacral junction there is a high correlation between the direction of the spinal curvature and the short leg with the lateral curvature, most frequently occurring toward the short leg side. Pelvic rotation most commonly occurs contralateral to the short leg side, and sacral involvement most often is on the same side of the pelvic orientations. The most common presentation is lateral curvature toward the short leg side with pelvic rotation toward the long leg side.

Consider the following example of pelvic unleveling and the associated compensation patterns. The patient presents with a high right hip:

- Head: right tilt

- Cervical spine: right flexion

- Shoulders: right low

- Scapulae: adducted, right low

- Thoracic spine: thoracolumbar curve convex toward the left

- Lumbar spine: thoracolumbar curve convex toward the left

- Pelvis: lateral tilt high on the right

- Hip joints: right adducted with slight medial rotation, left abducted

- Lower extremities: increased weight on long leg for stabilization

- Feet: pronation

- Weak left lateral trunk muscles, right hip abductors (gluteus medius), left hip adductors, right TFL

- Shortened right lateral trunk muscles, left hip abductors, and right hip adductors

Consider the possible presentation of pain patterns for a patient with a right high hip. They may present with left foot and ankle pain, right knee and hip pain and osteoarthritis, right shoulder pain, and left craniomandibular dysfunction and pain.

Gluteus medius weakness also contributes to pelvic unleveling. Habitually standing with the weight on one leg more than the other gives rise to stretch weakness that, if it persists, results in pain. The weakness of the gluteus medius usually presents on the high side of the pelvis and must be corrected to maintain good lateral alignment. The gluteus medius on the low pelvis side is shortened.

Leg length discrepancies also contribute to developmental changes of facial structure. Gelb (1994) found that over time, patients with a short right leg would develop left-sided loss of vertical dimension in the jaw. He found in these patients characteristic right-sided face changes that included a higher eyebrow, a higher and apparently larger eye, a higher ear, and an up-turning of the lips.

Pelvic Unleveling:

- Visual high hip

- Ipsilateral leg length discrepancy

SECTION REVIEW

1. From the anterior perspective, pelvic unleveling is evaluated by comparing the level of the *iliac spines* and the *pelvic crests*

2. Pelvic rotation most commonly occurs *contralateral* to the short leg side

3. The weakness of the *gluteus medius* muscle usually presents on the high side of the pelvis

PRONATION OF THE FEET

Foot pronation is the most common postural distortion pattern of the foot. Pronation means to turn or rotate the sole of the foot by abduction and eversion so that the inner edge of the sole bears the majority of the body's weight.

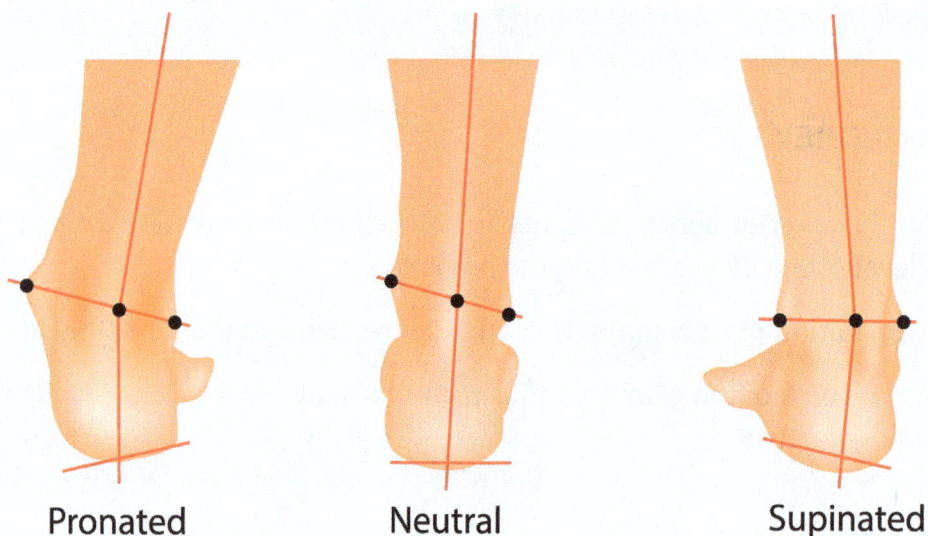

Pronated   Neutral   Supinated

It is most commonly bilateral, but if it is not bilateral, it is more commonly associated with the long leg. Pronation is characterized as abduction, dorsal flexion, and eversion of the foot. Visual postural analyses demonstrate a prominent ankle on the inside and a sunken one on the outside with weight distribution on the medial border of the foot.

In a normal gait cycle, the foot "rolls" inward about 15% as weight is transferred from the heel to the forefoot, comes in complete contact with the ground, and can support your body weight without any problem. Pronation is critical to proper shock absorption, and it helps you push off evenly from the front of the foot.

In the loading phase of gait, the lateral heel everts, causing ankle pronation. If you don't land on the lateral calcaneus, you are already everted so the acceleration of pronation is increased. As the ankle pronates, the tarsals rotate and unlock to absorb shock, and the tibia has internal rotation. The knees go from a neutral position to slight flexion and the pelvis has slight posterior rotation.

The spring ligament, which connects the calcaneus and navicular, is an important stabilizer for the foot. Pronation occurs when the spring ligament is stretched. Generally, you see coupled pronation and internal rotation with this instance. Once pronation becomes chronic, it continues to affect the ligament and can cause pain and associated symptoms.

It is very common that patients who have "flat feet" will over pronate. When the patient is standing, the Posture Expert should be able to place one finger under the arch of the foot. If you cannot do this, it is an indication that the patient has "flat feet" and over pronates. As the arches flatten, the muscles, tendons, and ligaments underneath the foot stretch, which can be asymptomatic or cause associated painful discrepancies.

The knees can be drawn together due to pronation. Although a full genu valgum or "knock kneed" appearance is an extreme case, the knees are drawn medially with the medial rotation of the tarsals. Patients will demonstrate more "wear and tear" on the medial aspect of their shoes.

Chronic pronation may lead to associated conditions of Posture Quadrant 4 including shin splints, anterior compartment syndrome, patella-femoral pain syndrome, plantar fasciitis, Achilles tendonitis, and tarsal tunnel syndrome.

Statistics demonstrate that 50–60% of runners exhibit mild to moderate over-pronation and up to 20–30% of runners exhibit severe over-pronation, whereas only about 3% of runners present with supination.

SECTION REVIEW

1. What is the most common postural distortion pattern of the foot? *Pronation*

2. The *spring* ligament, which connects the calcaneus and navicular, is an important stabilizer for the foot

3. Patients with pronation demonstrate more "wear and tear" on the *medial* aspect of their shoes

PRIMARY POSTURAL DISTORTION PATTERNS WHILE SEATED

The primary postural distortion patterns while seated differ from standing postural presentations in the lumbopelvic region of the spine. The primary reasons for a different postural pattern while seated are non-ergonomic chairs and sedentary lifestyle patterns, which affect the position of the pelvis and lower back.

Primary Postural Distortion Patterns While Seated:

- Forward head posture
- Kyphotic thoracic spine
- Anterior pelvic translation
- Posterior pelvic tilt

ANTERIOR PELVIC TRANSLATION WITH POSTERIOR PELVIC TILT

A decreased curvature, or flexion, of the lumbar spine characterizes anterior pelvic translation with posterior pelvic tilt. Posterior pelvic tilt is also referred to as a sway-back postural presentation. The pelvis is tilted posteriorly but deviates anteriorly in relation to the feet.

An increased posterior curvature of the upper back compensates for forward deviation of the pelvis. The hip joints are extended with anterior displacement. Muscular imbalances include weak hip flexors, external obliques, upper back extensors, and neck flexors. Weakness of the iliopsoas is often misdiagnosed for lordosis, a common mistake that Posture Experts should be aware of. The hamstrings and the lumbar paraspinal muscles are shortened and tight.

Here is a quick reference of what to look for when the common postural distortion patterns are noted.

This section will outline what muscular dysfunction and kinetic chain dysfunction patterns to consider when certain postural distortion patterns are revealed via posture imaging and visual postural analyses.

Forward Head Posture:

- When forward head posture is detected, consider evaluating the patient for weakness of the following areas: neck flexors, rhomboids, and mid and lower trapezius

- Consider tightness in the following areas: upper trapezius, pectorals, SCM, and latissimus dorsi

Thoracic Hyperkyphosis:

- When a hyperkyphosis is present, anterior displacement of the shoulders is very common. This involves the shoulders being elevated with medial rotation of the shoulder joints

- Patients with medially rotated shoulders have shortened pectoral muscles and weak rhomboids

- For patients presenting with elevated shoulders and scapulae, they also need to stretch the trapezius musculature and evaluate for the presence of trigger points

- With medial rotation of the shoulders, consider excessive elbow pronation leading to tendonitis or epicondylitis

- Muscle imbalances of the thoracic region demonstrate weak upper back erector spinae, external obliques, anterior abdominal muscles, and hip extensor muscles

- Trunk flexion is very common which will lead to a decreased zone of apposition, causing diaphragmatic strain

Anterior Pelvic Tilt:

- Anterior pelvic tilt with a lumbar lordosis is commonly seen when patients are standing

- With anterior pelvic tilt, check patients for tight hip flexors and lumbar paraspinal musculature

- Check for weakness of the hip extensors including the gluteus maximus, the hamstrings, and rectus abdominis muscles

Posterior pelvic tilt:

- Posterior pelvic tilt, commonly seen in sitting, occurs when the pelvis is tilted posteriorly but deviates anteriorly in relation to the feet

- Check patients for the following muscular imbalances: weak hip flexors, external obliques, upper back extensors, and neck flexors
- The hamstrings and the lumbar paraspinal muscles are shortened and tight

Pelvic Unleveling:

- Pelvic unleveling causes whole body postural compensations
- Ipsilateral to the hip with superiority, it is common to find visual leg length discrepancy, weakness of gluteus medius
- Contralateral high shoulder with ipsilateral trapezius tightness on the side of the high shoulder
- The weakness of the gluteus medius and the TFL usually presents on the high side of the pelvis. The gluteus medius and the TFL on the low pelvis side are shortened

Pronation:

- When patients present with pronation, it is commonly bilateral
- If not bilateral, it is more commonly associated with the long leg
- Check your patients for fallen arches, internal rotation of the tibia, and vastus medialis weakness

OTHER POSTURAL DISTORTION PATTERNS

In addition to the primary postural distortion patterns while the patient is standing and seated are postural asymmetries that patients may present with, but which will be much less common. Patients are not textbooks. Although statistically the above mentioned postural distortion patterns are the most common, patients may present with any combination of postural distortion patterns. For this reason a standardized plan of postural correction will not be adequate for all patients. Treatment plans should be specific to the needs of the postural presentation of each patient individually.

Lateral pelvic tilt

The first postural distortion is lateral pelvic tilt. This mechanical problem is chiefly due to compression at the articulating facets of the spine on the high side of the pelvis. The corresponding pain is in the areas with the greatest compression, usually over the articulating facet of the fifth lumbar vertebra on the high side of the hip. Leg abductors and the TFL are tighter on the low side of the pelvis. The leg is in adduction on the high pelvis side and the abductors, such as the gluteus medius, are weak.

Whole body anterior translation

The next postural distortion to consider is whole body anterior translation. When you are evaluating posture images, patients may present with anterior deviation of the body over the feet. Anterior translation occurs when the weight is shifted forward over the balls of the feet. Calluses may form on the balls of the feet over time, metatarsal arch supports may be indicated. This postural presentation is most common among tall, slender individuals. The ankle joint is in slight dorsiflexion due to the forward inclination of the leg and slight knee flexion. Posterior muscles of the trunk and lower extremity tend to be contracted.

Handedness postural patterns

Handedness postural patterns are the next posture distortion pattern. Handedness postural distortion patterns commonly develop due to repetitive ipsilateral motions. Detailed below is the handedness postural distortion pattern of a right-handed individual who has not experienced significant trauma.

- The right shoulder is low

- The right hip is high

- Slight deviation of the spine toward the left

- Tight left TFL

- Weak right gluteus medius

Dental occlusions

Posture Experts should also consider postural distortions of the craniocervical mandibular junction, and its global effect on posture. For balance to be maintained at this junction, there must be proper dental occlusion. Class II occlusion, or an overbite, is associated with cervical lordosis and forward head posture. Class III occlusion, or an underbite, is associated with a straightening of the normal anterior cervical curvature with a posterior head posture.

Strachan and Robinson (1965) showed that they could correct abnormal muscle firing sequences of masticatory muscles found in patients with malocclusion by correcting their leg length discrepancies with heel lift pelvic alignment techniques. The mandible tends to deviate in the same direction as the teeth and also toward the same side as the long leg. Huggare (1991) studied the effect of scoliosis on head posture. He found a high incidence of malocclusions in the scoliotic population, especially lateral malocclusion, or a crossbite.

Supination

Now consider other possible posture distortions of the lower extremity. By far the most common postural distortion pattern of Posture Quadrant 4 is pronation of the feet. However, patients may also present with supination of the feet or misalignment of the knees.

Supination is characterized as abduction, plantar flexion, and inversion of the foot. External rotation of the leg and thigh with subtalar joint varus is common. Supination is predominately associated with the short leg when pelvic unleveling is present. A supinated foot causing external rotation of the lower extremity will result in ipsilateral rotation of the pelvis.

Knee hyperextension and knee flexion

Misalignment of the knees is commonly a result of misaligned feet or hips. Patients may present with knee hyperextension, or less commonly with knee flexion. They may also present with bowed legs or knocked knees. Hyperextension of the knee is when the knees are extended past zero degrees. Knee flexion, more common in the elderly population, is when the knees are flexed forward beyond a neutral position. Bowed legs occur when the knees bow out laterally, and knocked knees occur when the knees come together laterally.

SECTION REVIEW

1. Which postural distortion pattern is chiefly due to compression at the articulating facets of the spine on the high side of the pelvis? *Lateral pelvic tilt*

2. *Handedness* postural distortion patterns commonly develop due to repetitive ipsilateral motions

3. Class II occlusion, or an *overbite*, is associated with cervical lordosis and forward head posture

SPINAL MISALIGNMENT PATTERNS

Common spinal misalignment patterns are related to cortical and cerebellar firing patterns. A common presentation for a patient with left cortical lateralization and right weakness of cerebellar activation is a right upper cervical misalignment and left mid cervical misalignment.

Spinal misalignment patterns often present in the spinal transition zones. The cervicothoracic transition area is an important transition zone, and a common area where patients will feel pain. This area of spinal transition is considered to be the "on/off" switch to the sympathetic nervous system, the area of the sympathetic chain ganglia. If a patient presents with a misalignment of this transition zone, effective postural correction is focused upon spinal realignment. Firing mechanoreceptors in this area to decrease nociception facilitation will benefit the patient; they will have better alignment and have less pain.

Spinal misalignment patterns of the thoracolumbar transition area are also common. Sedentary individuals present with increased pressure at this transition area because the lordosis is reversed. Thus, that stress is absorbed at the T12/L1 junction. In cases of increased kyphosis and increased lordosis, there is often counter rotation of the vertebrae at this level.

The lumbopelvic area is also integrated. It has been noted in the literature that when the ilium is misaligned posteriorly and inferiorly, it is correlated with an L5 misalignment on the same side. When the pelvis is misaligned anteriorly and superiorly, a corresponding misalignment on the opposite side of L4 is common.

Pain patterns of patients will vary based upon case presentation. However, in general, pain is located at the transitional zones of the spine and oftentimes considered to be chronic and/or recurring if not corrected. For postural correction, focusing on restoring postural symmetry at the transitional zones will help restore postural alignment of the spine and at the areas of compensation.

Zink (1979) describes postural distortion patterns in terms of "compensated" or "uncompensated." He explains that 80% of the population has a compensated pattern of the body in which "usually a rotational bias in one transition zone is accompanied by an opposite fascial rotation in the next zone throughout the body. Compensated postural distortion patterns are to counter balance the body."

Uncompensated postural distortion patterns demonstrate random and unpredictable misalignment patterns. This is in the minority of patients, but patients will present with unpredictable postural presentations. Unnatural postural distortion patterns are commonly due to traumatic injury or pathology.

SECTION REVIEW

1. Spinal misalignment patterns often present in the spinal *transition* zones

2. The *cervicothoracic* transition area is an important transition zone, and a common area where patients will feel pain

3. Sedentary individuals present with increased pressure at the *thoracolumbar* transition area because the lordosis is reversed while they are seated

EVALUATING MUSCULAR DYSFUNCTION PATTERNS

Muscular adaptations of postural distortion patterns tend to be chronic and develop due to prolonged, repetitive stress over time. The postural muscles tend toward hypertonus, meaning they are tight and in a state of contracture. Dynamic muscles tend toward overstretch, or hypotonic muscular presentation.

When evaluating muscular dysfunction patterns, consider the areas where the body folds. The pelvis, for example, most commonly folds forward (while standing) as the knees, legs, and the feet fold medially. Moving up the body, another common area of body "folding" is at the shoulders. The shoulders roll forward and the thumbs turn medially. At the level of the cervical spine, the head juts forward.

Forward head posture is one of the most common postural distortion patterns. As the scaleni and sternocleidomastoid (SCM) become tight, this contributes to forward head posture. The scaleni originate at the transverse processes of cervical 2–7 vertebrae, ending at the first and second rib. Tight scaleni draw the neck into a forward position. Tight SCMs contribute to forward head posture and decreased rotation of the cervical spine.

Tight pectoral muscles promote forward head posture and are inhibitory to breathing. The pectoralis causes anterior depression of the scapula. Posterior depression of the scapula is desired. This allows for functional scapula stability, shoulder mobility, and cervical relaxation. Anterior depression does the opposite motion, which can predispose patients to injury such as rotator cuff injuries. When the subscapularis becomes shortened, it causes protraction of the scapula and internal rotation of the shoulder. Stretching this muscle helps increase shoulder mobility. The trapezius muscles elevate the scapula and inhibit thoracic extension.

Consider the muscular dysfunction patterns of the upper extremity. The shoulders are commonly anteriorly drawn with internal rotation, resulting in tight pectoral muscles and weak rhomboids and latissimus dorsi. Trigger points are present in the trapezius muscles and the pectoral muscles. Pectoral trigger points can cause poor lymphatic drainage of the axillary region, which creates higher levels of acidity. This is a problem, especially for women. For patients presenting with elevated shoulders and scapulae, you need to stretch the trapezius musculature and evaluate for the presence of trigger points.

Patients with excessive elbow pronation have a weakened annular ligament around the radial head, leading to lateral and medial epicondylitis. Elbow pronation is easier to correct than foot pronation, however, because the elbow is non-weight bearing. An altered kinetic chain of movement of the upper extremity affects the stability of the shoulder and the postural presentation of the spine.

The abdominal muscles play an interesting role in postural correction. When the upper abdominals pull down on the sternum, this contributes to a rounded thoracic spine, making proper posture essentially impossible. This also affects the ability to expand the ribcage to full capacity. Repeated trunk flexion exercises may contribute to continued postural collapse.

Trunk muscular dysfunction patterns are seen with weakness on the leg-lowering test. In most cases, the trunk-raising test will be normal, indicating strong rectus abdominis muscles, but the leg-lowering test will be weak, indicating weak external obliques and hip flexor tightness. When the patient is performing the leg-lowering test and has an inability to keep the lower back flat, this is due to elongation of the external obliques and tight hip flexors.

Regarding the lower extremity, the majority of individuals have tight hip flexors and hamstrings. Patients who present with sciatica have tight piriformis muscles (usually unilateral tightness). Muscular dysfunction patterns of the TFL can commonly be misdiagnosed as sciatica.

With anterior pelvic tilt, the TFL becomes restricted, so it draws the hip into further anterior rotation. When the rectus femoris is tight, it too draws the pelvis into anterior tilt. As the rectus femoris is a large muscle, it absorbs a great deal of load stress from improper postural patterns.

The iliopsoas muscle is of utmost importance to postural correction. A properly functioning iliopsoas promotes efficiency in movements at the level of the spine, the hip, and the leg. Chronic iliopsoas tightness may be a primary reason for postural asymmetry, or postural asymmetry may be the reason for a tight iliopsoas.

Consider the affect that the iliopsoas has on postural alignment. When the psoas is contracted, it causes trunk flexion. Having a tight iliopsoas promotes trunk flexion, negating the holding pattern of the postural correction.

The iliopsoas is shortened in anterior pelvic tilt, meaning it increases the lumbar lordosis. An increased lordosis creates increased stress to the spinal discs, which will degenerate with load, stress, and time as variables. Long-term correction of pelvic unleveling is difficult to achieve with iliopsoas tightness. Asymmetric psoas strain can increase pelvic unleveling and lumbar strain.

As the pelvis is the base of the spine, chronic asymmetric postural patterns of the pelvis will lead to sustained compensation patterns, including scoliosis in more severe and prolonged cases. When you are analyzing your patients, be sure to evaluate for tightness of the iliopsoas muscles.

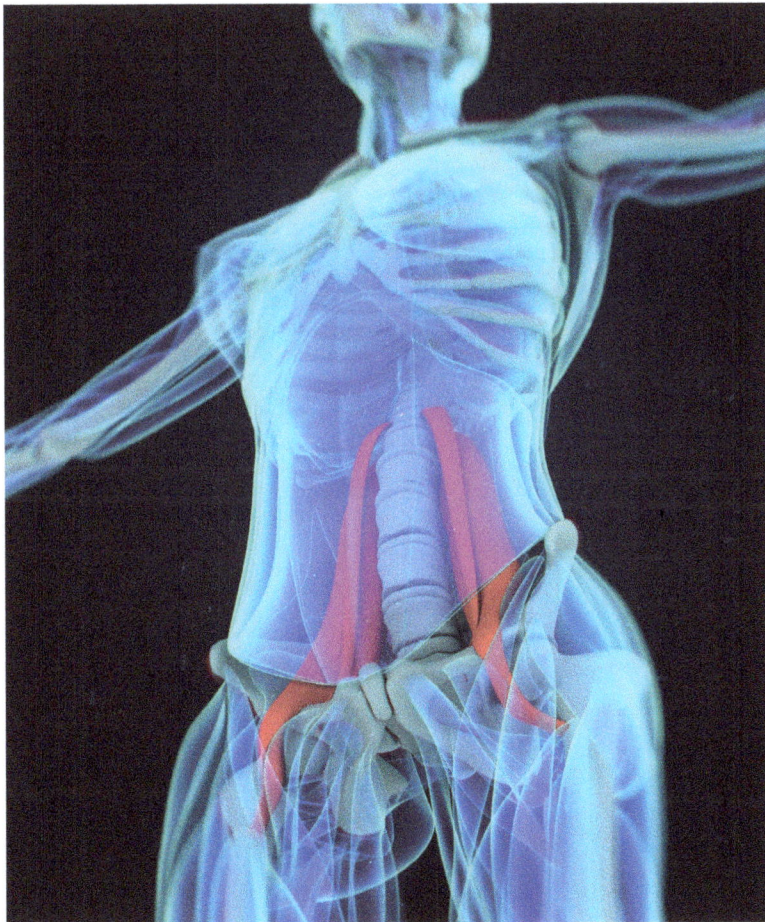

Patients presenting with pronation, or external foot flare, may also present with fallen arches, patellar approximation, internal rotation of the tibia, and vastus medialis weakness. Women who wear high heels on a consistent basis will present with gastrocnemius and soleus muscle shortening.

SECTION REVIEW

1. Trigger points of the *pectoral* muscles can cause poor lymphatic drainage of the axillary region, which creates higher levels of acidity

2. Elbow *pronation* can cause a weakened annular ligament around the radial head leading to lateral and medial epicondylitis

3. A tight *iliopsoas* promotes trunk flexion, negating the holding pattern of the postural correction

ALTERED MOVEMENT PATTERNS

With a strong understanding of the common postural distortion patterns, it is easy to see the biomechanical consequences of improper spinal and pelvic alignment and the associated muscular dysfunction patterns. The posture system is connected, meaning a misalignment in one posture quadrant will cause compensation patterns in the other posture quadrants. The overall effect of misaligned posture also contributes to modern day health discrepancies and common pathologies.

With chronic postural distortion patterns, the patient begins to move in distorted movement patterns that become the new "normal" for that patient. They stabilize painful joints and recruit other muscles to move the injured tissue. This creates muscle amnesia for the injured areas. Just as patients develop muscle memory from doing repetitive motions, such as learning a new sport, they also develop muscle amnesia when they do not use certain muscles that are stabilized. Muscle amnesia is due to the all-or-none firing patterns of muscles. Muscles either fire or they don't. Muscles that continue not to activate will atrophy with time, and will have muscle amnesia patterns.

In addition to altered movement patterns due to muscle amnesia, a patient with improper posture will also have altered proprioception. According to Haavik (2014), when a spinal segment doesn't move properly, it influences how the brain perceives and responds to all other sensory information. Dysfunction of the spine disrupts the brain's ability to sense what is going on accurately in the rest of the body (Holt, 2013).

Slifles et al. (2009) have shown that patients who present with mechanical low back pain have a lack of feed-forward activation of selected trunk musculature, resulting in a period of inefficient muscular stabilization. Weak trunk musculature leads to postural collapse. This should be considered in the postural rehabilitation program.

SECTION REVIEW

1. *Muscle amnesia* is due to the all-or-none firing patterns of muscles

2. Patients who present with mechanical low back pain have a lack of *feed-forward activation* of selected trunk musculature, resulting in a period of inefficient muscular stabilization

POSTURE ANALYSIS OVERVIEW

As a Posture Expert, once you know what postural patterns to look for, you then need to have a standard systematized postural evaluation. It is important to follow a system when evaluating patients to be accurate and efficient. As a Posture Expert, you will be trained how to do the following complete postural analysis.

The complete postural analysis consists of three important components: a structural analysis, a functional analysis, and a neurologic analysis that are all necessary for a complete understanding of the postural presentations of patients. Each of the components of the complete postural analysis is listed below.

Please note that some patients will require further analysis due to problem-specific or traumatic case presentation. This should be noted during the patient history. Inconsistent results may be due to old injuries or diseases that have altered the alignment pattern.

According to Kendall et al. (2005), "It is advisable to keep photographic records of posture to attain a really worthwhile evaluation of postural changes in growing children" (p. 88). This provides valuable insight into the need for ongoing posture images over the course of the patient's lifetime.

Complete postural analysis:

- Posture images
  - Anterior, posterior, and lateral views

- Visual postural analysis
  - Anterior, posterior, and lateral views

- Muscle strength tests
  - Rhomboids, external obliques, transversus abdominis, gluteus medius, and the TFL

- Muscle length tests
  - Pectoral muscles, diaphragm, lumbar paraspinal muscles, iliopsoas, hamstrings, and the gastrocnemius muscles

- Muscle hypertonicity
  - Suboccipital muscles, trapezius, and the thoracic and lumbar paraspinal musculature

- Range of motion
  - Cervical spine, thoracic spine, lumbar spine, shoulder, and feet

- Spinal motion palpation
  - Cervical spine, thoracic spine, lumbar spine, pelvis, and sacrum

- Spinal push test
  - Thoracic spine and lumbar spine

- Gait analysis
  - Anterior, posterior, and lateral gait patterns

- Leg lengths
  - Prone visual check and supine actual leg length

- Bilateral weight scales
  - Evaluate weight distribution bilaterally

- Functional movements
  - Squat, plank, deadlift, scapula retraction, floor press, static jump, arms overhead

- Zone of apposition evaluation
  - Diaphragmatic function

- Postural balance
  - One leg balance test

- Postural sway
  - Romberg's test

- Eye movement evaluation
  - Eye convergence and cardinal fields of gaze

- Vestibular evaluation
  - Vestibulo-ocular reflex and Fukuda's test

- Cerebellar dysdiadochokinesia
  - Coordination of limb movement

Structural analysis:

- Posture images
- Visual analysis
- Muscle strength
- Muscle length
- Muscle hypertonicity
- Leg lengths

Functional analysis:

- Spinal motion palpation
- Spinal push test
- Range of motion
- Gait analysis
- Functional movements
- Bilateral weight scales
- Zone of apposition

Neurologic analysis:

- Fields of gaze
- Eye convergence
- Vestibulo-ocular reflex
- Fukuda test
- Cerebellar dysdiadochokinesia

STRUCTURAL ANALYSIS

To view the overall structure and posture symmetry of the patient, it is important to do posture imaging as well as a visual postural analysis. The most important part of each of these components of the structural analysis is to get accurate clinical findings. When patients know that they are being evaluated, they will have a tendency to try and stand up straight and "fake" good posture. They may even find it difficult to find their normal posture because they are so unaware of their posture on a daily basis. For best clinical findings, systematize how you do the posture image analysis as well as the visual posture analysis with your patients.

Posture imaging

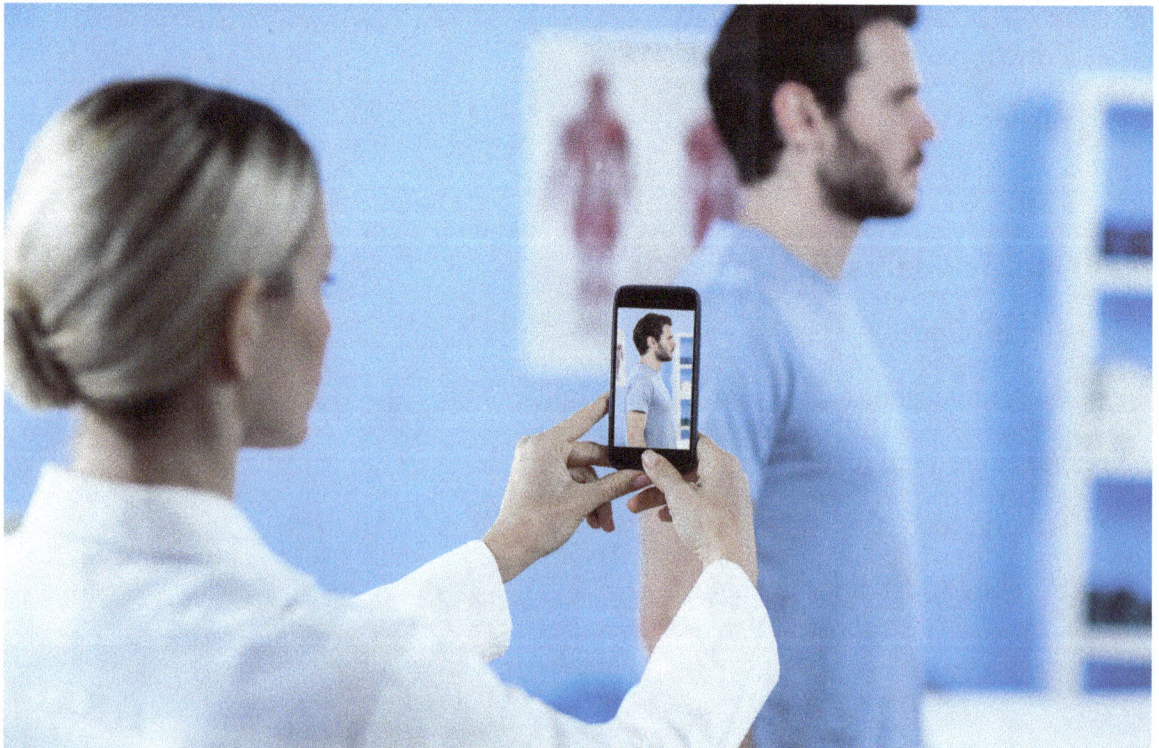

Posture imaging is an excellent tool for accurate clinical findings as well as patient education. As the saying goes, "A picture is worth a thousand words." When a patient can physically see their body analyzed with a posture image, they take an abstract concept and make it real. When patients can see their posture in a photo, they make the connection with what you are telling them. They understand that they really are suffering from postural distortions and that if they do not make a decision to change, the structure of their body will continue to decline. They are no longer just trusting what you say; they can see objective evidence supporting their need to correct the postural design of their body.

Posture imaging provides the Posture Expert and the patient with critical information that they need to know regarding the structure and function of the patient's posture system. Posture Experts analyze posture images to make an accurate analysis of the postural distortion patterns that the patient presents with.

Research supports that doing posture imaging is not only more efficient than manually measuring posture angles, but that it is also clinically accurate (Fortin et al., 2011). An accurate posture image provides practitioners with the information that they need to quickly analyze posture, reinforcing what was clinically noted on the visual posture analysis. Silva et al. (2009) found that visual analysis is not supported for determining head posture findings. A standard is necessary for objectivity. Posture images are a reliable and objective standard to utilize.

Structural correction can and should be objectively measured. Posture imaging provides you with a precise way to measure clinical outcomes. On each re-evaluation throughout their postural correction program, you can monitor the patient's progress objectively, demonstrating functional posture correction.

Taking a proper posture image includes two important participants, the Posture Expert and the patient. The Posture Expert must have a system, and tell the patient exactly what to do in order to get an accurate clinical reading of the patient's postural presentation. Also, the Posture Expert must have the proper tools.

To do an accurate posture analysis, the Posture Expert should have a posture grid hanging that the patient will stand in front of each time the posture image is being taken. They should also have the proper posture imaging technology to analyze postural measurements. It is important to mark exactly where the patient needs to be standing for the posture image, and exactly where the Posture Expert should be to take the photo.

Prejudging this distance will provide ease in the end. To avoid moving the iPad or camera while taking the posture image, have a stand or a tripod to hold it in place.

Once the Posture Expert has the proper materials in place, it is then important to have the proper system and proper communication with the patient. For instant validation of all posture evaluations, utilize the Wade Technique for Posture Analysis. The Wade Technique is the standard for posture evaluations because it demonstrates a natural state of posture. If it is not done properly, the Posture Expert risks not having accurate findings. Have the patient repeat this sequence for anterior, lateral, and posterior posture images and visual analyses.

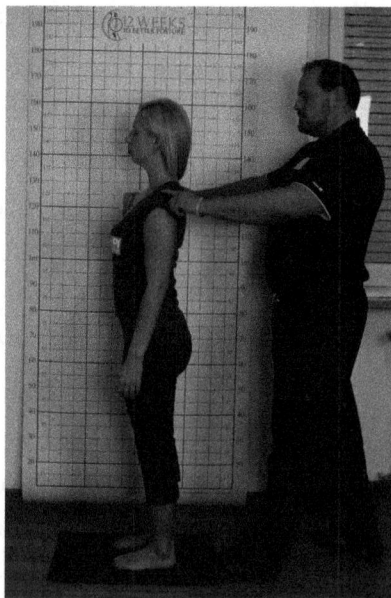

Posture Image Checklist:

1. Determine where to take posture images in your clinic

2. Place a posture grid on the wall

3. Get posture imaging software for accurate analysis

4. Mark a place where the patient will stand so that they are centered in front of the grid

5. Mark a place where the Posture Expert will take the image

6. Place a camera or iPad holder in the designated spot where the image will be taken from

7. Ensure that the camera or iPad is positioned correctly:
   a. The camera is straight
   b. It is aligned with the posture grid
   c. You can see the whole postural presentation of the patient

8. Begin implementing posture images on all initial examinations and re-evaluations

9. Place the patient in the proper position for every posture image. They will stand in the designated area, centered in front of the grid

10. The Posture Expert is in their designated area to take the posture image

11. Explain to the patient how to perform the Wade Technique for Posture Analysis before they perform it

12. Cue the patient to perform the Wade Technique for Posture Analysis
    a. The patient closes their eyes
    b. They take a deep breath in
    c. Breathe out completely
    d. As they breathe out, cue the patient to collapse their shoulders

13. As the patient breathes out and relaxes in real posture, take the posture image

14. Print the posture image

15. Store the posture image in your database as a pre- and post-comparison on future re-evaluations

16. Engage the patient on their report of findings by asking them what they see on the posture image

17. Begin postural correction treatment with the patient

18. Repeat these steps on the re-evaluation

19. Compare the results of the patient's first posture image to their re-evaluation

The Wade Technique for Posture Analysis

The Wade Technique for Posture Analysis instantly validates your posture analysis, both for visual posture exams and with the utilization of posture imaging. The greatest objection with posture analyses is that when patients know their posture is being evaluated, they tend to fake good posture. Whether it is consciously or subconsciously, patients have a tendency to stand up straighter than normal because they are being evaluated.

The fundamental reason this is incorrect is that when a patient tries to fake their posture, even if it's subconscious, your evaluation becomes clinically inaccurate. When the patient is then asked to repeat the posture on a follow up examination, they are unable to duplicate that exact same position. So, there is no way to accurately and objectively compare the changes that have taken place from pre- and post-treatment posture images.

It is impossible to correct the patients' postural distortion patterns if inaccurate information is collected during the initial evaluation. The purpose of the Wade Technique for Posture Analysis is to bring the patient from an active posture to a passive posture, or their real posture.

How do your perform this technique? First you have the patient close their eyes. Then have them breathe in fully and breathe out fully. As they exhale, instruct them to collapse their shoulders, allowing their body to fall into normal posture. As soon as they breathe out, this is when the analysis should take place.

By closing their eyes, the patient eliminates the visual perception of their body in their environment, now relying on their vestibular system and proprioceptive sense of the posture system to hold themselves upright. Proprioception is how we perceive our bodies in space.

Patients who present with postural distortion patterns can more easily compensate for these postural distortions with their eyes open because their eyes always seek to be parallel with the horizon. When their visual field is removed, their body position will be aligned within their environment based upon their faulty body sense.

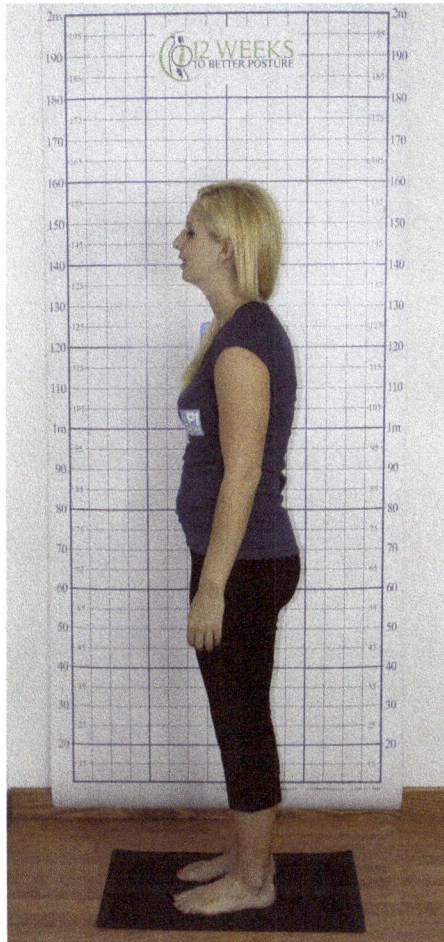

Why is breathing so important during this posture check? By exhaling and allowing the shoulders to relax, the patient is no longer engaging their ancillary respiratory muscles, primarily the scaleni and the sternocleidomastoid muscles bilaterally. When you see people take a big breath in, you watch them raise their chest, demonstrating an upright chest position. When they breathe out, they present with trunk flexion, a common postural distortion that we want to correct. If you took a posture image on the inhalation versus the exhalation, you would have completely different findings.

To be accurate and have reproducible findings, you must see the patient in their most relaxed state. Multiple things happen to a patient's physiology when they walk in your door. If the patient feels nervous and knows that they are being evaluated, their physiologic presentation is to demonstrate dominance, which means that they will stand up taller and straighter with their chest forward.

Humans have what is called "mirror neurons", meaning we have a tendency to mirror physiologic body language of the people around us. Have you ever noticed that if one person yawns, so will other people? Of if one crosses their arms for long enough, so will others?

Because you as a Posture Expert have proper posture yourself, your patients will have the natural tendency to mirror your posture. These subconscious changes in posture are minute and can't be replicated. Because it knows this is likely to happen, the Wade Technique for Posture Analysis eliminates error and ensures objective accuracy from one posture image to the next.

How do we know if we have done the posture evaluation correctly? The analysis is considered correct when the patient is in real posture, not active posture. Real posture is replicable because the patient needs no extra energy expenditure to hold the body upright.

Active posture is not natural, meaning there is an over utilization of energy. When the patient fatigues, they will go back into real posture. To check for active posture, look for the following: as the patient sticks their chest out, the elbows go back and are often behind midline of the body. This is an indication of excessive muscle contraction to hold the body upright. When you see this with the elbows and chest, you may see it to the point of the shoulders being behind the pelvis. Also check the position of the head. The eyes should be level, not looking up or down.

With relaxed posture, the eyes will be parallel with the horizon, the elbows will be in line with the shoulders or drawn anteriorly, the chest drops with exhalation, and there is no apparent muscle contraction.

Two types of errors may occur when performing the Wade Technique for Posture Analysis. A false negative is due to user error. For example, the Posture Expert is holding the iPad for posture imaging at the wrong angle. This will skew the accuracy of the postural evaluation.

The standard in posture analysis is to evaluate the posture with a fixed plumb line against a posture grid, or for purposes of a technologic analysis utilize the centerline on the iPad with a posture grid. The body itself is not a valid standard for measurement because it is not a fixed object; it moves in space.

A false positive is when it appears as though the patient has proper posture because they are in active posture at the time of the evaluation, not real posture. Remember, your ability to make lasting postural corrections as a Posture Expert is dependent upon the quality of the analysis that is performed.

Visual posture analysis

To perform an accurate visual posture analysis, you will have the patient perform the same instructions described above for the Wade Technique of Posture Analysis. Still have the patient placed in front of a posture grid.

For purposes of systemization, always evaluate the postural presentation of the patient from the head down to the feet, and always do so anteriorly, laterally, then posteriorly. By following a pattern, the Posture Expert will be well trained in performing an efficient and accurate visual postural analysis.

Listed below are the anatomical markers that the Posture Expert should utilize for comparison and measurement while performing a visual posture analysis and while analyzing posture images.

Anatomic markers for postural analysis of the patient anteriorly:

- Head: to determine if it is in a neutral position (no lateral flexion or rotation)

- Eyes: to determine if they are parallel to the horizon

- Ears: to determine if they are level with one another or if there is lateral flexion of the head

- Chin: to determine if the chin is centered or if there is rotation of the head to one side or the other

- Shoulders: to determine if they are level bilaterally (not elevated or depressed), have even muscular development, and are back (not rotated forward)

- Arms: to determine if they are in a neutral position, at even lengths, with palms toward the lateral aspect of the body and the thumbs pointed forward

- Pelvis. To determine if the pelvis is level, evaluate if both anterior superior iliac spines and pelvic crests are in the same transverse plane

- Hip joints: to determine if the hips are in a neutral position or if there is abduction or adduction

- Patellae: to determine if they are level and pointed forward, or if the knee is rotated medially or laterally

- Feet: to determine if they are parallel with slight out-toeing. Evaluate if the medial malleoli are in the same vertical plane or if there is evident pronation or supination

Anatomic markers for postural analysis of the patient laterally:

- Head: to determine if the head is in a neutral position or if there is flexion or extension of the cervical spine

- Eyes: to determine if the eyes are parallel to the horizon

- Ear: to determine if the ear is aligned over the shoulder or if the head is anteriorly placed in relation to the shoulder

- Cervical spine: to determine if there is a normal curve with slight anterior convexity, or if the curve is increased or decreased

- Thoracic spine: to determine if there is a normal curve with slight posterior convexity, or if the curve is increased or decreased

- Shoulders: to determine if the shoulders are back or rotated forward, and if they are aligned over the hips

- Arms: to determine if they are in a neutral position, at even lengths, palms facing toward the lateral aspect of the body with the thumbs pointed forward

- Lumbar spine: to determine if there is a normal curve with slight anterior convexity, or if the curve is increased or decreased

- Pelvis: to determine if the pelvis is in a neutral position, with the anterior superior iliac spines in the same vertical plane as the pubic symphysis

- Hip joint: to evaluate if there is a neutral position of the hips, or if they are extended or flexed

- Knee: to evaluate if the knees are in a neutral position, or if they are extended or flexed

- Ankle: to determine if the ankle is in a neutral position where the leg is vertical and at a right angle to the sole of the foot

- Feet: to determine if the feet are pointed forward or if there is in-toeing or out-toeing

Anatomic markers for postural analysis of the patient posteriorly:

- Head: to determine if it is in a neutral position (no lateral flexion or rotation)

- Ears: to determine if they are level with one another or if there is lateral flexion of the head

- Shoulders: to determine if they are level (not elevated or depressed), have even muscular development, and are back (not rotated forward)

- Scapulae: medial borders are parallel and about 4 inches apart

- Arms: to determine if they are in a neutral position, at even lengths, with palms toward the lateral aspect of the body and the thumbs pointed forward

- Thoracic spine: to determine if there is a lateral deviation

- Pelvis. To determine if the pelvis is level, evaluate if both posterior superior iliac spines and pelvic crests are in the same transverse plane

- Hip joints: to determine if the hips are in a neutral position or if there is abduction or adduction

- Achilles tendons: to determine if they are parallel or if there is supination or pronation of the foot

- Feet: to determine if they are parallel with slight out-toeing. Evaluate if the medial malleoli are in the same vertical plane or if there is evident pronation or supination

Posture image cervical analysis

Before moving forward with the rest of the structural analysis of the complete postural analysis, we will examine in more depth how to evaluate cervical posture for correction via posture imaging. Harrison et al (2002) defined the ideal cervical curvature as an arc of 63 degrees from C1 to T1 with specific segmental angles.

Utilizing radiographs alone demonstrates a 3D object in a 2D manner from a static perspective. Using posture images along with visual analysis, we can accurately measure the position of the body. Fortin et al (2011) demonstrate that Posture Experts can more effectively measure posture angles on posture imaging than on the patient during a visual analysis.

When posture images are taken accurately, they provide the Posture Expert with the information they need to make appropriate clinical decisions. From posture images, posture angles can be measured, and Posture Experts can objectively evaluate the postural presentation visually. What you find on posture imaging and how you interpret it is the most important part of the analysis. Consider individual postural distortions and also coupled distortion patterns that arise from compensation patterns and coupled motions.

To determine the Burns Cervical Angle, a line is drawn perpendicular at the level of C7 on the posture image. This is taken from the shoulder neck junction—from the lowest part of the neck that arrives at the shoulder. A line is then drawn from this same point to the external auditory meatus. This angle is measured. This angle determines the amount of anterior or posterior head translation that is present.

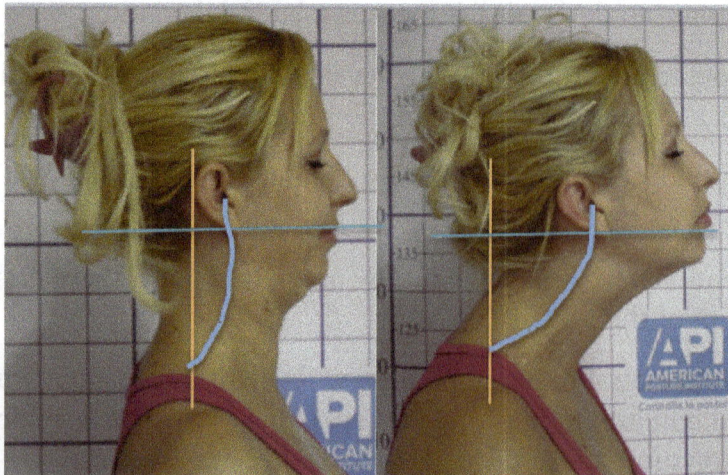

To determine the Lateral Flexion Angle, a point is placed in the middle of the eyes and in the center of the chin. A second set of points is placed on the posture image, one in the episternal notch and one in the center of the neck below the chin. A line is drawn from each set of points, the head being drawn inferiorly, and the neck being drawn superiorly. Where these lines intersect is the Lateral Flexion Angle. This will determine the side and degree of Lateral Head Flexion.

For the Burns Cervical Angle and the Lateral Flexion Angle, a decrease in the angle measurement will be associated with postural distortion patterns. The postural distortion patterns are commonly associated with pain and discomfort for the patient.

Muscle tests

The next component of the structural aspect of the complete postural analysis is to evaluate muscle strength. Muscle strength tests are done to evaluate for muscle weakness; muscle length tests evaluate whether the muscle length is shortened causing a decreased range of motion, or stretched causing increased range of motion.

Muscle strength tests are evaluated via a grading system from "zero", meaning no movement of the muscle, to "normal", meaning the patient can hold the position of the muscle against strong pressure. Muscle strength tests are performed of the following muscle groups: the rhomboids, external obliques, transversus abdominis, gluteus medius, and the tensor fascia latae (TFL). Muscle strength tests are active. The patient will resist pressure exerted by the Posture Expert.

Muscle length tests consist of movements that increase the distance between origin and insertion, elongating the muscle. Muscle length tests are performed for the following muscle groups: the pectoral muscles, the diaphragm, lumbar paraspinal muscles, iliopsoas, hamstrings, and the gastrocnemius muscle groups. Muscle length tests can be performed actively or passively, depending upon the preference of the Posture Expert.

Please note that you can perform muscle tests on other muscles too. This will be specific to the presentation of the patient and based upon your clinical decision-making.

Muscular hypertonicity should also be evaluated for the following muscle groups: the suboccipital muscle group, the trapezius bilaterally, and the thoracic and lumbar paraspinal musculature bilaterally.

Muscular hypertonicity is defined as "a condition in which there is too much muscle tone...Muscle tone is regulated by signals that travel from the brain to the nerves and tell the muscle to contract" (National Institute of Neurological Disorders and Stroke). To evaluate for hypertonicity, the Posture Expert should palpate the aforementioned muscle groups and evaluate for the presence of muscular rigidity, muscle spasms, and inflammation. Palpate the anatomy bilaterally to evaluate the difference.

Leg length analysis

The final component of the structural posture analysis is to evaluate the difference in leg lengths of the patient. Research demonstrates that between 53–75% of people have leg length discrepancies (Knutson, 2005). Common methods for performing leg length analyses are by doing actual and apparent leg length tests.

Actual leg lengths are measured from the anterior superior iliac spine (ASIS) to the medial malleolus. Apparent leg lengths are measured from the umbilicus to the medial malleolus.

The Posture Expert may also choose to do a visual leg length analysis. This can be performed with the patient supine or prone by visually analyzing the difference between the length of the legs. Evaluate visually by comparing if the heels are lined up bilaterally.

Studies of schoolchildren show that the majority of children show leg length discrepancies and the likelihood of the discrepancy increases with a child's age. Travell and Simmons (1993) reviewed radiographs of a group of 1,446 schoolchildren between 5 and 17 years of age; 80% had at least a 0.16cm (1/16-inch) discrepancy and 3.4% had a difference of 1.3cm (1/2 inch) or more. It was also demonstrated that 92% of senior high school students showed measurable leg length differences. This study suggests that differences in leg lengths tend to increase as children grow.

FUNCTIONAL ANALYSIS

Functional analyses determine the functional capacity of the posture system. By determining function, the Posture Expert will understand the level of fatigue of the posture system, and have a better understanding of the treatment plan necessary for postural correction.

Motion palpation

The first component of the functional analysis is spinal motion palpation. The purpose of spinal motion palpation is to evaluate for localized decreased range of motion of the spine. This is a passive test for the cervical, thoracic, and lumbar spine. Spinal motion palpation is performed with the patient seated, and the Posture Expert will perform the analysis at each spinal level.

Take note of which spinal levels have a decreased range of motion, and in what direction the range of motion is decreased.

Spinal push test

To determine the major and minor points of postural instability, the spinal push test is performed. It is important to note that when we refer to instability, we are referring to postural instability, or postural collapse. We are not talking about instability of the spine in relation to ligamentous damage, or fracture.

The spinal push test provides immediate feedback of dysfunction of the vestibular system, the system responsible for keeping the body upright in an extended position. When you challenge the spinal segment, you are testing the integration between the vestibular system and the myofascial and connective tissues surrounding the spinal segment.

When a healthy segment is challenged, or pushed forward into flexion, the otoliths of the vestibular system fire to reflexively oppose the anterior stimulus. This response keeps the patient upright against gravity by extending the spine.

With postural instability at that segment, the patient demonstrates anterior postural sway. This is indicative of breakdown in the integration of the myofascial spinal tissues and the vestibular system. It tells the Posture Expert exactly where to make the postural correction to restore proper alignment to the posture system. Immediately after the correction, the patient would be re-tested. You would expect to see immediate changes in which the patient is completely stable with no postural sway before leaving your office.

To perform the spinal push test, have the patient stand normally, then perform the Wade Technique for Posture Analysis. Stand behind the patient and tell them, "I am going to be touching your back, don't let me push you over, but don't resist backwards, OK?" It is not mandatory, but prompting the patient before performing the test can help improve accuracy. It is clearer where the points of postural instability are located.

When performing the spinal push test, you have your initial contact. This is the first contact your finger or thumb makes when touching the spinous process of the patient. This is a light contact, the lighter the better in terms of the information you want to take away from this test. There is no set distance that you are trying to push to other than to locate the point of resistance. As you push, it will be a light contact with a slow gentle follow through until the point of resistance is located.

During initial contact there are a few possibilities that may happen. If this is a new patient or a patient who is very unstable, they will most likely fall forward. This most often involves the patient's entire body shifting or moving forward with a slight push. In some instances, the patient will bend at the waist to keep from falling over, or take a step forward.

If the patient has a high level of postural stability, they will demonstrate very minimal anterior postural sway. When you locate a major or minor point of instability, the patient will shift forward, demonstrating anterior postural sway. The amount of sway depends upon the level of postural instability. Long-term patients will show a low level of sway whereas new patients will likely show increased anterior sway.

The motion forward is not the determining factor for a point of instability. It is a clue or signal that there may be a point of instability present.

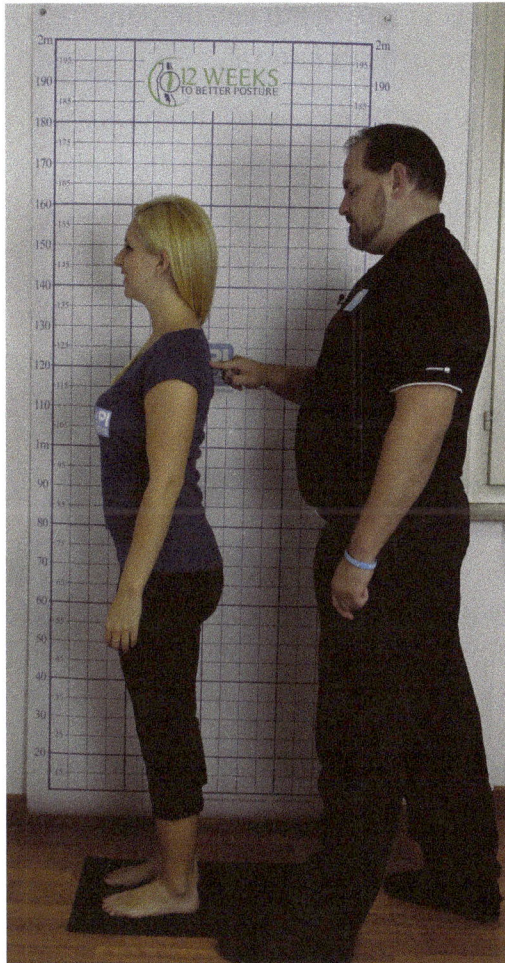

How you deduce the point of instability is based on the point of resistance. As you push through the initial contact, you will reach a point (either immediately or once the patient's resistance initiates) where it feels like the spine becomes more stable, or solid, or stronger. This is the point of resistance. The point where the postural stability of the spine can match the force that you are applying into the segment.

A stable segment will be strong and firm. This could be demonstrated by pushing your finger against a wall. An instable segment would be the equivalent of putting a pillow against the wall and then pushing through that pillow until it becomes firm or hard. Instable segments have a "spongy" feel.

For best practices of the spinal push test, avoid the following mistakes. Do not push too hard or use too much force. The patient may not be able to resist your pressure, or they will recruit other areas of the spine to compensate. Do not press on the next segment before the patient returns to neutral.

When the spinal push test is performed correctly, the patient will experience two feelings. As you push forward on a stable segment, the weight will stay primarily in the heels of the feet, and the posterior chain will activate. They will feel activation primarily of the hamstrings and the gluteals.

When you locate a point of instability, the weight of the patient will shift either slightly or completely to the balls of the feet. The quadriceps and the core will activate to compensate.

Range of motion

Global range of motion is performed at the cervical, thoracic, and lumbar regions of the spine as well as the shoulders and the feet. The standard for performing ranges of motion is with the use of goniometers to measure the precise degrees of movement.

Posture Experts may also choose to perform visual range of motion evaluations. When evaluating range of motion visually, compare the patient's range of motion from right to left. Take note of which side has reduced range of motion.

Although it is less common than having a reduced range of motion, also evaluate for the presence of hypermobility. With hypermobility, the patient brings their joint beyond the normal range.

According to Yochum and Rowe, the spinal curvature normal ranges of motion are the following:

Cervical spine:

- Flexion = 30–45 degrees

- Extension = 40–55 degrees

- Lateral flexion = 40–45 degrees

- Rotation = 70–80 degrees

Thoracolumbar spine: the thoracic and lumbar values are taken together as it is difficult to measure thoracic movement and lumbar movement separately. Also, local range of motion is taken through spinal motion palpation.

- Flexion = 90 degrees

- Extension = 30–35 degrees

- Lateral flexion = 30–40 degrees

- Rotation = 30–35 degrees

Accurate tests for range of motion of the spine should not include movement of the hips. For lateral flexion, if there is pelvic unleveling, the spine is in flexion toward the high hip, but overall flexion on the side of the hip will be reduced.

In flexion, the cervical spine moves in the direction of decreasing the normal forward curve. The thoracic spine moves in the direction of increasing the normal backward curve, and the lumbar spine moves in the direction of decreasing the normal forward curve.

In extension, the cervical spine moves in the direction of increasing the normal forward curve, the thoracic spine moves in the direction of decreasing the normal backward curve, and the lumbar spine moves in the direction of increasing the normal forward curve.

Lateral flexion, occurring in the coronal plane, is a movement in which the head and trunk bend toward one side while the spine curves convexly toward the opposite side. Rotation, occurring in the transverse plane, is considered to be clockwise or counterclockwise

Zone of apposition evaluation

The next component of the functional posture analysis is to evaluate the zone of apposition. The zone of apposition is the area of the diaphragm encompassing the cylindrical portion, which corresponds to the portion directly opposed to the inner aspect of the lower ribcage (Boyle, Olinick, Lewis, 2010).

The zone of apposition is important because it is controlled by the abdominal muscles and directs diaphragmatic tension. When the zone of apposition is decreased or suboptimal, it can cause inefficient breathing and diminished activation of the transverse abdominis muscle, leading to weakened lumbar stabilization.

To evaluate the zone of apposition, watch the patient breathe in and out while they are lying supine. Evaluate the movement of their diaphragm, ribs, belly, and upper chest. With efficient breathing of the patient, the Posture Expert will note fluid movement up and down of the belly with minimal to no movement of the upper chest cavity.

Gait analysis

Gait is the foundation of bipedal motion and the functional movement that we perform most often throughout the lifespan. Problems with gait can be detrimental. With improper gait, a patient's ground force reaction is multiplied, adding more stress to the posture system.

Here are some important neurologic considerations pertaining to gait. Posture Quadrant 4, or the lower limbs and feet, has a large amount of proprioception representation. Meaning that a significant amount of the information that we receive about the movement position of our bodies is due to our gait patterns. When that gait pattern is disturbed, the proprioceptive feedback to the sensory cortex is blurred.

The cerebellum plays an important role in coordinating gait by creating a synchrony between the flexor and extensor musculature. This synchrony allows coordinated movements with dynamic postural stability. With dysfunction of the cerebellum, the patient presents with a wide based gait. When they bring their feet closer together, they will likely feel instable.

The gait cycle is a repetitive pattern involving steps and strides. A step is one single step, a stride is a whole gait cycle. The step time is the time from one foot hitting the floor to the other foot hitting the floor.

The stance phase is the phase in which the foot remains in contact with the ground, and the swing phase is when the foot is not in contact with the ground.

Phases of Gait:

- Initial contact
- Loading phase
- Mid stance
- Terminal stance
- Pre swing
- Initial swing
- Mid swing
- Terminal swing

With the initial contact, the heel contacts the ground leading to the loading phase. During the loading phase, 90% of load is absorbed by the quadriceps when the knee is flexed at 20 degrees. With lack of knee flexion, the load will be distributed throughout the leg. This phase is characterized by load transmission and hip stability with forward motion.

The next phase is mid stance. In mid stance the weight of the body is shifted anteriorly and the hip extends, preparing the body for terminal stance in which the heel of the foot comes off the ground. This phase is driven by the plantar flexors of the foot. If the ankle is stiff and there is less dorsiflexion, the knee will hyperextend.

After terminal stance is pre swing. In pre swing the muscles of the anterior capsule of the hip are active and there is passive tension of the quadriceps and hip flexors. There is plantar flexion of the ankle. Following pre swing is initial swing with significant knee flexion so that the foot clears the ground.

The final phases of gait are mid swing and terminal swing. In mid swing it is particularly important that the gluteals fire to support the body upright. The ankle joint is in a neutral position. Terminal swing is preparation for the stance phase with the initial contact of the next cycle.

There are many components to analyze for an accurate gait analysis. Because there are many things to observe simultaneously, the best way of performing gait analysis is to film the patient walking. When they are recorded, you can watch the video in slow motion to see and measure the angles. For best practices, record them walking on a treadmill.

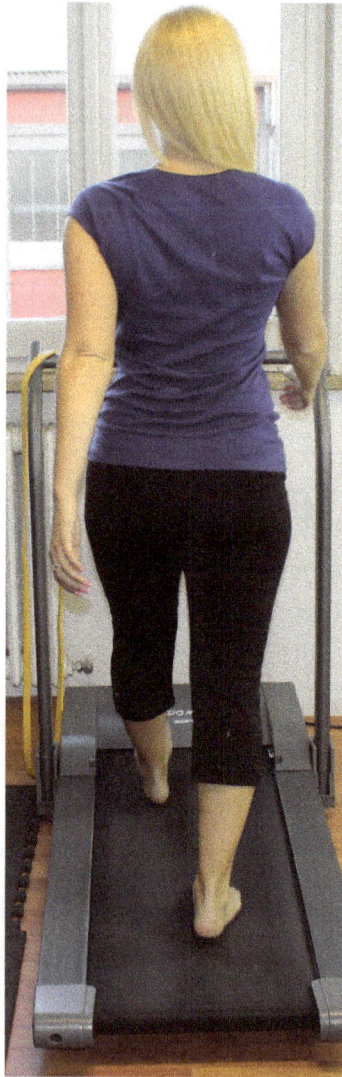

When filming the patient, you should record them from the posterior aspect and from the lateral aspect on the treadmill to see their gait pattern appropriately. Have them select their treadmill speed. They should be walking at their "normal" pace.

As the patient is walking, you are evaluating each posture quadrant, not just the feet. Take note if there is forward head posture or a head tilt of Posture Quadrant 1. Evaluate for postural hyperkyphosis of Posture Quadrant 2 and decreased arm swing. Analyze

Posture Quadrant 3 for indication of pelvic unleveling or pelvic rotation. You may also see an increased lordotic curve or a swayback presentation in which the hips are translated anteriorly.

For evaluation of Posture Quadrant 4, determine if pronation or supination is present. Evaluate for toe-in or toe-out foot flare. Watch the patient's knees to see if they bow out or come together as in a knock-kneed presentation.

If you notice that the patient has gait pattern faults during their strides, this can be due to muscular weakness or it can be due to joint dysfunction. It is important to then palpate the areas where you suspect dysfunction to confirm your analysis.

Test the range of motion of the joints to see if they need to be mobilized, and do muscle tests to test for strength of suspected muscle weakness. This will give you a precise correction protocol when doing posture rehabilitation.

This is a general statement and does not apply to all patients. However, it is a common presentation. The majority of patients will present with excessive pronation of the feet with toe-out foot flare and gluteal weakness that will impact their gait patterns. Although this doesn't apply to everyone, these are common patterns of dysfunction that you may see often in clinical practice.

If you aren't sure where to start with gait analysis, recognize that having a treadmill and recording the patient walking and actually measuring their angles are best practices. If this doesn't match your practice style, you can at least watch your patient walk in the office.

Watching their gait will show you their global gait pattern including toe-in or out foot flare, pronation and supination, excessive movement or stiffness of the hips, limping or pathological gait, chest flexion, forward head posture, and concentric arm swing.

Also watch the patient's head, trunk, and arms while they are walking. If the patient leans forward, the posterior chain is on. If they lean back, the posterior chain is off, decreasing activation of the gluteals. When gluteals are switched off, the femur is not stabilized.

Other compromised gait patterns include the patient holding their breath or lack of arm swing. They may also have a limp or pathologic gait pattern such as shuffling gait or hemiplegia. Pathologic gait should be treated for the pathology. For the majority of your patients, you will see biomechanic faults that can be corrected with posture rehabilitation.

Common gait analysis postural faults include the following:

- Pelvic hike ipsilateral to the high hip with pelvic unleveling during swing. This is increased with the presence of foot drop

- Pelvic drop ipsilateral to a weak gluteus medius during stance

- External hip rotation during termination of stance phase into swing. This can be muscular or structural

- Internal hip rotation from contact into midstance. This too can be muscular or structural

- Knee hyperextension in midstance. This is due to weak quadriceps or lengthened ligaments

- Supination or pronation will be evident by evaluating the position of the calcaneus in relation to the Achilles tendon during heel strike

- Limping gait in response to acute injury

- Antalgic gait in response to acute low back pain

Functional movements

The next component of the functional analysis is the basic human functional movements. The movements include a squat, plank, straight leg deadlift, scapula retraction, push up, arms overhead, and static jump. These movements are analyzed in a safe place (your practice) to see if they can be performed without postural collapse.

If the patient is unable to perform these movements in a safe environment, they will likely hurt themselves in a stressful situation. While they are performing these functional movements, if you see flexion or extension anywhere of the spine, consider it a postural fault. The patient should maintain a neutral spine during the movements.

The basic movements of human function simulate motions that humans perform on a normal basis. For example, the inability to perform a squat in your office means the patient can be injured when getting up from a chair or when squatting down to sit on a chair. They will also have weak postural stabilization while lifting.

The inability to perform a deadlift means the patient is more prone to injuring themselves when bending forward and lifting an object from the ground. Think of a mom reaching for her child or grabbing a package that is waiting on the doorstep.

If the patient cannot activate the proper musculature when pulling an item toward them or when lifting their arms overhead, they risk injuring their upper extremity, shoulder, and upper thoracic spine. This could occur when they are placing luggage in the luggage bins overhead on an airplane.

Do your patients have to be athletes to perform human functional movements? The answer is absolutely not. Yes, with athletes you want to ensure that they are able to perform functional movements accurately, too. But these movements are not reserved just for athletes to be doing in the gym. Any human who cannot properly perform functional human movements is likely to experience postural decline and has an increased likelihood of injuring themselves.

When evaluating functional movements, you are recommended to take a video of the patient performing the movements for two reasons. One, you can show the patient their progression as they improve throughout their treatment plan, and secondly, you can more specifically analyze the patient's dynamic posture.

When making the analysis, you want to evaluate each posture quadrant to see if postural collapse is present. Each movement has a possible score of 4, allotting one point to each posture quadrant. If the patient performs the functional movement without any postural collapse, they receive a score of 4. If they perform the movement but have forward head posture and a hyperlordosis of the lumbar spine, they receive a score of 2.

While you are performing the evaluation in your practice, also take note in which posture quadrants the patient's postural collapse was present. In relation to the previous example, if the patient has postural collapse of Posture Quadrants 1 and 3, it would be scored in the following manner: overall score of 2 with collapse of PQ 1 and PQ 3.

The first functional movement to be analyzed is a squat.

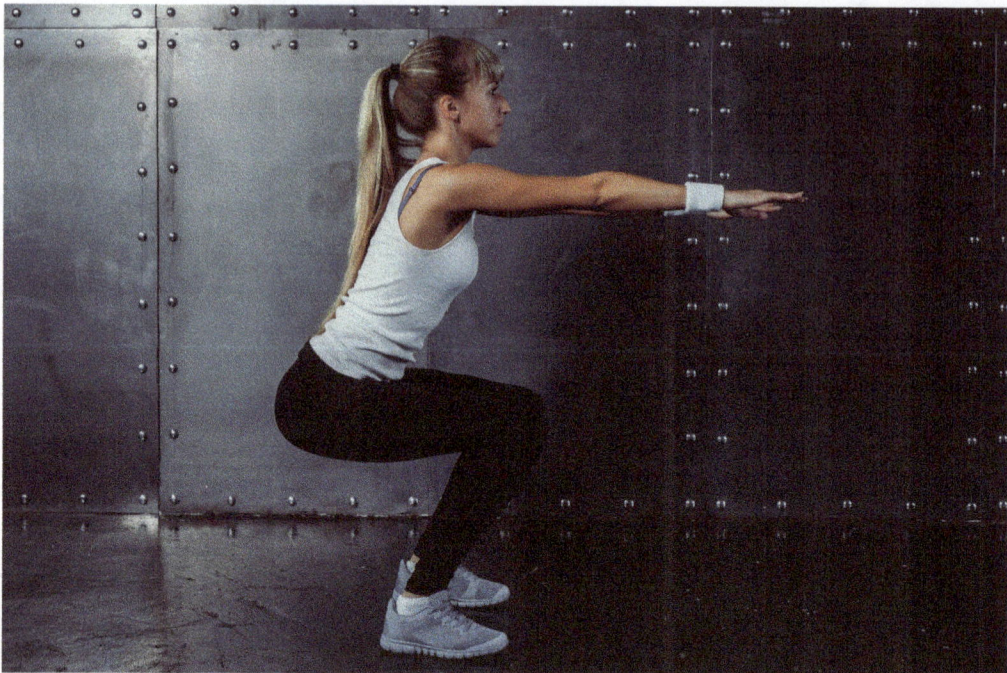

- In Posture Quadrant 1 the cervical spine is neutral and the eyes are parallel with the horizon. The most common mistakes are cervical extension and jaw clenching. Patients will commonly look up while performing a squat, putting the neck into extension, and they will commonly clench their jaw, especially if performing the movement with high weights in a gym setting

- In Posture Quadrant 2 the shoulders should be back with the back straight. As the patient does the squat, their chest should stay upright. The most common mistake of Posture Quadrant 2 is shoulder instability in which the shoulders are drawn anteriorly, resulting in chest flexion. This can also impact respiration

- In Posture Quadrant 3 it is fundamental that the pelvis stays neutral and is level from side to side. It is much more common to see an anterior pelvic tilt. You will almost never see a patient do a squat with a posterior pelvic tilt. You can tell that the patient has anterior pelvic tilt if there is a visual hyperlordosis of the lumbar spine.

- In Posture Quadrant 4 the shins should stay vertical with the knees over the ankles and both feet are pointed forward. As the patient goes into the deep squat, ensure that their knees and feet stay pointed forward and don't collapse to the midline. The most common postural faults of Posture Quadrant 4 are pronation of the feet, the knees are drawn forward in relation to the feet, or the knees collapse medially

The next functional movement is a straight leg deadlift.

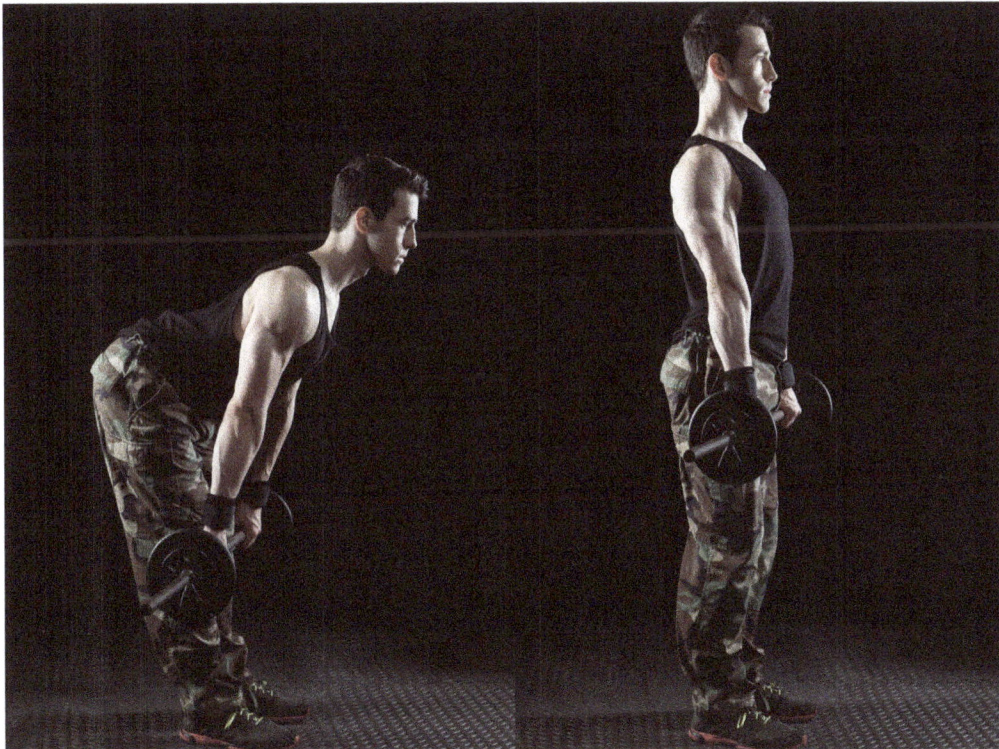

- In Posture Quadrant 1 the cervical spine should stay in a neutral position throughout the movement. Cervical flexion or extension as the patient drops down or raises up is considered a postural fault

- In Posture Quadrant 2 the thoracic spine and shoulders should be straight and in proper alignment. Indications of weak posture include scapula winging or shoulder anteriority with a rounded spine appearance. This will be most common as the patient lowers their upper body toward the floor

- In Posture Quadrant 3, pay attention to the position of the hips and the lumbar spine. If Posture Quadrant 2 was rounded into a C shape while the patient was lowering the upper body, a very common compensation will be to arch the lower back while raising back up, causing a hyperlordosis. These two postural faults are correlated with one another and should both be corrected. When the patient comes up, the movement should happen at the hips with the back straight and contraction of the core musculature

- In Posture Quadrant 4 the feet should be pointed forward, slightly apart, and the legs stay straight. They shouldn't be locked, but they should stay straight throughout the movement. The primary muscle contraction will be in the gluteal muscles

The next functional movement is a plank.

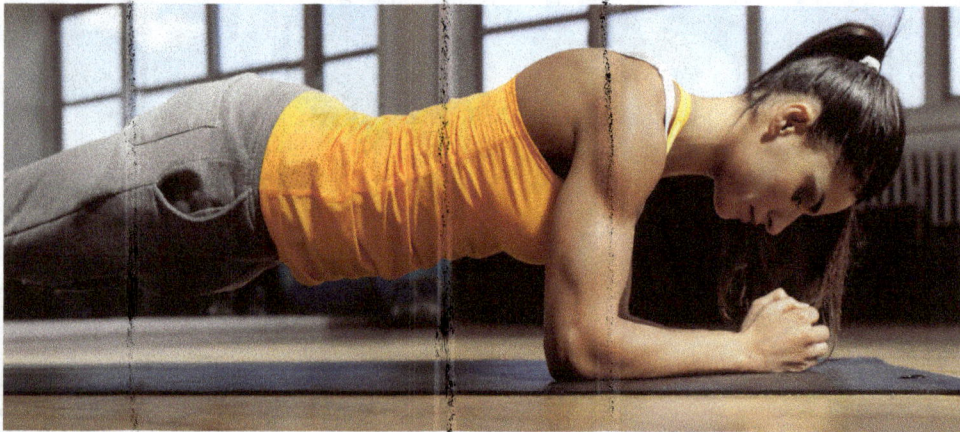

- In Posture Quadrant 1 the cervical spine should stay in a neutral position while performing the exercise. Cervical flexion or extension is considered a postural fault. You will commonly see that when patients fatigue, their heads drop into flexion and they clench their jaws

- In Posture Quadrant 2 the spine should be straight with no scapula winging and the shoulders should not be rounded. The elbows are under the shoulders with a 90-degree angle at the elbow. If the patient placed an imaginary rod along their spine, all places of the spine would be touching the rod, and the rod would be parallel to the floor

- Posture Quadrant 3 again works together with Posture Quadrant 2. The rod laid across the back should also be flat against the lumbar spine. If there is a gap then hyperlordosis is present. The patient should demonstrate a strong core activation with the hips level. Common mistakes will be dropping the pelvis down or arching the back and sticking their behind in the air

- In Posture Quadrant 4 ensure that the legs are straight and the knees are not bent. The heels stay perpendicular to the ground and do not collapse medially or laterally

Following planks are pushups. The postural presentation is similar to a plank, but the patient is on their hands, not their forearms. They will lower their body and push themselves back up instead of holding a sustained position as with the plank.

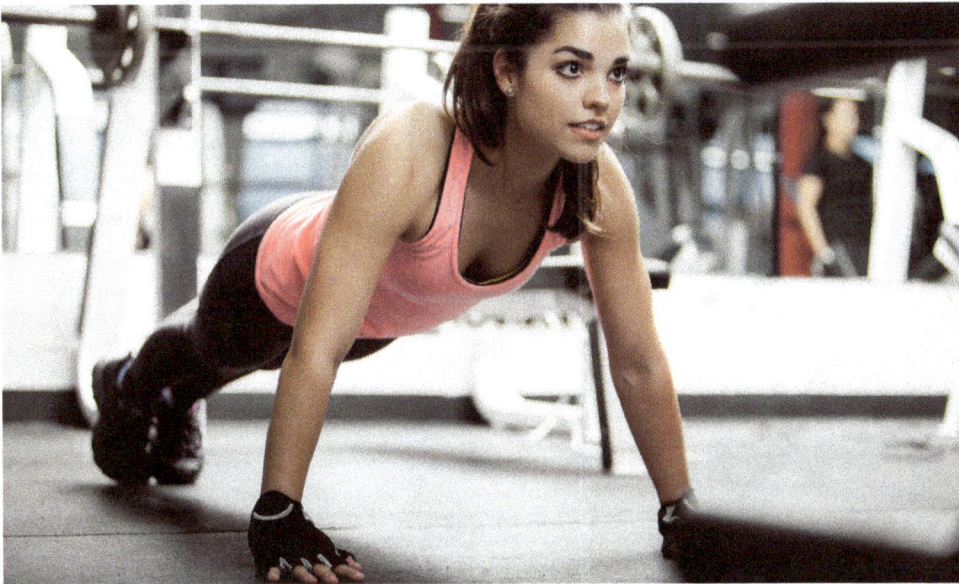

- In Posture Quadrant 1, check for the same position as you do with planks. The cervical spine should stay in a neutral position while the patient is performing the exercise. Cervical flexion or extension is considered a postural fault

- In Posture Quadrant 2, watch the patient's elbows. The wrists are aligned under the shoulders and the back is straight. You shouldn't see a C shaped curve. A common mistake is that the elbow will go out laterally instead of staying close to the body. Also the hands should be facing forward, and not turned out. External hand rotation indicates shoulder immobility patterns

- In Posture Quadrant 3 the lower back is flat without anterior or posterior pelvic tilt. With weak core musculature you will see a curve of the lumbar spine

- In Posture Quadrant 4 ensure that the legs are straight and the knees are not bent. The heels stay perpendicular to the ground and do not collapse medially or laterally

In the next functional movement of scapula retractions, your patient will primarily be working their upper body. However, the overall posture is very important.

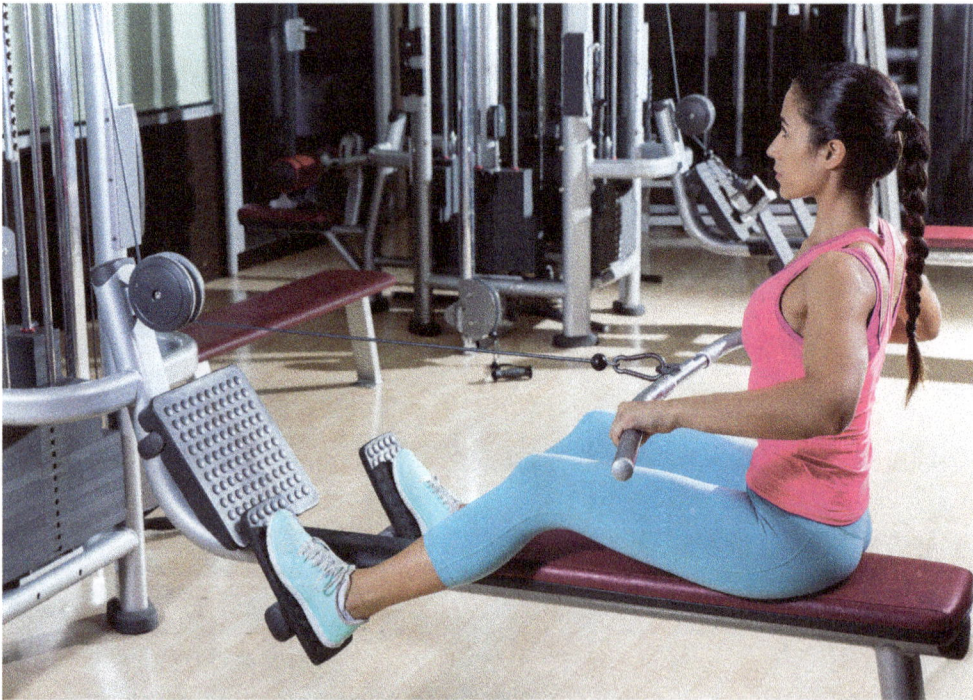

- In Posture Quadrant 1 the cervical spine should be in neutral position with the eyes parallel to the ground and ear in alignment with the shoulder. As the patient loses the strong neutral position of the cervical spine, the upper thoracic position and shoulders shift forward. You may see forward head posture

- In Posture Quadrant 2 the shoulders should be pulled back, the back straight, and the elbows close to the body. With shoulder instability, the shoulders will round forward or be pulled far forward with the initial movement. Another common postural fault is that the elbows are too wide apart and do not stay close to the body

- In Posture Quadrant 3 the pelvis should be neutral with no anterior or posterior pelvic tilt. Also, the patient should not rotate their hips as they pull the band back. They should have the power to keep the pelvis pointed forward with equal weight distribution on the right and left sides

- In Posture Quadrant 4 make sure both feet are facing forward and slightly apart

The next functional movement to evaluate is arms overhead. During this movement the patient raises their arms over their head while keeping their back against the wall.

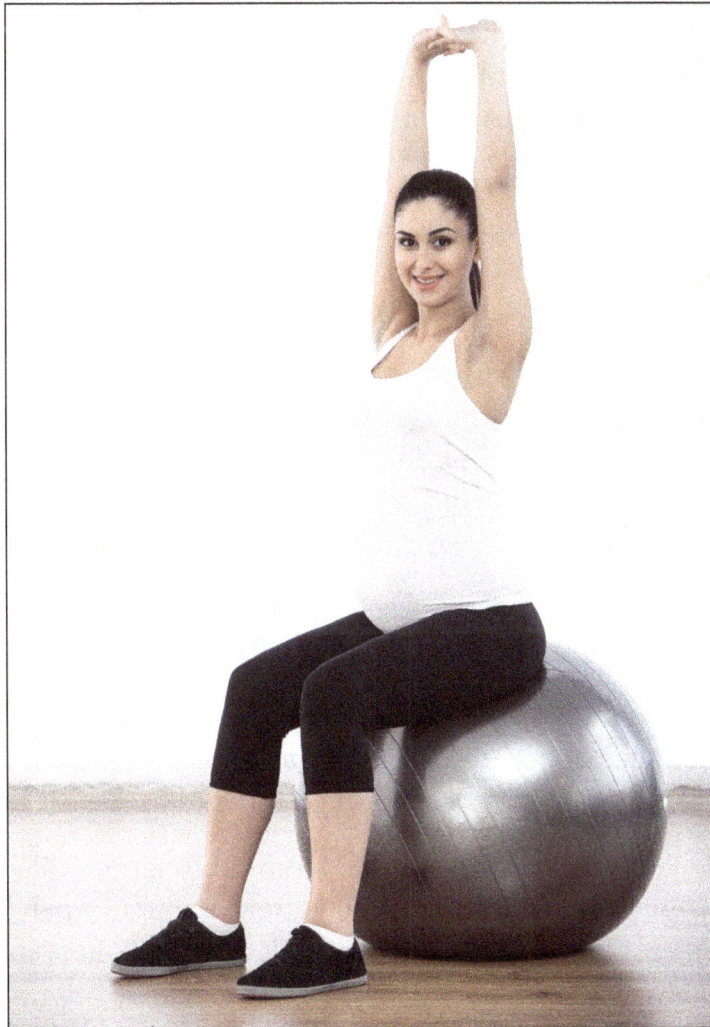

- In Posture Quadrant 1 you want to see a nice neutral spine of the cervical region with the back of the head against the wall, and the head level so that the eyes are looking forward parallel to the floor. You do not want to see forward head posture, or the patient looking up to keep their head against the wall.

- In Posture Quadrant 2 the shoulders are pulled back and the thoracic spine is against the wall. When patients present with hyperkyphosis this will be very difficult for them.

- In Posture Quadrant 3 the lower back is flat against the wall and the pelvis is neutral. Patients who present with anterior pelvic tilt will have difficulty flattening their back. As the patient raises their arms over their head, watch the patient's lower back. They may struggle to keep their back against the wall. If there is a gap between the wall and the patient's back, there is postural collapse of this posture quadrant

- In Posture Quadrant 4 look to see that the heels of the feet are against the wall and the toes are pointed forward. If the patient cannot perform the exercise with their feet against the wall, have them take a small step forward so that their back is flat

The last functional movement that we emphasize at the American Posture Institute is static jumps, meaning that the patient performs a jump from a static position. This is very important because if the patient does not know how to jump and land, they can easily be injured performing normal daily activities such as jumping to catch something. If they land with improper form, it can cause multiple problems to the posture system.

- In Posture Quadrant 1 the cervical spine should be neutral, and as the patient lands they should instantly be able to orient their eyes parallel to the floor

- In Posture Quadrant 2 the thorax is strong, meaning that the chest doesn't collapse when the patient lands. The thoracic spine is straight, the shoulders are back and they do not round forward as the patient lands

- In Posture Quadrant 3 the pelvis stays neutral throughout the jump and landing. A common postural distortion pattern is anterior pelvic tilt, seen as a lumbar lordosis as the patient swings their arms back in preparation for the jump. They should be able to keep a neutral pelvis

- In Posture Quadrant 4 we want to see proper bending in preparation for the jump. Meaning that as the knees bend, the shins should stay vertical with the knees over the ankles. The feet are pointed forward when the patient is in pre-jump stance and when they land

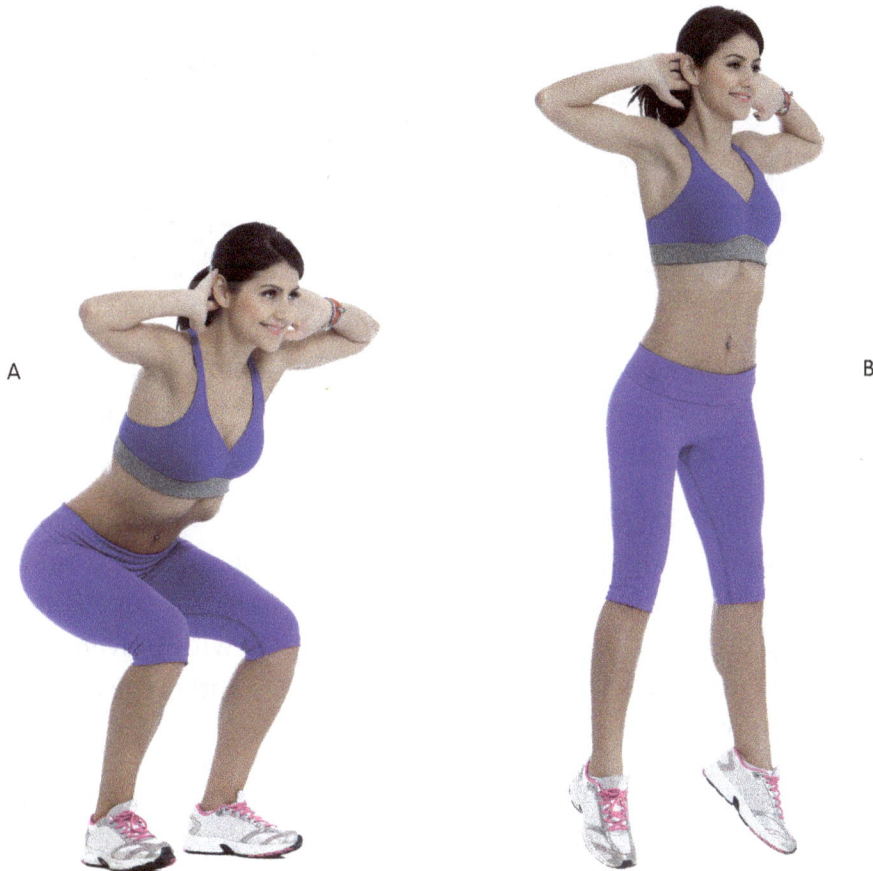

Bilateral weight scales

The final aspect of a functional posture analysis is to have the patient stand on bilateral weight scales. Have the patient stand with one foot on each scale and look forward without moving. Compare the weight of the left and the right side of the body to see if the weight distribution is equal or if there is a deviation of weight distribution from the right to the left side of the body.

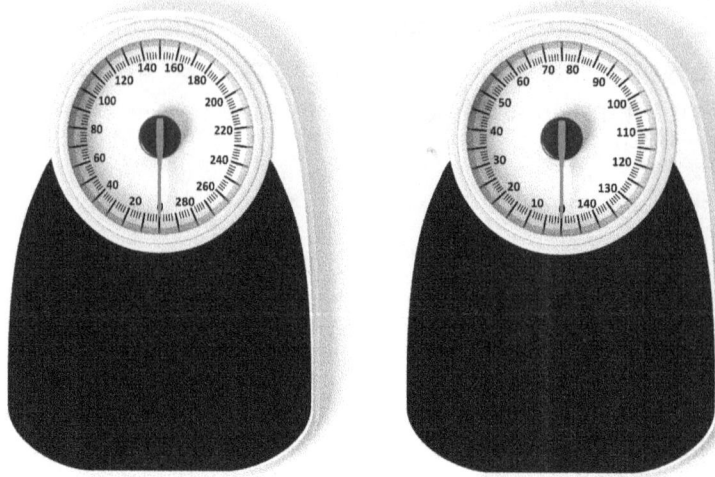

Patients who present with pelvic unleveling and a leg length discrepancy will likely have a difference in weight distribution bilaterally. Typically, patients present with more pressure over the long leg side (Morscher, 1972).

Lewitt (1993) demonstrated that articular dysfunction at the craniocervical junction can cause an unequal distribution of weight between the lower extremities. When weight distribution was measured by instructing a patient to put equal weight on both feet while standing on a pair of matching scales, patients with movement restriction at the craniocervical junction showed that one limb consistently registered at least 5kg (2.3lb) heavier than the other limb.

Mechanisms that can cause asymmetric pressure upon the legs in Posture Quadrant 4 include postural distortion patterns of the cranial base induced by the birth process, and the functional control mechanism in which people primarily use only one leg for postural support.

NEUROLOGIC ANALYSIS

In this section you will learn the main neurologic examinations for performing posture analyses. This section includes tests of the visual, vestibular, proprioceptive, and cerebellar systems.

As we mentioned in Module 2, the nuclei of the cranial nerves that control the visual and vestibular system live in the brainstem. The brainstem also houses the center that controls posture, the pontomedullary reticular formation. We want to identify any visual and/or vestibular insufficiencies because their output will be affecting the posture system.

We also know that the cerebellum plays an important role in posture by coordinating agonist and antagonist function. Locating cerebellar weakness is fundamentally important for postural correction.

Please note that although this is termed the neurology section, technically all tests that have been performed are dependent upon neurology. The spinal push test for example is a test of vestibular function to localize the level of postural instability. Proprioception, or knowing where our body is in space, has been tested throughout the entire complete posture analysis.

Also please recognize that this is not a full neurologic exam. This section is relative to posture and gives you the information to be a Posture Expert. If you want to learn more about neurology I recommend doing the advanced Postural Neurology course too. And of course, while performing the complete posture analysis, if you do see significant neurologic signs or red flags, always consider the necessity of referring a patient to a neurologist.

Eye movements

The receptors in the cervical spine have important connections to the vestibular and visual apparatus as well as several areas of the central nervous system. Dysfunction of the cervical receptors in neck disorders can alter afferent input, subsequently changing the integration, timing, and tuning of sensorimotor control. Measurable changes in cervical joint position sense, eye movement control, postural stability, and reports of dizziness and unsteadiness by patients with neck disorders can be related to such alterations to sensorimotor control (Treleaven, 2008).

The eyes and the head move together. Either the rotation of the eyes is opposite of the direction that the head moves to keep the head straight, or the eyes move with the head as if looking over the shoulder. The effect of horizontal gaze direction on neck musculature, as viewed with an EMG, is augmented. These observations provide evidence of increased interaction between eye and neck muscle activity with cervical rotation (Bexander and Hodges, 2012). This will be especially apparent with patients who have experienced whiplash.

What this means for practical purposes is that when patients have eye movement dysfunction, you will see increased rigidity and/or postural distortions of the cervical spine. There is a neurological connection in the brainstem that connects the neck muscles with the eye muscles. Proprioception from the cervical spine influences the autonomic response to head position and changes in head posture.

To test the function of the eyes, you will test each field of gaze and convergence. To test the fields of gaze, stand in front of the patient holding a pen or pointer about 14 inches from their eyes. Ask the patient to follow the pen with their eyes without moving the cervical spine. You can do this in two ways—you can make a broad circle with the pen, stopping at each field of gaze, or make an H shape.

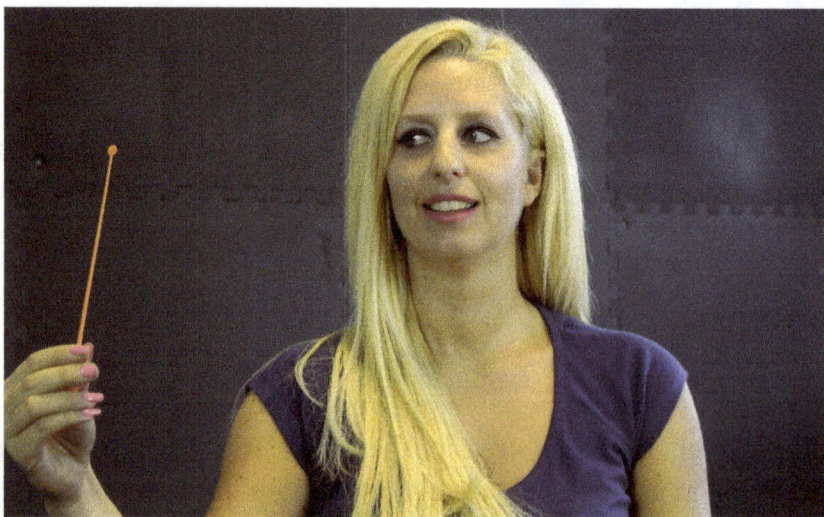

What are you looking for? Watch the patient's eyes. If they cannot focus, if they move their head, or if you see a saccade or nystagmus then you know that the eye muscle controlling that movement is weak and further attention is needed.

When the patient looks up, they are activating the superior rectus and inferior oblique. When they look down, they are activating the inferior rectus and the superior oblique. When looking laterally, they are activating the lateral rectus of the lateral eye and the medial rectus of the medial eye. For example, when they are looking left, the left lateral rectus is activated of the left eye and the right medial rectus of the right eye. When they are looking right, the opposite is true.

When they are looking up to the right, they are activating the superior rectus of the right eye and the inferior oblique of the left eye. The opposite occurs when they are looking up and to the left.

When they are looking down and to the right, the inferior rectus of the right eye and the superior oblique of the right eye are activated. It is the opposite when they are looking down to the left.

It is also important to check convergence of the eye muscles. Convergence is the ability of both the eyes to simultaneously demonstrate inward movement to midline. This is essential for clear focus of near objects.

Three reactions occur simultaneously: the eyes adduct, the ciliary muscles contract, and the pupils become smaller. This action involves the contraction of the medial rectus muscles of the two eyes and relaxation of the lateral rectus muscles. The medial rectus attaches to the medial aspect of the eye and its contraction adducts the eye. The medial rectus is innervated by motor neurons in the oculomotor nucleus and nerve.

An asymmetry of eye convergence means that the body is in constant compensation, with the most prominent effect on head posture, cervical range of motion, and shoulder posture.

To test convergence, we will do three tests. For the first, stand in front of the patient with a pointed pen at a 45 degree angle. Bring the pen forward and watch the eyes converge medially. Both eyes should converge and they should be able to hold the converged position for 10 seconds. Watch to see which eye does not converge medially or if they fatigue quickly. The eye that diverges laterally is the weak eye.

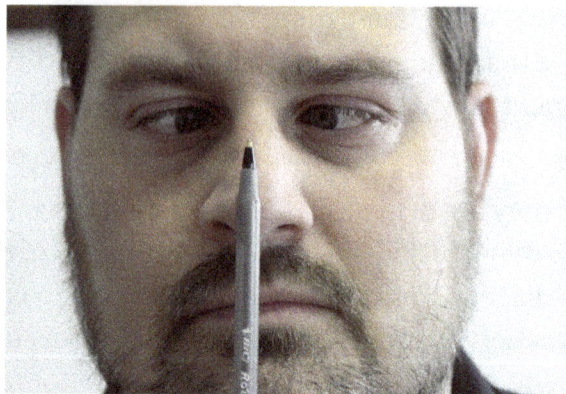

Next we will test the convergence reflex by holding the pen between the patient's eyes, the tip at eye level. Tell the patient to look into the distance, then converge the eyes centrally by looking at the pen. Look into the distance, then converge again in the center. Again watch to see which eye is divergent.

The final convergence test is to see each eye individually and to test for a exophoria which means that the eye turns out when covered. We want to see an esophoria where the eye is turned in even when covered. To perform this test, stand in front of the patient with the pen 15cm from the patient's eyes. Place the pen tip at their nose, and tell the patient to look at the pen, and uncover the eye. Watch to see how the uncovered eye responds. If they have an exophoria, then the eye will quickly saccade to midline when uncovered. If they have an esophoria, both eyes will be converged. Perform this test on both eyes.

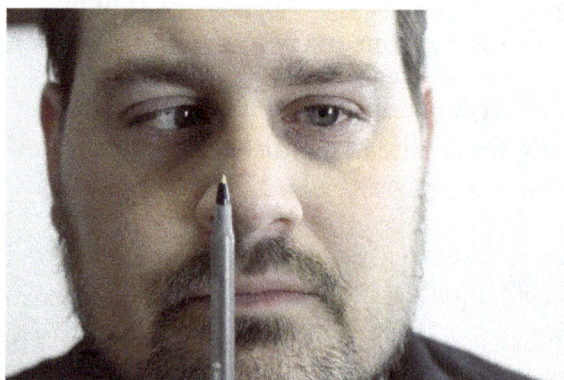

Take note of the divergent eye of the first two convergence tests and the eye with the exophoria on the cover test. This will be important for our correction purposes.

VOR analysis

There are extensive anatomical connections between neck proprioceptive inputs and vestibular inputs. If positional information from the vestibular system is inaccurate or fails to be appropriately integrated in the CNS, errors in head position may occur, resulting in an inaccurate reference for head and neck position sense. Conversely, if neck proprioceptive information is inaccurate, then control of head position may be affected (Armstrong, NcNair and Taylor, 2008).

To test vestibular function you will perform the vestibulo-ocular reflex to evaluate gaze fixation with movement of the head.

The vestibular system is made up of three different semicircular canals bilaterally. As human beings we have advanced communication among the vestibular and the visual system in which we can hold our head upright while looking at different stimuli.

This intricate connection between the 6 muscles controlling the movements of the eyes and the 3 semicircular canals is evaluated through the vestibulo-ocular reflex. Your patients should be able to keep their gaze fixated at a target while moving their head from side to side, up and down, and diagonally.

If the patient is unable to do this, it demonstrates weakness of the vestibular system which will directly impact the posture system, because remember the vestibular system controls your extensor response. With a decreased extensor posture, your patients will go into flexion. Which is exactly what we don't want to happen.

You will test the patient's horizontal canals by holding a pen and asking them to focus their gaze on the point of the pen while moving their head back and forth. You, the Posture Expert, will evaluate their ability to keep their gaze focused on the pen while rotating their head and moving their cervical spine.

Signs of vestibular dysfunction include quick eye saccades, inability to focus, changes in posture, and the feeling of dizziness.

Test the patient first by evaluating their ability to focus their gaze with horizontal rotation of the head. Then test at a 45-degree angle to the right and left.

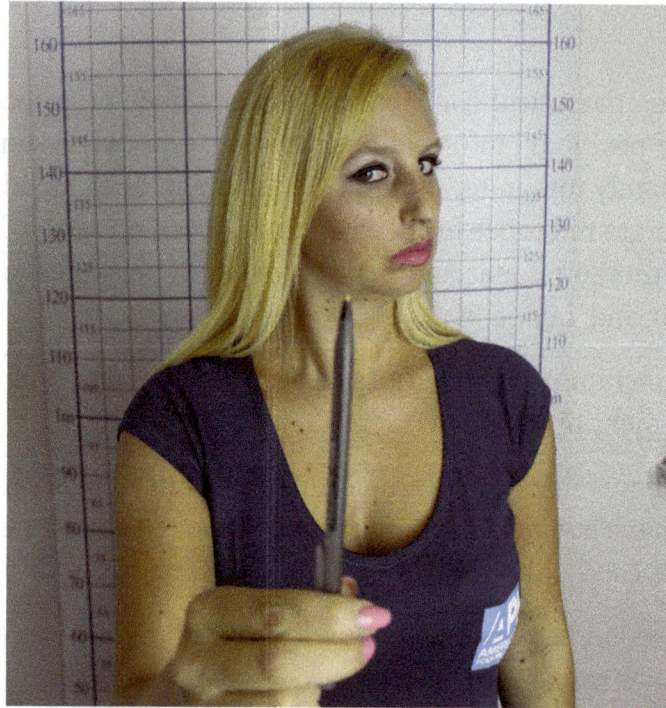

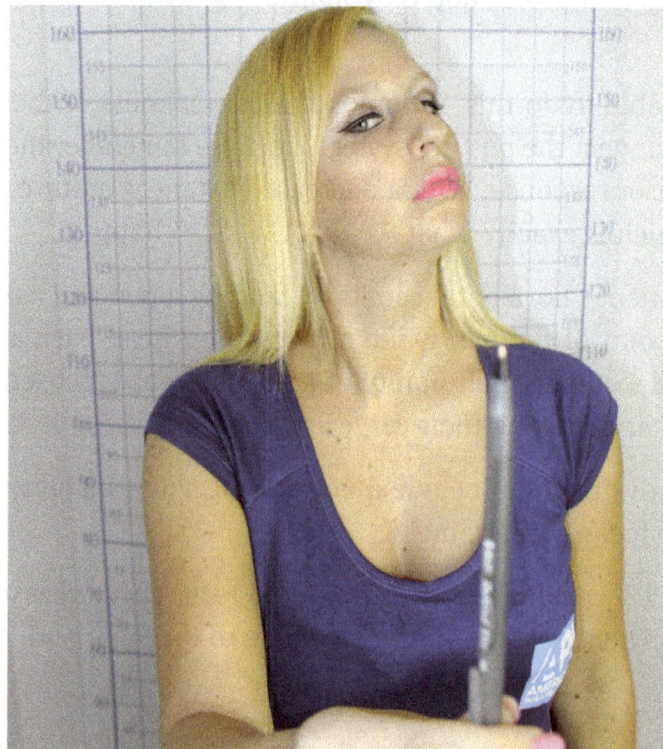

While turning the head to the left, the patient should be able to keep their gaze fixated. Get the patient to move their head down to test the right anterior canal and back to evaluate the left posterior. By getting the patient to turn their head to the right, you are testing the left anterior and right posterior canals.

If you prefer to be hands on, you can test the canals with a quick movement in which you tell the patient to gaze at you, looking right in between your eyes. With their gaze fixated, hold their head on either side and quickly move it to the left and the right. As you move the head, keep your eyes on theirs to see if the patient can maintain their gaze or if their gaze pursues to the direction of turn and then quickly saccades back to midline. This will be an indication that the patient needs to work on VOR exercises and build neuroplasticity of their vestibular system.

Posture balance scale

The purpose of the posture balance scale is to determine the level of postural balance that the patient presents with. Based upon which level the patient is in, they will perform specific balance training to improve their balance and postural stability.

How to perform:

Step 1. To perform step 1 of this assessment, you will have the patient take their shoes off, stand with aligned orientation within the room, place both feet together, hands by their sides, and close their eyes.

- The Posture Expert stands in front of the patient with one arm out ready to catch them if they fall

- The Posture Expert watches to see the direction of initial posture sway, to what degree the patient sways, if the patient falls or has to take a step to feel stable

Step 2. To perform step 2 of this assessment, have the patient begin in the same position, then raise one leg up to the point where the thigh is at a 90 degree angle with the hip joint. Their eyes are open.

Posture balance scale levels:

Level 1. Excessive postural sway and one leg balance fail. The patient reports they feel like they are falling, are nauseous, or have vertigo. They take a step or fall. The patient cannot stand on one leg with proper posture for more than 5 seconds. They demonstrate sway, put their leg down, or fall.

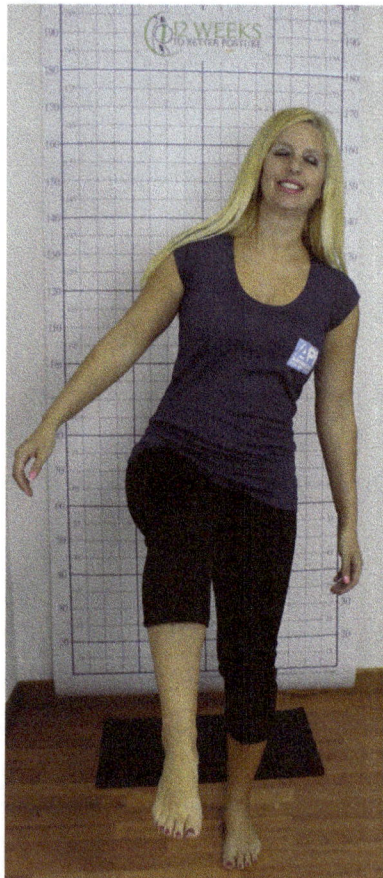

Level 2. Minimal postural sway with one leg balance minimal fault. The patient sways with their eyes closed, but not more than 6 inches of sway. Patient does not take a step, does not feel like they are falling or feel dizzy. The patient is able to perform one leg balance without postural distortions or excessive sway for up to 15 seconds.

Level 3. Stable posture with one leg balance stability. The patient does not demonstrate postural sway of more than 2 inches. The patient is able to perform one leg balance without postural distortions or excessive sway for up to 30 seconds.

Fukuda test

The Fukuda stepping test is a vestibulospinal test to measure asymmetrical labyrinthine function. The purpose of the test is to determine if there is vestibular system weakness on one side of the body.

To perform the Fukuda stepping test, you should first make sure there is plenty of space around the patient to perform the evaluation. To start the test, stand in alignment with the room. Place a marker on the floor or on the wall that the patient is centered around as their starting position. You can also have them centered in front of your posture grid.

Have the patient close both eyes and hold their arms outstretched directly in front of them. Now, have them start stepping in place.

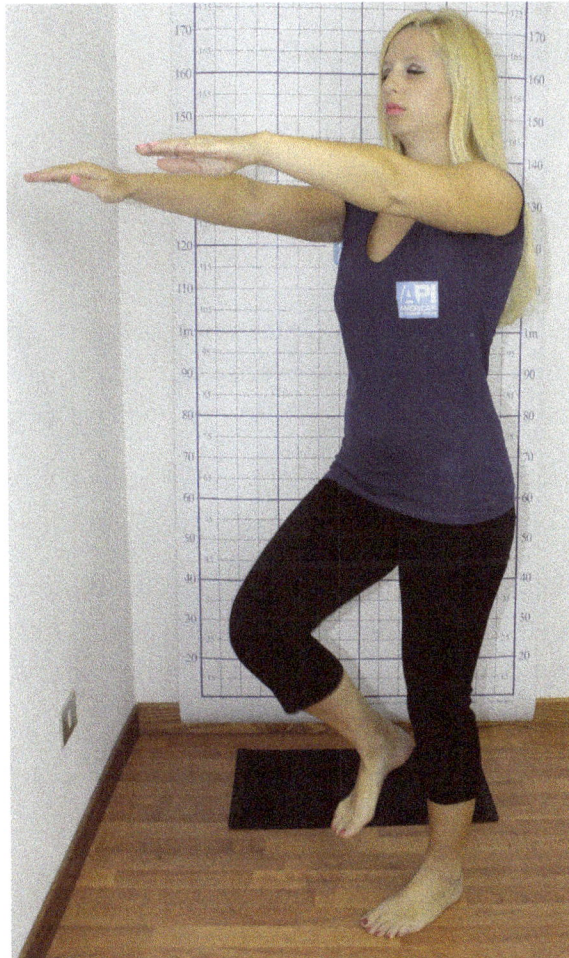

The patient's pace should be comfortable, but as if they are taking a brisk walk. Watch the patient and make sure they don't bump into anything. They remain walking in place for about 50 steps. Then prompt them to open their eyes and determine how much their body has rotated to one side or the other.

After the patient has performed the Fukuda stepping test, mark where they have stopped marching, and compare the angle to the initial starting position. An angle of 30 degrees or more may indicate vestibular weakness to the side their body deviated. The patient walks to the side of their vestibular lesion.

Now I do want to note here that in literature on the subject there is debate of the reliability of the Fukuda test. Which is why we are also testing the VOR of the vestibular system to be more specific. Both are useful tools for our postural analysis.

Cerebellar dysdiadochokinesia

Next the patient will perform a cerebellar test, giving you an idea of the side of decreased cerebellar function. If you were doing a full neurology test, this would not be the only test you did, but for a posture analysis it is very useful in determining the side of cerebellar weakness.

Dysdiadochokinesis is an impaired ability to perform rapid alternating movements such as bilateral forearm pronation and supination. Performing rapid alternating pronation and supination movements steadily and quickly requires significant cerebellum coordination.

With cerebellar weakness, the patient's rapid alternating movements will become weaker or irregular and one limb will be slower than the other limb.

To perform this test, you can have the patient seated or standing with their elbows by their sides. Have them start with their arms facing down. Instruct them to perform movements of pronation and supination as fast as they can while looking forward. Have them repeat this until you tell them to stop.

As the patient is performing rapid alternating movements, watch to see which side, if any, begins to lag or become uncoordinated. The side of lag and uncoordinated movements is the side of cerebellar weakness.

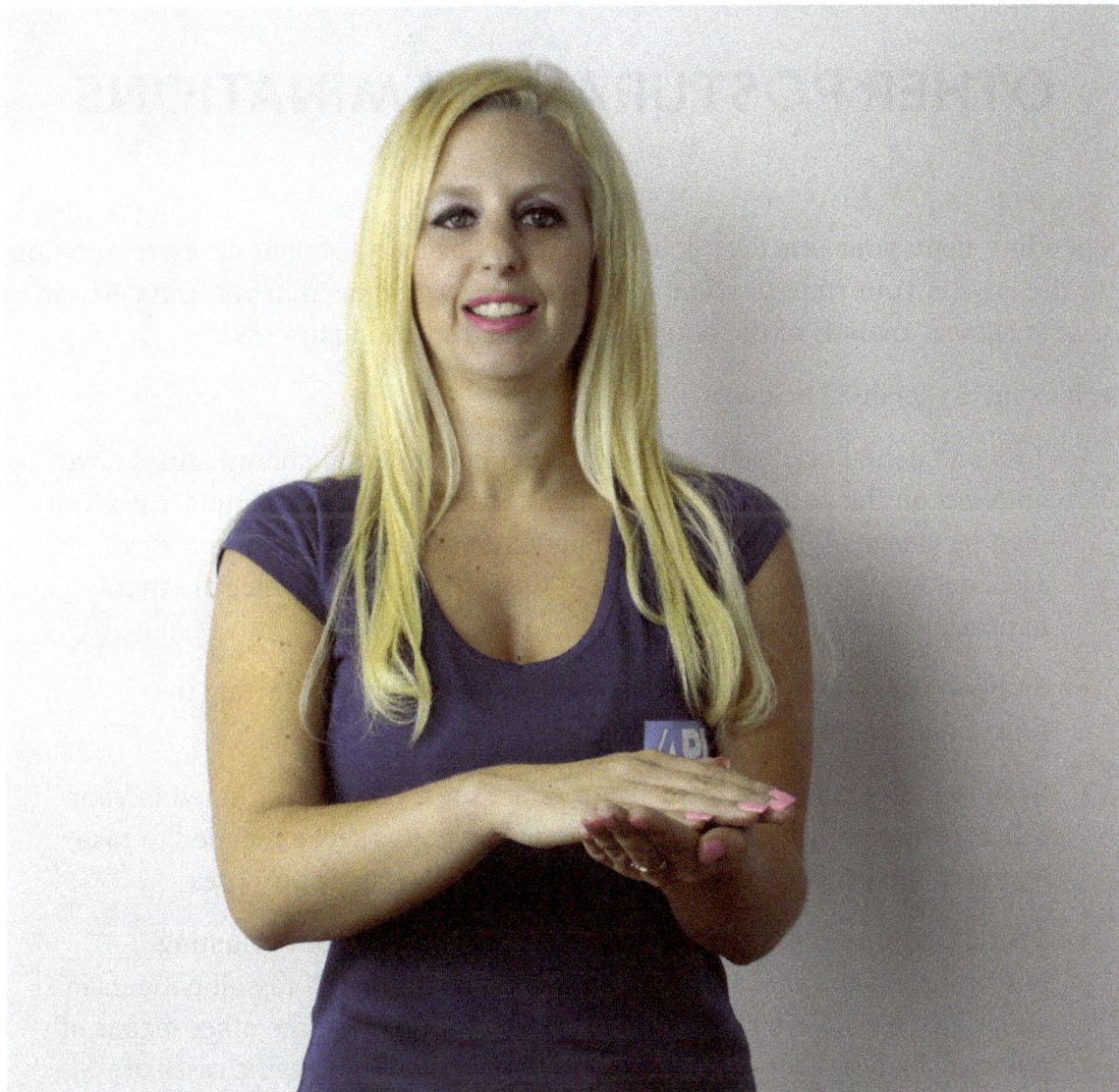

OTHER POSTURAL EXAMINATIONS

Depending upon your practice, your healthcare specialty, patient case presentation, and the laws in your state or country, there are other exams that you can perform to assist in clinical analysis of the patient's postural distortion patterns.

Each exam is explained below:

- TMJ and dental occlusion analysis to evaluate if dental abnormalities have an effect on the postural presentation of the patient. For example, there is a high incidence of malocclusions in patients with forward head posture. Also, among the scoliotic population, there is a high incidence of lateral malocclusion, or a crossbite

- Sensory and muscle tests to evaluate for abnormalities affecting the function of the spinal nerves and the peripheral nerves

- Scoliosis tests can be performed. An Adam's test can be performed in your office. If there is indication of a scoliotic curve, it is recommended to take X-rays of the patient's spine for confirmatory diagnostic purposes

- Specialized imaging, such as X-ray, is highly valuable for evaluating postural presentations. However, if it is not possible to X-ray all patients in your clinic considering the laws and regulations, utilize the other means of postural analysis for primary diagnostic purposes. For specific cases of faulty posture, you can consider referring out for an X-ray examination, such as to confirm the presence of scoliosis

- Orthopedic exams may also be indicated to decipher differential diagnoses. Orthopedic examinations should be utilized at the Posture Expert's discretion, based upon their clinical knowledge and goals as a practitioner

Module 4

CLINICAL APPLICATION FOR POSTURE CORRECTION STRATEGIES

INTRODUCTION

Welcome to Module 4 where we will be discussing the clinical application of the American Posture Institute's Complete Postural Correction system. Up until this point we have done an in-depth analysis of why postural correction is the new paradigm of healthcare for movement and structural specialists in the field.

In Module 2 we examined the structure and the function of each of the posture quadrants within the posture system. Each posture quadrant is related to the others, working together in symmetry and synchronicity to move the body, hold the body upright, and to provide life-sustaining functions. Proper posture supports maximum efficiency and optimization of human performance.

Then in Module 3 an emphasis was placed on the practical application of doing a proper postural evaluation. This module covered each component of the complete posture analysis, including the structural, functional, and neurological assessments.

Each human being presents with a unique postural presentation. The complete postural analysis allows the Posture Expert to thoroughly analyze their patients' posture, identify postural distortion patterns and areas of postural collapse due to weak postural compensations, and determine the treatment plan necessary to correct the postural distortion patterns so the patient can live a healthier life.

Module 4, like Module 3, will be highly applicable. You can implement this information into your practice immediately. The module will begin with an engaging conversation about the three components of API's highly advanced and clinically tested postural correction system. Each component is necessary for sustaining long-term postural correction.

By implementing this system, you will ensure your patients reap the benefits of sustained postural correction to optimize their human performance. They will look better, move better, and feel better. The three components of the complete postural correction system includes spinal alignment, posture rehabilitation, and posture habit re-education.

API's postural correction system can be implemented in any office or practice, with low overhead expenditure. The initial investment of additional postural correction equipment is minimal, with minimal time commitments necessary to train your staff and patients to utilize the equipment.

When you utilize the knowledge you have gained of the Posture Principles and position yourself as the Go-To Posture Expert in your community, you will have a blue ocean market of new patients waiting for complete postural correction. You will likely experience a high level of fulfillment in practice, and patients will have improved compliance for better retention in your practice. The implementation of postural correction in your practice will render high performance with objective clinical outcomes.

This module will provide you with the information necessary to correct postural distortion patterns with a proven technique. In this module, we will begin by discussing the 3 components of the system, including spinal alignment, posture rehabilitation, and posture habit re-education.

Each component will be fully explained with clinical application protocols provided. Remember, if your goal as a practitioner is to optimize human performance for your patients, you are recommended to implement all three components of the postural correction strategies together. This system was specifically designed to advance human function by improving structure and function of the posture system. No shortcuts are warranted when you are addressing human health and vitality.

API POSTURAL CORRECTION SYSTEM

Postural treatment protocols are designed to restore and preserve proper postural biomechanics and dynamic postural movements. By aligning the body, you ensure external stressors are absorbed equally throughout. A strong postural framework allows your patients to interact more efficiently within the environment in which they live and function.

Not all postural correction programs are created equal. Many are highly specialized in correcting one aspect of the posture system, such as just focusing on increasing flexibility. For long-term corrective health benefits and optimal human performance, a 360-degree correction approach is necessary. Correcting one aspect of the posture system is not enough. Solely focusing on flexibility without increasing mobility will create unnatural flexibility patterns that contribute to postural collapse.

API's postural correction system is a highly researched and advanced system. This is the only system in the world to integrate the 3 key components of complete postural correction, including spinal alignment, posture rehabilitation, and posture habit re-education. This correction system is targeted at improving function of the entire posture system, then creating new cognitive habit loops to increase postural fitness.

Best recommendations for care are broken down into 4 different stages of postural correction, generally recommended at 12 weeks for each phase of correction. However, it is always important to consider patients' individual case presentation and healthcare needs when advising treatment plans. For example, asymptomatic children are likely to respond much faster than an adult with advanced postural degeneration. Be mindful of the patient's needs and do regular re-evaluations to evaluate the patient's progress throughout the postural correction process.

API POSTURAL CORRECTION PROGRAMS

The 4-program approach ensures that the patient learns the basics of postural correction, and is able to sustain proper posture without postural collapse. These programs are designed to improve the patient's posture in a sequential fashion that their bodies can handle without overwhelming them. When done correctly, the API Correction Programs will re-educate the patient's human physiology patterns while maintaining static postures and during dynamic movement.

Each of the programs utilizes the 3 key components of complete postural correction: spinal alignment, posture rehabilitation, and posture habit re-education. These components are used in different ways with each program.

The patient begins at a basic level to improve their posture while static. It is necessary to see objective changes in static posture before moving to the second program, Dynamic Posture. The patient learns how to maintain proper posture while performing the foundational movements of human function. Once they can perform these movements and maintain proper postural design, they advance to the third program which is Brain-Based Postural Correction to correct the neurology controlling the posture system. The final program, Postural Fitness, challenges the body to resist postural collapse during complex movement patterns over the lifespan.

Four phase posture program progression of complete postural correction:

- **Posture program 1**: structural postural restoration for static postural correction changes seen on posture imaging

- **Posture program 2**: dynamic postural correction to perform human functional movements without postural collapse

- **Posture program 3**: brain based postural correction to improve the function of the neurology controlling the posture system

- **Posture program 4**: lifetime posture to maintain postural fitness and prevent postural collapse throughout the patient's lifespan

Static Postural Restoration

The first correction program is Static Postural Restoration, which is generally recommended for 12 weeks (this is patient specific; always make recommendations based upon your analysis) and is the first aspect of the 12 Weeks to Better Posture correction progression series.

The objective of this program is to see correction of postural distortion patterns on posture imaging. Watch the patient stand, and watch them sit. Can they maintain proper posture in these positions? The recommended outcome measure is to evaluate their pre- and post-posture images to see measurable change.

The posture rehabilitation that they will do in this first phase will support their upright posture so they can resist gravity in an efficient manner for prolonged periods of time whether seated or standing. The exercises performed in this phase are the foundation for their postural correction experience. Each patient will purchase a Posture Kit in the initial program that has the tools necessary for them to perform the "at home" posture rehabilitation.

Unless indicated otherwise, patients will do Complete Posture Correction treatments for spinal alignment, in-office cervical traction, in-office vibration therapy, at home reverse posture exercises that are specific to their cervical postural distortion patterns, and at home postural ABCS exercises to improve their alignment, balance, and core control.

Dynamic Postural Correction

After the patient has completed the first program and has objective results demonstrating improvement of postural distortion patterns on posture imaging, the patient moves to the second program, Dynamic Posture.

Dynamic Posture is posture in motion; patients are evaluated for objective changes while performing functional movements and during the gait cycle. After performing

Dynamic Posture, the patients will have a clear understanding of how to perform each of the functional movements and will be able to perform them with proper posture.

The patient is recorded on video pre and post to demonstrate objective changes during their re-evaluation. Document their progress in video format so the patient can physically see their postural improvements. During the program, the patient will continue to get Complete Posture Correction treatments over a 12 week period, perform in-office cervical traction if necessary, in-office vibration therapy, and at home postural ABCS exercises to improve their alignment, balance, and core control in motion.

The exercises that the patient performs in this phase will be more dynamic, more complex, and will emphasize improvement of functional human movements.

Brain-based Postural Correction

The third progression of the 12 Weeks to Better Posture Series is Brain-based Postural Correction with the intention of creating neuroplastic changes of the posture system. The purpose of this program is to perform brain-based movements that stimulate important neurology controlling the posture system.

Posture rehabilitation integrates musculoskeletal movements with brain-based activities. The main neurologic centers that will be stimulated include the motor cortex, the sensory cortex, the visual system, the vestibular system, the PMRF, and the cerebellum. In this phase of postural correction, the Posture Expert gains a further understanding of postural neurology. This allows them to identify the principal location of postural dysfunction and will provide inputs into the system to make neuroplastic changes of the posture system.

In this phase patients are performing postural neurologic rehabilitation such as eye movement drills, VOR drills, complex movements, and balance training to improve their brain-based posture.

Lifetime Posture

After obtaining measurable improvements in the Dynamic Posture and Brain-based Posture programs, the patients are encouraged to stay active with their postural fitness.

They are then advanced to the fourth program of the API system, which is called Lifetime Posture.

At this point the patient should be able to perform all basic movements of human function. To continually improve the integrity of the patient's posture system, the Posture Expert will now challenge the patient to maintain proper posture and prevent postural collapse during complex multiplanar movements.

In the Lifetime Posture Program the patient will continue to do Complete Posture Correction treatments for spinal alignment but at a lesser frequency, in-office cervical traction if necessary, at home reverse posture exercises if necessary, and at home postural ABCS exercises. During the Lifetime Posture Program, the patient will do many of the exercises on the vibe plate to increase the amount of stimulation to the posture system.

Patients will perform complex multiplanar exercises on the vibe plates. They will continue to use the JBIT for gait, plus they will perform the functional human movements against varying levels of resistance. Posturally fit patients have achieved the highest level of postural correction and are encouraged to maintain this level of postural fitness throughout the course of their lives.

PATIENT COMPLIANCE

Postural correction will help improve patient compliance because patients "get" posture and they can see measurable and objective changes. Posture is easily and effectively communicated by Posture Experts, making it relevant to the patient.

In healthcare, the most commonly used definition of compliance is when "patients' behaviors (in terms of taking medication, following diets, or executing lifestyle changes) coincide with healthcare providers' recommendations for health and medical advice" (Sackett, 1976). Therapeutic non-compliance, therefore, occurs when a patient's lifestyle behaviors lack congruence with the recommendations of their healthcare provider.

Patient non-compliance is a serious obstacle to achieving full postural correction results. Being mindful of patient compliance strategies is important when working in the healthcare sector. Research demonstrates that in some disease conditions, more than 40% of patients sustain significant risks by misunderstanding, forgetting, or completely ignoring healthcare advice (Martin et al., 2005). Further research shows that lifestyle changes have the lowest patient compliance rates, of only 20%–30% adherence.

What your patients do outside of the office is as important as what they do at your office. At the American Posture Institute, we utilize a 3 component system for complete postural correction. Daily posture rehabilitation exercises and posture habit re-education are vital components to correction that the patient does almost exclusively outside of your office.

For patients to obtain optimal results, they must adhere to their treatment recommendations. Yet, the research tells us that only 20–30% of patients adhere to long-term lifestyle changes. How can we, as healthcare professionals, bridge this gap and improve patient adherence to improve postural correction results?

Simply put, the treatment plans need to be exciting, have a clear objective, and be measured in short enough intervals that the patient doesn't lose interest. When the treatment plans are shorter, research tells us that adherence is between 70–80%, which is much higher. When recommending postural correction programs to the patient, you want to keep their initial program of care to a small amount of time—approximately 12 weeks—with a clear and measurable objective that the patient can work toward and achieve.

When patients commit to postural correction programs, they are buying an idea: the idea that when they finish, they will have better posture and will be healthier. When the patient receives a tangible item in addition to the idea of better health, it will feel more real to them and help them stay motivated longer. Tangible items bring an abstract idea to reality. Providing patients with Posture Kits is a great way to stimulate motivation through the power of tangibility.

Jin et al. (2008) evaluated the primary factors affecting patients' therapeutic compliance. The main factor contributing to patient non-compliance was the patient's perception of side effects or pain when using the therapy for a long duration. Posture Experts can easily address this factor of non-compliance by communicating with their patients each time a therapy is recommended—both for posture habit re-education and for posture rehabilitation. Explain the benefits of the therapy and how minimal the threats or side effects are.

The second factor contributing to patient non-compliance is related to patient satisfaction with the healthcare facility and accessibility (Jin et al., 2008). If patients experience long wait times, or find it difficult to reach the healthcare facility, they are shown to be less compliant. This can be avoided by having efficient procedures in which the patient is not treated as a number. They are taken care of, but the procedures in your office support clinically precise and efficient work. If a patient has to wait 30 minutes for a 3-minute treatment, their satisfaction will drop, and likely affect their compliance.

The third factor contributing to non-compliance is related to chronicity. Acute patients have better compliance than chronic patients (Jin et al., 2008). When you are dealing with chronic patients, take this into consideration. Utilize the communication strategies that we just discussed, and help them see the benefits of your treatment. They don't need all of the features, they just need hope. They need to see the benefit they will receive from complete posture correction.

SPINAL ALIGNMENT: COMPLETE POSTURE CORRECTION

Spinal alignment is the first component of the Complete Posture Correction system. Functional spinal alignment corrects the osseous and articular postural faults limiting the performance capability of your patients. Postural alignment protocols are designed to restore and preserve proper postural biomechanics, allowing patients to fluidly perform dynamic postural movements. By aligning the framework of the body, you ensure external stressors are absorbed equally throughout the body. This keeps the patient in a state of postural fitness in which the posture system does not collapse or weaken when environmental stressors are present.

The Posture Expert will identify levels of major and minor postural instability by performing the spinal push test and a posture scan with the Wade Technique for Postural Analysis (this clinical evaluation is explained in greater detail in Module 3). Once the postural faults and the levels of major and minor instability are identified, the Posture Expert can begin the correction.

API's spinal alignment technique is called the Complete Postural Correction (CPC). The CPC is performed by the Posture Expert to immediately improve spinal biomechanic function and postural alignment. The CPC corrects local posture faults and points of postural instability. It is not a high force thrusting or rotational technique.

The CPC of the thoracic spine is based upon the alignment of Posture Quadrant 2. In Posture Quadrant 2, the Posture Expert will evaluate the patient for anteriority of the clavicles and shoulders, asymmetric rib movement with respiration, and decreased joint proprioception of the thoracic spine from the spinal push test.

Anteriority of the clavicle and the shoulders will be corrected with a clavicle push. The thoracic spine will be corrected at the levels of instability by leveraging movement into the spinal segments that have postural instability. Unbalanced rib motion is corrected with an anterior to posterior impulse to open the thorax while the patient is lying supine.

The CPC restores spinal alignment and joint motion. This is achieved by leveraging motion into the fixed segments of the thoracic and lumbar spine from inferior to superior. In this manner, the correction takes place in a direction that promotes upright stability because the angle of correction is opposite to that of gravity.

Why is the anti-gravity correction protocol the key to postural correction? Because it reverses flexor dominant posture associated with sickness and postural collapse. When the body is stressed, sick, or weak, it naturally assumes a flexor dominant position. The purpose of the CPC is to reverse this sick posture. This cannot be achieved by thrusting straight posterior to anterior or anterior to posterior. It requires the inferior to superior component in relation to line of drive.

To perform the correction, the patient begins in trunk flexion, and then the correction takes place from inferior to superior over a lever to bring the patient to extensor upper body posture. Upright posture is the most healthy and most intelligent posture, allowing the anatomy of each of the posture quadrants to perform their organic functions.

The CPC was designed based upon accuracy and immediate correction of posture and joint position. Each patient will also be re-tested after the CPC is performed to ensure that his or her alignment has improved.

The expected outcome is immediate, sustainable postural realignment with an increase in proprioception of the posture system. The outcome measure of each CPC performed will be a posture scan, the Wade Technique for Posture Analysis, the spinal push test, and visual leg length analysis. These outcome measures provide the Posture Expert with immediate feedback if alignment has been restored to the posture system.

SPINAL ALIGNMENT: MUSCLE CORRECTION

As each patient presents with a unique postural presentation, evaluate them for muscular dysfunction patterns that are causing postural collapse. Proprioceptive neuromuscular facilitation stretching (PNF) and trap and release muscle therapy are highly effective techniques that can be inserted throughout the CPC protocol to correct muscular dysfunction compensation patterns that are contributing to misalignment of the posture system. Muscular correction, when rendered necessary, is highly beneficial for patients and should be accounted for.

The Posture Expert may perform PNF and/or trap and release muscle therapy as they move through the sequence of the CPC for efficiency. However, if the Posture Expert chooses to do the whole CPC sequence then correct muscular dysfunction patterns, this is also an adequate strategy. Muscular dysfunction patterns are evaluated in depth during the complete posture analysis. Muscular dysfunction patterns may also be noted during the posture scan at each visit.

PNF is a contract-hold-passive stretch. Both isometric and concentric muscle actions are completed immediately before the passive stretch to achieve autogenic inhibition, which is a reflex relaxation. You are recommended to utilize PNF stretching on the following muscle groups for postural correction: the hamstrings, the iliopsoas, the gluteus medius, and the pectoral musculature. Remember, each patient is different, so the spinal alignment muscle correction should be specific to the needs of each patient.

Trap and release muscle therapy is a functional correction method for postural distortion patterns. The Posture Expert applies pressure to the shortened muscle fibers and the patient engages full range of motion of that muscle. Trap and release muscle therapy is highly effective in releasing muscle tension. For optimal results, consider evaluating the following muscle groups for hypertonic muscle patterns that need trap and release muscle therapy: the trapezius muscles, the latissimus dorsi, the sternocleidomastoid, and the lumbar extensors. When palpable hypertonicity is detected in these muscle groups, trap and release muscle therapy is a highly effective correction strategy.

SPINAL ALIGNMENT: REVERSE POSTURE EXERCISES

In Module 3 you learned how to evaluate head posture distortion patterns on posture imaging. Once you have determined the primary postural distortion patterns, you have multiple correction options that the patient will progress through in their treatment plan.

The progression of correction will be reverse posture exercises, reverse posture exercises with resistance, traction, then traction with weight. Reverse posture exercises are exactly as they sound. They reverse the primary head posture distortion patterns. For example, if the patient presents with anterior head translation as seen in many presentations of forward head posture, the purpose of the reverse posture exercise will be to reverse this distortion by posteriorly translating the segments of the cervical spine.

With anterior head translation, the patient will do posterior glides or neck retractions. The patient should perform the reverse posture exercise in one set of 10–20 repetitions through the range of motion without pain, and hold each repetition for a count of five.

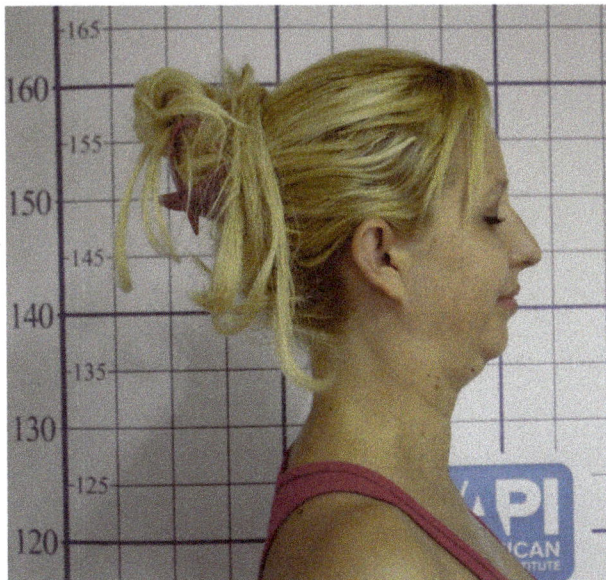

At the initial stages, no resistance is to be used. The intensity is increased by advancing the number of repetitions and sets until a maximum of 7 sets of 20 is reached.

The exercises should be performed daily to achieve maximum results. The patient must be able to perform these reverse postural exercises correctly under supervision before being allowed to perform them at home.

Once the patient is able to perform this exercise with proper posture and without pain, they progress to doing the same reverse posture exercise, but now with resistance. Increasing the resistance activates the co-contraction of the remote muscles. The exercises follow the same progression of repetitions.

One of the simplest ways to perform exercises against resistance is to use an elastic bungee band or cord. A quick and easy set up could be established by having the Posture Expert hold the band/cord while the patient performs the exercise. More permanent set up for these is established by placing an eyehook into a board that is then securely attached to the wall. A head harness could be utilized, or if the band is wide enough, it can be placed directly around the head.

The next progression is to perform cervical traction in the reverse posture position. After the patient can perform cervical traction comfortably, they advance to the use of head weights with cervical traction.

SPINAL ALIGNMENT: HEAD WEIGHTS AND SPINAL TRACTION

In addition to the CPC and functional muscle care for the correction of postural alignment, head weights and spinal traction are also recommended for the majority of patients. Cervical head weights and spinal traction are highly effective in spinal curve correction and restoration, especially when patients present with forward head posture. The CPC corrects the localized level of postural instability; head weights and spinal traction contribute to correction of the spinal curves.

Patients should wear cervical head weights for a minimum of 20 minutes per day. For best use, the head weights should be worn while the patient is standing and active. The patient should be instructed to look forward, keeping their eyes level with the horizon. Looking down will increase weight on the head and cervical spine in the direction of gravity. For best results, the patient wants to maintain an upright posture.

Head weights are effective in correcting the cervical curvature because the frontal head weighting system activates the body's righting reflexes. As this occurs, it causes the patient's body to reposition forward under the weighted head. The patient finds an aligned postural presentation under these conditions. Cervical head weights retrain the soft tissues of the cervical spine to maintain proper posture of Posture Quadrant 1 in relation to Posture Quadrant 2.

Spinal traction is also highly effective and necessary for spinal curve correction. Spinal traction decompresses the spine to reduce pressure on the spinal nerves. Traction is effective in correcting forward head posture and swayback postural presentations. The Posture Expert can choose to perform spinal traction for the patient, or have spinal traction machines in which the patient can perform traction on their own in the office or at home as a part of their Complete Postural Correction strategy. If the patient is instructed to perform spinal traction on their own, they should be shown how to utilize the traction devices correctly to ensure safety and best results.

Why is traction a beneficial aspect to postural rehabilitation? Postural distortion patterns of your patients arise from time and stress. In order to correct these postural distortion patterns in an efficient manner, it is important that you apply a safe and specific stress to reshape the anatomy in a positive way.

With the use of traction, predictable outcomes can be applied to patient care. The most obvious starting point for patients with cervical postural distortion patterns will be with exercises to strengthen musculature as needed, and correct the faulty curvature. Progression of structural rehabilitation will be cervical traction with head weights. Weighted cervical traction will start with less weight and time, moving into more weight for longer periods of time to correct the patient's anatomy further.

The fundamental concept behind tractioning is a simple one. To correct the postural distortion patterns, we must bring the head back to correct posture under the premise that the head has become misaligned due to time and stress. We will then try to correct it using time and stress through tractioning. Therefore to correct the head posture through tractioning, we will do the reverse posture position to counter the postural distortion pattern.

The goal of cervical traction is to produce a deformation force that will return the spine and spinal tissues to normal alignment and resting length. The force from the traction will produce strain in the tissues, which have become pathologically shortened due to abnormal posture maintained for months or years.

The main ligament involved is the anterior longitudinal ligament along with the anterior annular fibers of the intervertebral discs. However, all muscles and ligaments must deform for complete correction of abnormal alignment. A sustained force is necessary to get past the elastic range and into the permanent deformation range of plasticity.

Patients suffering from a history of stroke, high blood pressure, spurring of the posterior aspect of the spine, spinal stenosis, or space occupying pathologies will be considered high risk, and care needs to be taken when you're applying any forces to their spine. Traction can still be pursued, but never compromise the integrity of the spinal cord or its blood supply.

To correct the head posture through cervical traction we will do the reverse posture position to counter the patient's primary postural distortion pattern. This methodology is utilized with all head posture distortion patterns. The patient will be placed in the reverse postural position, and apply the reverse posture range of motion without recruiting any secondary movements from other areas of the body (e.g. head, thoracic spine, shoulders, etc.). To begin with, the patient will hold this position for 5–25 minutes.

Once they can hold the position for up to 25 minutes, weight will be applied. Weights are based upon patient capability but can be started at 1lb upwards of 30/40lb. Please note, there should never be a large jump in weight and the maximum starting weight should be no more than 5lb.

If you don't have a traction system with a fulcrum and weights, your patients can wear head weights while performing cervical traction. Also in this situation, the patient will gradually increase the amount of weight for correction of the head posture distortion patterns.

At the American Posture Institute we are firm advocates of the utilization of head weights. The patients use them at home and in your practice while doing vibration therapy. If the patient wears the head weights for just 5 minutes with vibration therapy, it has been shown to be as useful as the patient wearing them for up to 20 minutes without.

Research demonstrates that the utilization of anterior head weights improves forward head posture and restores the lordotic cervical curve. Anterior weighting of 3–5lb is adequate. The patient will start with 3lb and advance to 5lb as they progress through their treatment plan. They are instructed to wear the head weights 20 minutes per day while standing upright and/or walking.

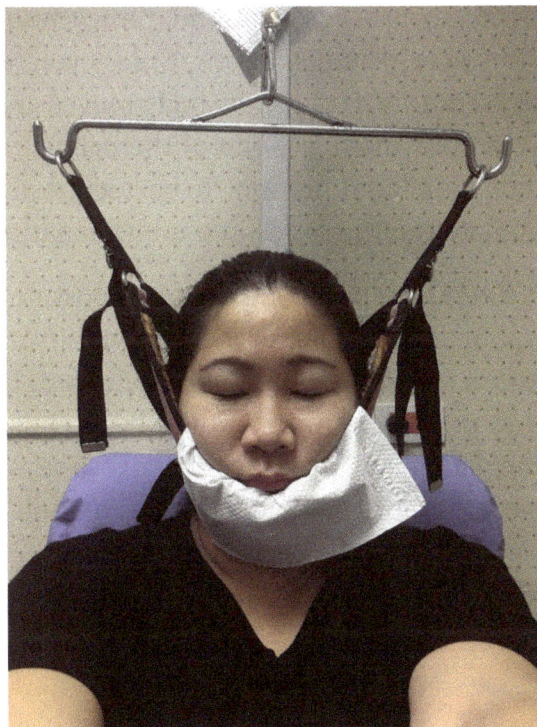

POSTURE REHABILITATION

Posture rehabilitation is the second component of the Complete Postural Correction system. The purpose of posture rehabilitation is to correct muscular dysfunction patterns that inhibit efficiency in function of the posture system. Correction of postural faults involves examination of alignment and tests for muscle length and strength. Preservation of good alignment depends on establishing and maintaining good muscle balance. Exercises designed to strengthen weak muscles and stretch tight muscles are the way to restore muscular balance and support the proper alignment of the spine.

Due to Specific Adaptation of Imposed Demand (SAID) it is important to change exercise protocols regularly. Challenge patients by changing or adding exercises to their postural rehabilitation plan throughout their treatment. Muscles strengthen only when they are stressed. If the patient does the same routine for too long, the musculature of the body will adapt to this pattern of exercises, thus they will have less benefit.

Functional posture correction focuses upon muscular integration. In daily activities we don't emphasize isolated muscle group exercises. Unless you're going to the gym and specifically targeting specific muscle groups, the body moves and functions as an entire system. As discussed in previous modules, one of the primary causes of postural distortion patterns is repetitive uniplanar motion. To correct postural distortion patterns, utilize exercises that stimulate their muscles in a multiplanar fashion.

Functional exercises are a fundamental component of postural correction and useful in the treatment of neck pain and back pain. The National Institute of Health revealed that exercise is underutilized for chronic back and neck pain. Fewer than 50% of subjects presenting with neck or back pain in a study by Freburger et al. (2009) were prescribed exercise. Of the patients who were told to exercise, 46% were given the recommendation by a physical therapist, 29% by a physician and 21% by a chiropractor.

POSTURAL ABCS

API's system of posture rehabilitation is based upon the ABCS of posture. The ABCS is a postural correction strategy to correct the following dimensions that support postural fitness: alignment, balance, core control, and stretching and strengthening targeted muscle groups. For complete postural correction the patient should be doing rehabilitation with exercises for each category in addition to the CPC alignment protocol and posture habit re-education.

Posture rehabilitation can be performed in the office, at home, or both (depending upon the practice setup that the Posture Expert chooses). When you are beginning posture rehabilitation, it is always important to show the patient how to perform the rehabilitation therapies and exercises before they perform them on their own. Demonstrate to them how to perform each exercise with proper posture. If they experience postural collapse while doing exercises, it will not improve their posture, and may even make it worse. Take time to work with the patients so that they understand how to perform each exercise correctly. They will have much better clinical results, will move with better precision, and will not overstress the posture system.

As a Posture Expert it is important to remember that as patients begin different phases of posture rehabilitation, they should feel their muscles working. They may describe it as muscular pain or soreness, just as they would feel if they started a new workout program. This is a normal response. However, if the patient feels radiating pain, intense pain, nausea, headaches, shortness of breath, dizziness or extreme fatigue, this is a red flag that they need to stop the exercises immediately and be monitored before being given approval to continue.

POSTURE REHABILITATION: ALIGNMENT EXERCISES

Alignment exercises reinforce the musculature necessary to support the postural re-alignment that was done with the CPC protocol. Once the articulations and the osseous components of the posture system are aligned and moving properly, muscle work is necessary to sustain proper postural design. Alignment exercises should not be used alone to correct postural alignment; they should be utilized in addition to the spinal alignment techniques discussed previously.

Patients who present with diaphragmatic dysfunction will perform the 90/90 exercise to correct the zone of apposition and improve respiration. They will also be instructed how to perform diaphragmatic breathing allowing full range of motion of the diaphragm and increased pulmonic capacity. Diaphragmatic breathing cannot be performed with trunk flexion. For full range of motion of the diaphragm, it is necessary to hold Posture Quadrants 1 and 2 upright with proper alignment. This is an important consideration of postural correction.

To improve alignment of Posture Quadrant 3 in relation to Posture Quadrants 2 and 4, patients will utilize the posture cushion. The posture cushion is utilized for rehabilitation purposes to strengthen core muscles that support the lumbar spine, and to improve mobility of the lumbar vertebrae. Utilization of the posture cushion is highly recommended, especially for patients with low back pain, to improve hydration of the lumbar spinal discs. Proper movements on the posture cushion assist in pain management of herniated discs and improved circulation of the CSF (cerebrospinal fluid). In addition to the rehabilitative purposes that the posture cushion serves, it is also utilized for ergonomic use in daily life. Patients can sit on the posture cushion at work for a postural ergonomic workspace.

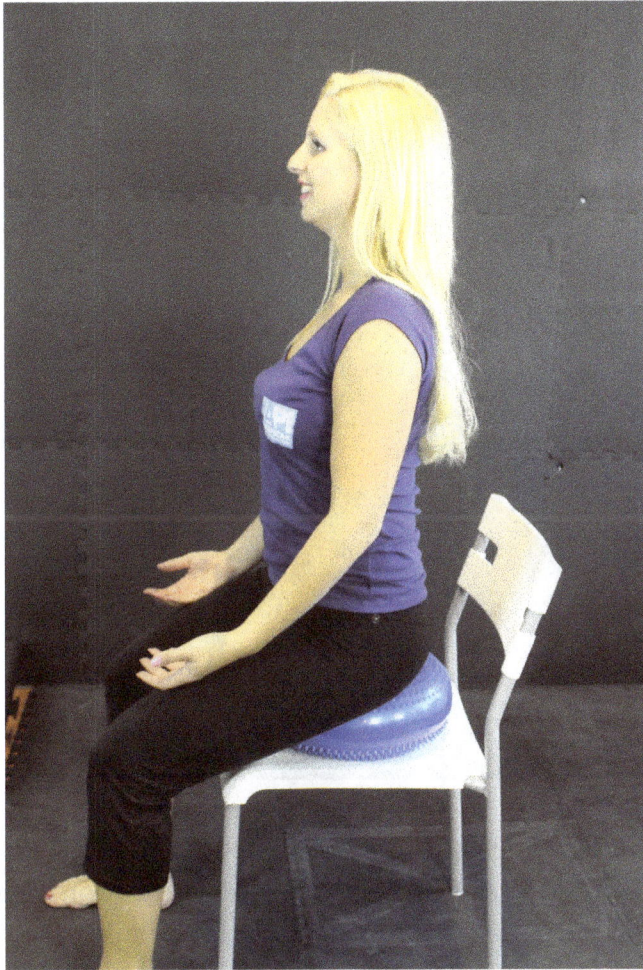

For improved muscular alignment of each posture quadrant, the patient will perform each of the following exercises: wall posture, neck retractions, and posture angels. Wall posture is utilized specifically to support proper lumbopelvic alignment. This exercise is fundamental for sustained posture correction of Posture Quadrant 3 because it targets movement of the iliopsoas muscle that supports proper alignment of the pelvis and the lumbar lordotic curve. The patient should be instructed to make small, controlled movements of their pelvis without bending their knees. They should primarily feel movement of the core posture quadrant during this exercise.

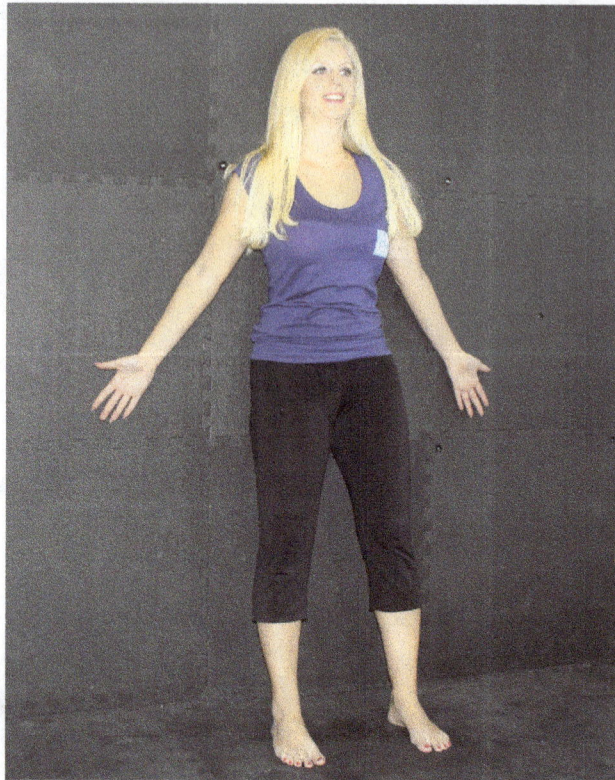

Neck retractions are a necessary exercise for patients who present with forward head posture. Forward head posture and any other postural distortion patterns of the cervical spine are identified on the patient's posture image. Based upon their case presentation, the patient will then perform neck retractions and reverse posture exercises to support correction of the cervical spine in the opposite direction of their misalignment. As the patient develops postural fitness, they will also perform the exercises against resistance and with weights. During these exercises, patients are encouraged to keep their eyes parallel to the horizon, looking straight ahead.

For improved postural alignment of Posture Quadrant 2, the posture angel exercise will be performed. This exercise reinforces the alignment of the thoracic spine while reducing trunk flexion and anterior displacement of the shoulders. The patient should feel a strong contraction of the muscles that retract the scapulae medially. The patient is again instructed to keep their eyes parallel with the horizon, looking straight ahead. They are also instructed to keep their shoulders against the wall to prevent anterior displacement.

POSTURE REHABILITATION: BALANCE EXERCISES

Postural balance training improves stability and equilibrated function of the posture system, helping to support stable postural balance and to decrease vulnerability of preventable injuries. There is not a day in your patient's life in which their postural balance is not important. Many postural correction programs reserve balance training for athletes and geriatric patients. Please note that postural balance is fundamental throughout the lifespan of your patients and is recommended for all patients, regardless of their current level of postural fitness.

A principal component of postural balance training is the utilization of vibration plates. The patient will utilize a vibration plate when they come into your office, unless they have a vibration plate at home. The energy transferred through vibration causes the muscles of the posture system to contract and relax quickly. This creates a great overall workout for the body while stimulating joint proprioceptors to improve proprioception. The length of time and velocity of the vibration therapy will differ from patient to patient based upon their level of postural fitness. As their posture improves, they should be able to utilize the vibration plates for increased amounts of time and an increased speed of contraction.

Please note there are contraindications to vibration therapy on vibration plates. Contraindications include advanced osteoporosis, a pacemaker, cardiovascular disease, pregnancy, vascular thrombosis, and epilepsy. If the patient is unable to perform vibration therapy, they can still do the other postural balance training exercises provided below.

The principal exercise for postural balance training is one leg balance. This exercise requires that the patient maintain proper posture while standing on one leg. The non-support leg is brought up to the point where the knee is in alignment with the hip joint and is bent to 90 degrees. The patient is instructed to hold this position for 30 seconds with proper alignment of all posture quadrants without postural collapse.

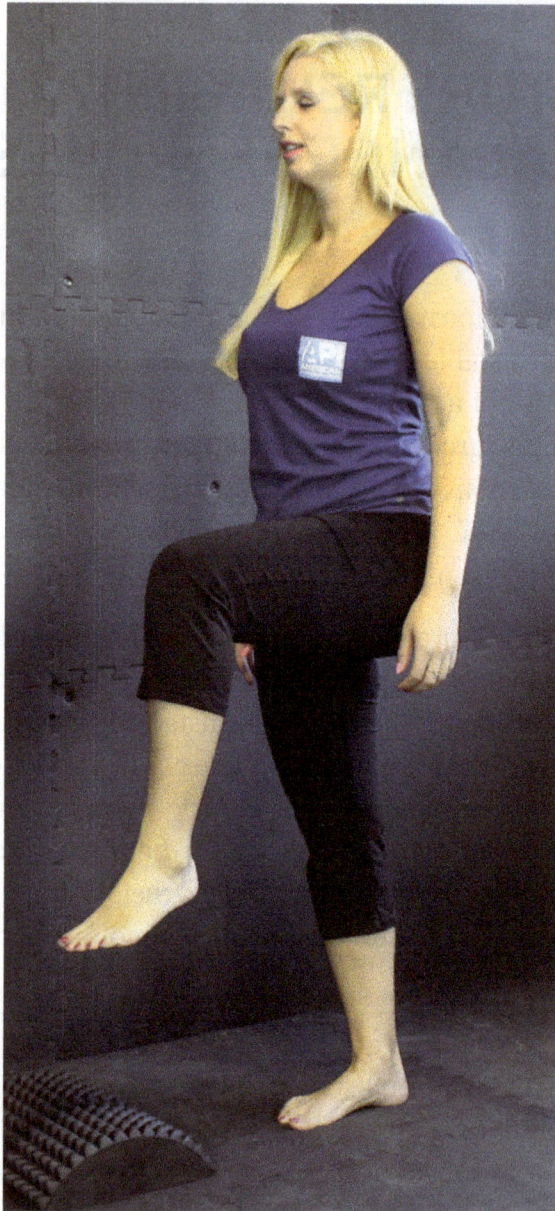

Sustaining the proper postural position of the body without postural sway is difficult. In fact, it is oftentimes more difficult for patients to maintain proper posture while static. The reason that muscles fatigue from being still is that they are stabilizing the body and never get a rest. When walking, or in motion, certain muscles rest while others are activated. When standing still, we utilize bilateral muscle groups continuously.

As the patient improves their postural fitness with 1 leg balance, meaning they can stand on 1 leg for 30 seconds or more with proper posture, have the patient advance to performing 1 leg balance with an instable surface such as on a wobble board. As they advance beyond this point, have them perform one-legged squats, first on a stable surface, then for highly advanced patients on an unstable surface. Challenging the patient's physiology will help them continue to improve their postural balance.

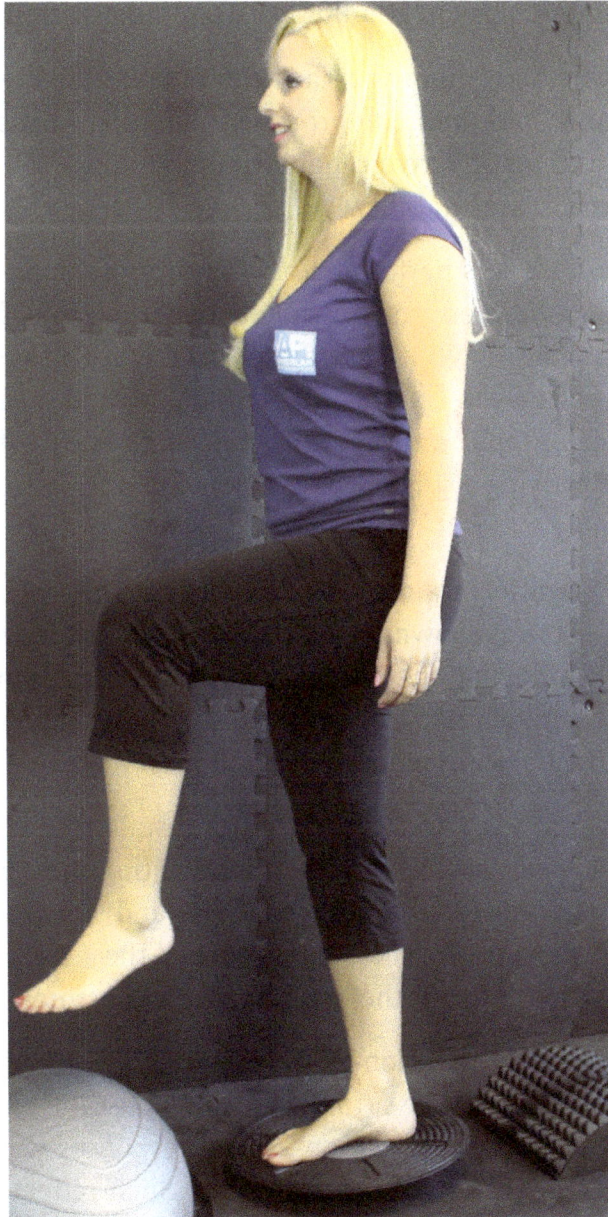

Whole body vibration

Whole body vibration is a neuromuscular training method that uses a low to moderate vibration stimulus to improve muscular strength and power. During whole body vibration training, the patient stands on a platform while maintaining a static position or performing dynamic exercise. The vibration creates an extra load, simulating the effects of resistance exercises. Patients will use whole body vibration for durations ranging from multiple 1-minute sessions to continuous 30-minute sessions.

The utilization of whole body vibration has been proven effective in improving postural stability for young, old, and compromised patients. In research, it is evident that vibration therapy is an effective rehabilitation strategy to utilize with patients who need to improve postural stability.

A 4-week study on posture was performed on 4 groups of young males to determine both the short- and long-term effects of whole body vibration. Of the 4 groups, 3 exercised on a vibration platform with different parameters. The subjects were exposed to vibrations 3 times each week (Piecha, 2014). The method measuring postural stability was with a stabilograph, a device that measures body sway. Body sway was measured pre-study, following a single whole-body vibration session, 1 week later, and 4 weeks after all training ended.

Over the long term, vibration training significantly shortened sway and trembling motions in the frontal plane as shown on the stabilograph. The lengths of these motions decreased significantly following the 1-week post-study measurement. Based on these results, researchers concluded that long-term vibration training improves posture stability of young men in the frontal plane (Piecha, 2014).

How does this mechanism work to improve postural stability? Studies have revealed the influence of ongoing sensory discharge on modulating the central representation of muscle afferents from individual limbs. Vestibular and somatosensory inputs arise from such whole-body movement. The convergence of these two modalities is important in motor control, especially for the maintenance of postural stability.

Researchers measured the perturbation-evoked responses following displacement of a chair that research participants were sitting on pre and post the utilization of vibration therapy. The amplitude of the perturbation-evoked responses was reduced following whole body vibration by 56% of the control group. Such reduction of perturbation-evoked responses was comparable to the attenuation of somatosensory evoked potentials and nerve stimulation. The researchers concluded that muscle-spindle discharge in extensor musculature leads to gating of both of the afferent pathways. These results have potential implications to the understanding of the central nervous system control of stability during ongoing movement (Staines, et al., 2001).

You are recommended to utilize vertical triplanar whole body vibration machines for postural correction. This type of whole body vibration plate is also recommended for patients who desire performance-based results such as increased strength, postural correction results, an increase in bone density to prevent osteoporosis, and an improvement in balance and stability. This will be the most common type of whole body vibration plate for postural correction practices.

The technology applied to deliver vertical vibration is rather complex and thus these machines are often expensive to produce. The platform that the patient stands on moves up and down in one solid continual motion. Intense high frequency upright micro-vibration moments with a small range of motion or amplitude 1–4mm are generated using these types of machines.

Due to the fast motion of the triplanar vertical vibration, patients will actually move up and down and front to back all at the same time. This three-dimensional range of movement is where the term tri-phasic or tri-planar originates. Patients will feel an even distribution of vibration frequency, not a back and forth movement as is expected with oscillating vibration. When utilizing vertical vibration, your patients will likely feel the vibration throughout their entire body, from their feet to their head. The "feeling" of vibration tends to be more profound with vertical than it is with oscillating.

Triplanar whole body vibration machines have less motion than the oscillating machines. However, the triplanar machines have speeds that are considerably higher than their oscillating counterparts. Speed ranges between 20 Hz to 50 Hz. The difference in speed makes triplanar machines more effective at increasing muscle strength as opposed to burning fat with oscillation. You would still get a great workout on the triplanar machines, but if weight loss is the primary concern, the oscillating machines will perform considerably better.

The triplanar machines are also going to be more effective at achieving bone density increases because they put a bigger load on the muscle groups. The triplanar machines are typically more expensive than the oscillating machines. However, due to the results, most rehabilitation facilities, physical therapists, osteopaths, chiropractors, and doctors utilize the triplanar style of machines.

Postural Correction: Vibration Therapy:

Type of vibration: vertical triplanar vibration, whole body vibration

Frequency: 15–25 Hz

Time: 10 minutes

Special instructions: the most important consideration is that the patient maintains proper posture throughout the duration of vibration therapy. Instruct them to look forward and avoid looking down during the therapy. There will be different exercises to perform if the patient is in static or dynamic phases of postural correction.

Protocols:

- Forward head posture: the patient will utilize head weights during vibration therapy to help correct their cervical curvature

- Flexor dominance and anterior shoulder displacement: have the patient open their chest with their hands facing outwards for 30 second intervals, perform an iliopsoas stretch, hamstring stretch and perform 5 pelvic tilts

- Shoulder unleveling: patient will hold weight in their hand on the side of the superior shoulder. They can also wear shoulder weights

- Dynamic posture: the patient will perform functional movements during whole body vibration, including planks, pushups, squats, arms overhead, deadlifts, and scapula retraction

POSTURE REHABILITATION: CORE CONTROL

Core control exercises strengthen the core musculature that supports and protects the lumbar spine. These specific core control exercises are targeted at strengthening the inner corset musculature for proper postural alignment of Posture Quadrant 3. Functional core control exercises work the inner corset core musculature, not just the rectus abdominis, a very common mistake that patients make when "working the core".

The principal muscle to strengthen of the core posture quadrant is the deep transverse abdominis muscle that runs horizontally. As mentioned previously, the transverse abdominis will only activate if the lumbopelvic region of the spine is in proper alignment. Core control exercises should therefore be done in conjunction with CPC treatments for proper spinal alignment.

Core control exercises include the following: core planks, core bracing, and abdominal hollowing. For proper form while performing each of these exercises, please refer to the photo below.

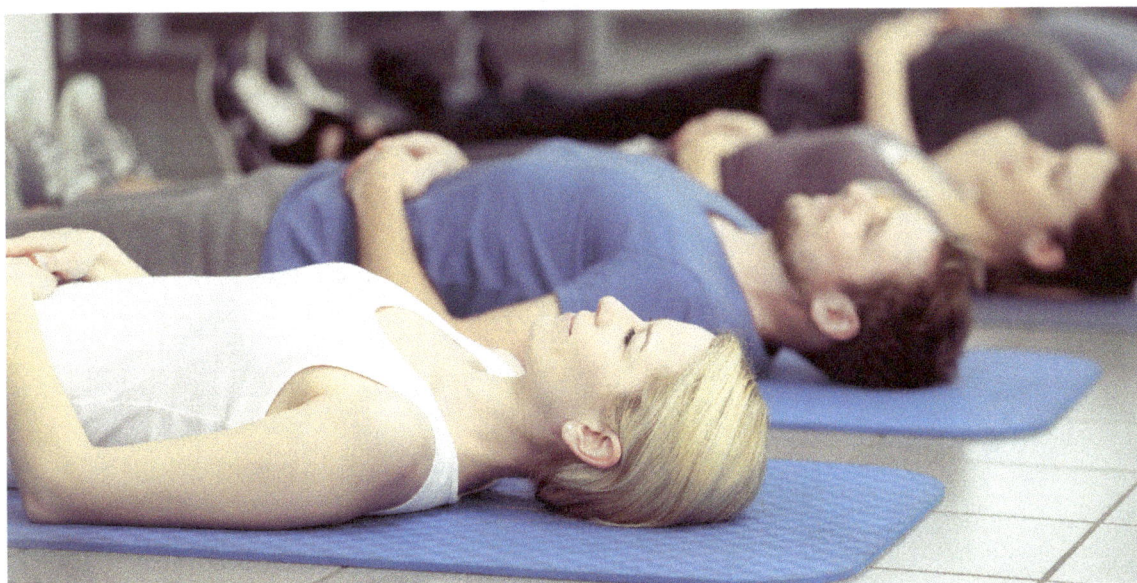

To perform core bracing, the patient will brace their core musculature as if they were to be punched in the stomach. This is global activation of the abdominal muscles. Abdominal hollowing is when the patient focuses on drawing their umbilicus back toward their lumbar spine without drawing the thorax forward. This form of core stabilization is commonly used in yoga and Pilates practices.

POSTURE REHABILITATION: STRETCHING AND STRENGTHENING

The final component of the ABCS is stretching and strengthening. Stretching is performed for shortened muscle groups that pull the body downward with gravity. Strengthening is recommended for weak, elongated muscle groups that prevent the patient from being able to hold themselves upright against gravity. Stretching and strengthening will be unique to the patient based upon their postural presentation; this is a critical component of sustained postural correction.

There are many different recommendations for proper stretching protocols in the literature. According to Baechle and Earle in the publication *Human Kinetics* (2000), patients should perform stretches slowly, and hold the stretch for 15–30 seconds. Stretches should be repeated 2–3 times per muscle group. With pre and post tests, the patient should be able to move easier and better immediately after a stretch.

The muscles that patients need to stretch to improve their posture will vary based upon their case presentation. The majority of patients will benefit from stretching the following muscle groups, so be sure to evaluate your patients for tightness in these areas: the hamstrings, the pectoral muscles, the piriformis, and the iliopsoas. Always instruct your patients how to do the stretches while maintaining proper form. If they experience postural collapse during these stretches it will be counterproductive.

For strengthening exercises, evaluate your patients for the need to strengthen the following muscle groups: the thoracic paraspinal musculature and the rhomboids with scapula retractions and posture angels, and the gluteus muscles with squats.

When you are focusing on strengthening muscles for the purpose of postural correction, be sure to discuss the importance of proper form with your patients. The goal is not to perform a lot of repetitions, nor is it to utilize heavy weights. The objective is to have the patients perform a small number of exercises with proper form and controlled contractions of the muscle groups. While performing any of the strengthening exercises, patients should focus on diaphragmatic breathing for proper respiration and abdominal hollowing to engage the core musculature.

In addition to the exercises noted above for strengthening, the patient will also perform the functional movements that they were unable to perform during the posture analysis. These functional human movements will be performed until the point of postural collapse. The purpose of the patients performing these exercises is to build their postural fitness so they are able to perform the human functional movements without injuring themselves.

The gluteals are one of the most important of the extensor group of muscles. However, in most people they are weak. In Module 3 you learned how to test for muscle strength and how to evaluate for glut weakness in gait. If either of these tests demonstrate weakness, it is clinically appropriate to do glut strengthening exercises.

We discussed functional movements. One of the main functional movements you will work with patients on is squats. Recognize when they are doing functional movement training that the patient should focus on glut activation during squats.

In addition, we are going to go through a couple of exercises that are really important for glut activation. While the patient is doing these exercises, you aren't focused on them doing a lot of repetitions, rather the quality of the contraction and the quality of the patient's posture during the exercise.

The goal is to localize the gluteus muscles and to only activate those muscles. What you will commonly see when patients start to fatigue while doing these exercises is that they will compensate by activating their quadriceps, lumbar paraspinals, and even their upper body while gritting their jaw. To minimize this, you want to do the exercises with the patient in your office so they feel how to do them correctly, and they can replicate them at home.

You want the patient to hold the gluteal contraction for 30–90 seconds. In the beginning they will likely only be able to do so with proper posture for about 30 seconds. As they develop more postural fitness, have the patient increase the amount of time.

The patient will perform each exercise at home. In the office, they can perform the exercise with or without whole body vibration. Whole body vibration will increase the level of difficulty of the exercise even further. Vibration will be a progression of the exercise.

The first exercise is the clamshell. The patient will lie on their side with or without a band around their legs. The patient will hold an isometric contraction with their heels together; they don't arch back and have relaxed paraspinal musculature of the lower back. They hold the contraction for 30–90 seconds.

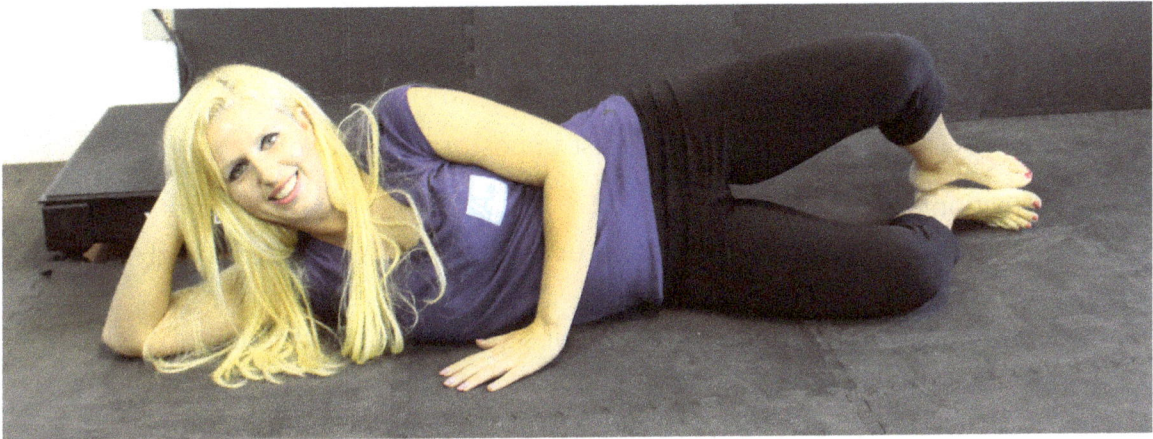

The next exercise is the fire hydrant, which is again performed with a contraction of 30–90 seconds with the patient wearing or not wearing an exercise band. The patient is in the quadruped position with their hips level, relaxed lower back and no scapula winging. They raise one leg up and to the side and hold the contraction, then repeat with the other side.

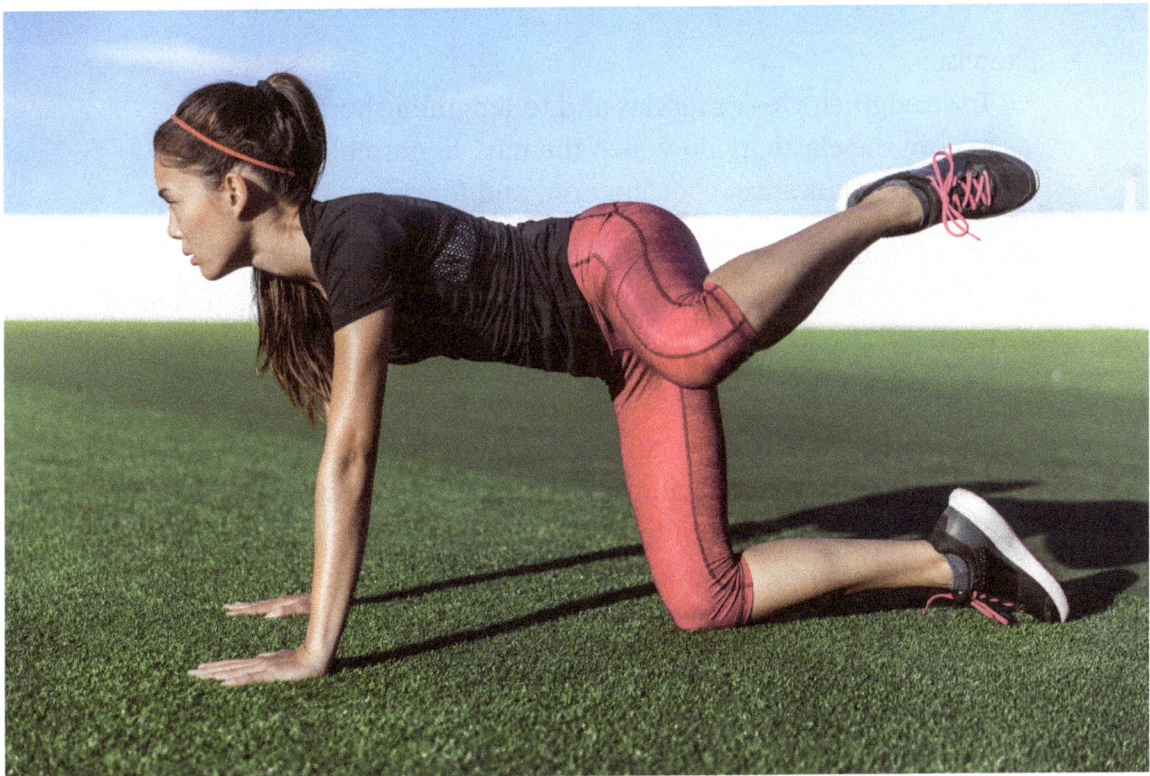

Ancillary Posture Rehabilitation Therapies

These ancillary therapies indirectly assist in postural correction.

- Traction:
  - A force to produce elongation or stretch of joint structures and/or musculature
  - The force pulls in the direction of separation of distraction of extremity joints or vertebral bodies
  - Therapeutic effects: pain and spasm relief, adhesion reduction, improved circulation, stretches tight muscles

- Massage:
  - Improves circulation, promotes relaxation of muscles, helps loosen scar tissues, stretches tight musculature and fasciae
  - Appropriate in reducing excessive edema that restricts ROM (range of motion)
  - Prior application of heat generally increases the response

- Exercise:
  - To strengthen weak muscles and to lengthen short muscles to restore the elasticity on which the muscle normally functions
  - Increase endurance, coordination, and function

- Electrical Stimulation:
  - Utilized for pain control, muscle re-education, and management of edema

- Supports:
  - To immobilize a part, to correct faulty alignment, to relieve strain on weak muscles, to facilitate function, and to restrict movement
  - Not effective in correcting stretch weakness if the opposing muscles are tight—the tight muscles will continue to pull the muscle past normal neutrality

- Heat:
  - Relief of pain and muscle spasm, decreased joint stiffness, increased extensibility of collagen tissue, increased blood flow
  - Should *not* be used for muscle weakness, as the goal is *not* to relax the muscle
  - Should *not* be used in acute situations or areas where sensation and circulation are impaired

- Cold:
  - Vasoconstriction to reduce pain and swelling following trauma
  - Inhibits spasticity, facilitates muscle contraction, useful for muscle re-education
  - Cold and heat reduce muscle spasms, but cold is more effective because cooling of the muscle allows sustained voluntary contraction
  - Cold should *not* be used with hypertension, Raynaud's syndrome, rheumatoid arthritis, ischemia, vascular impairment, cold allergies

BRAIN-BASED EXERCISES

Cerebellar exercises

The primary function of the cerebellum is to coordinate movements by establishing synchrony among the flexor and extensor musculature. In Module 3 you evaluated dysdiadochokinesia by having the patient perform rapid movements with their arms simultaneously. The arm that was slower, or showed lag, is on the side of cerebellar weakness. The relationship is ipsilateral.

To improve cerebellar function, perform complex movements. On the side of cerebellar weakness you can perform figure 8 movements with the distal extremities, specifically the hand and the foot.

Have the patient start by performing 10 repetitions of figure 8s, then re-test. Please realize that any input to the system is a neurologic stimulus. We can re-test immediately to see that a change has been made.

As the patient progresses, you increase the level of difficulty. For example, they can close their eyes, stand on one foot, or perform Figure 8s on whole body vibration. These are all appropriate progressions to increase the level of difficulty and build neuroplasticity.

Eye movements

Correcting the eye convergence is very important to sustained postural correction. This is done by literally working out the eyes. The patients should do this for one minute per day, 30 seconds in the mornings and 30 seconds in the afternoons.

When teaching patients how to do eye exercises, be aware of their level of fatigability and their posture. This is delicate anatomy; you don't want to drive the patient too hard in the beginning or they will have a headache. Also, you don't want to see them moving their cervical spine. They should just be moving their eyes.

Before and after doing an eye exercise session, the patient should rub or massage their eyes to stimulate sensory activation. They will begin by doing small circles to improve convergence. If the patient presents with a divergent eye, then you want to work that eye more. For example, if the patient has a divergent left eye, you want to do more circles off to the right, forcing the left eye to converge. Do small eye circles for about 30 seconds.

Then, to improve eye movements, do large eye circles to stimulate gaze in all directions. Perform this for about 30 seconds. If the patient was unable to perform a smooth pursuit in one direction—meaning that as they were looking in that direction, their eyes did a saccade back to the center—then you want the patient to hold their gaze in that direction for at least 10 seconds. For example, if you noticed weakness when the patient drew their eyes up and left, then when they go up and left again, they will hold that gaze for 10 seconds before moving in the next direction.

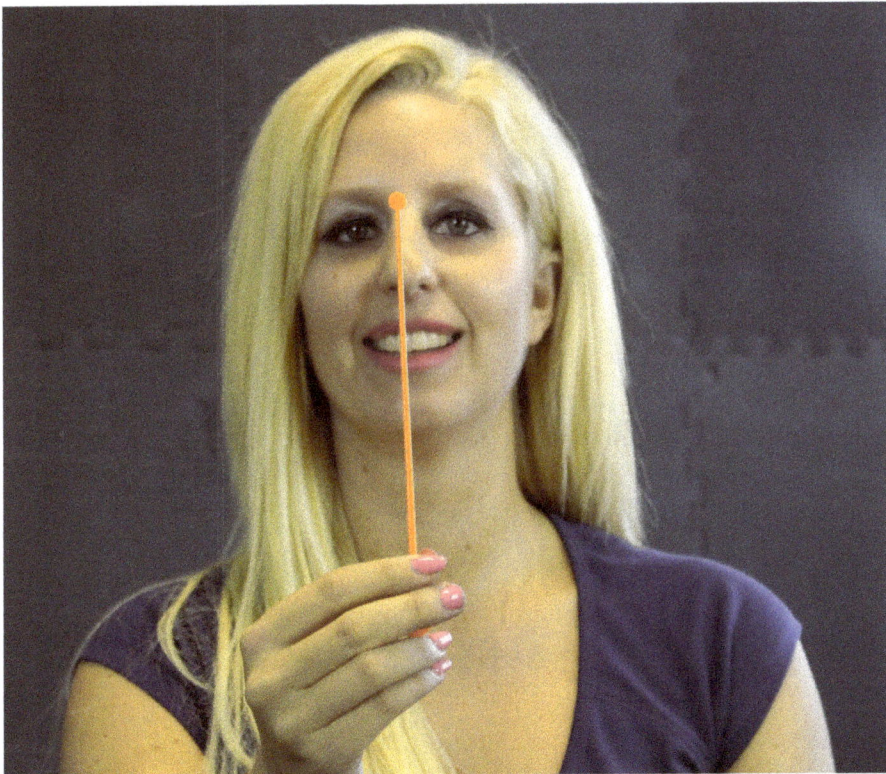

Doing these exercises each day will have a profound effect on the patient's posture system.

Vestibulo-ocular reflex

Based upon the patient's VOR analysis, which canals showed fatigue or weakness? These are the motions you want to strengthen.

To perform these exercises, have the patient stand with their finger or a pen in front their face, centered between their eyes. You can also put a mark on the wall for them to focus on.

The patient will keep their gaze focused on the point while moving their head in different directions. They will move their head back and forth performing no-no exercises with their gaze fixated centrally. This exercise is utilized for patients who need to activate the lateral canals.

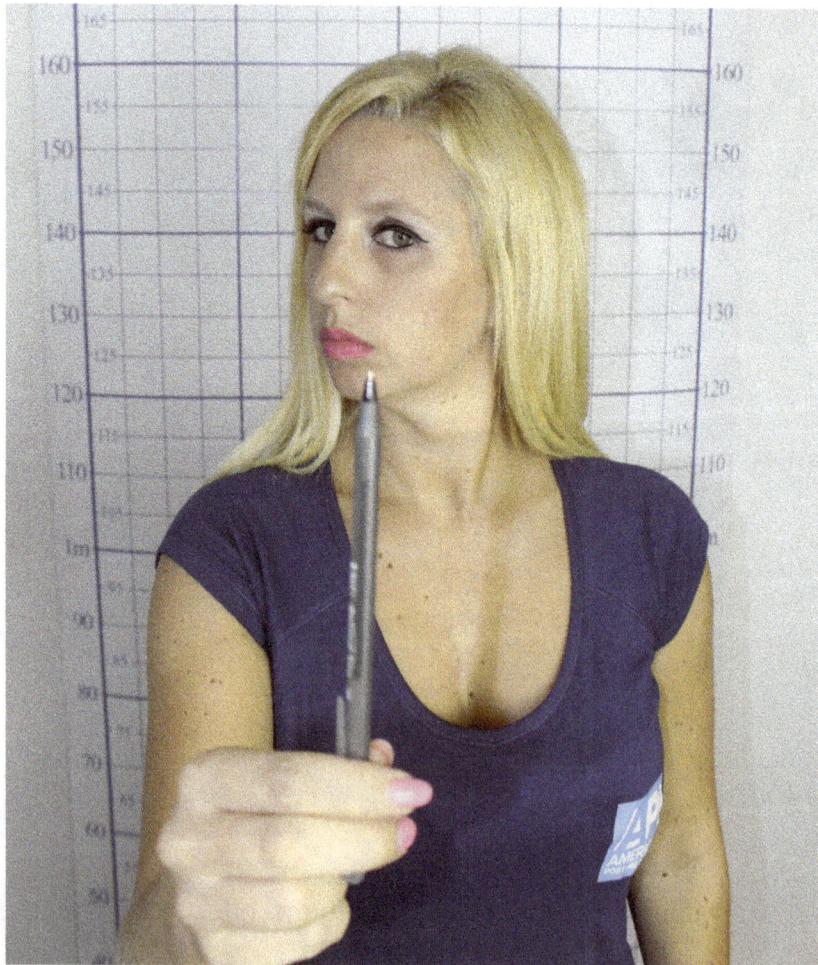

The patient can also perform yes-yes exercises for vertical activation. Keeping their gaze fixated on a central point, they will move their head up and down.

The patient can move their head down diagonally at a 45-degree angle and back at a diagonal of 45 degrees to activate the anterior and posterior canals. As they are turning their head to the left, they keep their gaze fixated. Have them move their head down to test the right anterior canal and back to evaluate the left posterior. By having them turn their head to the right, you are testing the left anterior and right posterior canals.

Now, please be aware that this is a very powerful exercise; you don't want to over-stimulate the patient. Signs that the patient is being over-challenged are redness, dizziness, sweating, and postural changes.

Watch your patient perform this the first time to gage their level of postural fitness and to prevent working them beyond their current vestibular capacity. In general, patients will be able to perform 5 repetitions side to side, up and down, and along the diagonal line of activation. Patients can increase repetitions as they progress through their treatment plan.

POSTURE HABIT RE-EDUCATION

The final component of the American Posture Institute's 3-component postural correction system is Posture Habit Re-education. The purpose of re-educating postural habits is for intentional postural awareness and mindfulness of the body in its surrounding environment. Through posture habit re-education, the patient creates new neural pathways that support proper postural design. The goal of posture habit re-education is to retrain the dysfunctional posture patterns of the body through neuromuscular re-education.

> **"Habits are defined as actions that are triggered automatically in response to contextual cues that have been associated with their performance."**
> **Neal et al., 2012**

Habits are cognitively efficient actions because the automation of common actions frees mental resources for other tasks. However, the process of creating new habits, or healthy habits, is a mindful process.

A focus on posture habit re-education should be performed daily to create efficient muscle memory sequences. Posture habit re-education is fundamental for long-term postural changes to be maintained. In order to change habits, patients must commit to a change in lifestyle. If the patient is not committed, it will be much more difficult, or even impossible to change their postural habits.

POSTURE HABIT RE-EDUCATION: HABIT FORMATION

Gardner et al. (2012) explain the relevance of habit-formation principles in achieving desired health outcomes. They suggest the formation of new habits is a simple formula. It may not be easy to adhere to—this requires motivation and mindful dedication in achieving the outcome, but the formula itself is simple.

To create a new habit, Gardner et al. (2012) suggest a patient repeats an action consistently in the same context. The habit formation attempt begins at the "initiation phase", during which the new behavior and the context in which it will be done are selected. Automaticity develops in the subsequent "learning phase" of habit formation during which the behavior is repeated in the chosen context to strengthen the context-behavior association. The last step in habit formation is the "stability phase" in which the habit has been formed and persists over time with minimal effort.

Duhigg (2012) presents similar ideas about habits and habit creation. The process of creating new biological habits is intentional, not accidental. Every habit re-education process has a specific cycle, called the Habit Cues and Response Cycle, for creating new habits. The Habit Cues and Response Cycle is controlled by the basal ganglia. Every single habit is created in this sequence, through a cue that stimulates a certain behavior, and the behavior is directly associated with a reward (Duhigg, 2012).

To change habits, focus on changing the behavior associated with a particular cue. For example, a posture habit cue for a particular patient could be a posture bracelet in their gym bag. When they arrive at the gym and put on their posture bracelet, they have created a cue that triggers the associated behavior. The associated behavior is proper posture while exercising. If the patient has proper posture during their workout, they should then intentionally reward themselves. The patient will decide on an appropriate reward that they desire. Rewards can be big or small, but they must be intentional. For example, each time the patient does the exercise with proper posture, they reward themselves with a drink of water. The Habit Cues and Response Cycle for this patient is the posture bracelet in the gym bag as the cue, the behavior is proper posture while exercising, and the reward is a drink of water.

NEW HABIT FORMATION

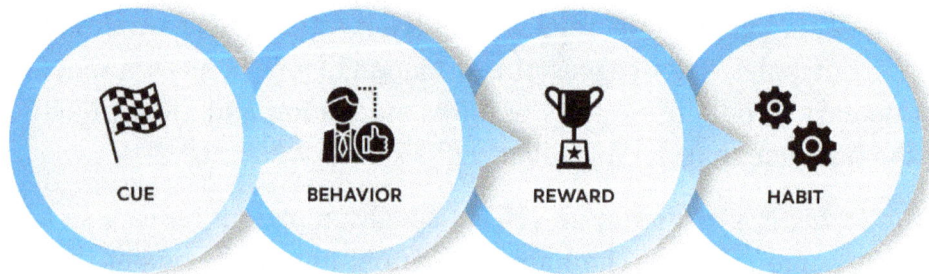

CUE · BEHAVIOR · REWARD · HABIT

Keystone habits, as explained by Duhigg (2012), are habits that are emotionally driven. The basis of keystone habits suggests that as a patient changes one habit, that one single habit then affects the rest of their life. Patients will often experience this, but may not realize that they have created a keystone habit.

Felicia, a patient at the American Posture Institute, commented on her re-evaluation that postural correction had changed her life completely. After beginning a postural correction treatment plan due to severe low back pain, she felt better and could finally live without pain. Because she didn't experience pain with exertion, she began working out five days per week, which she hadn't done in nine years, since her first son was born. She felt that the only time she had to work out was early in the mornings before the kids woke up for school. So now she wakes up one hour earlier per day for exercise. Because she wants to replenish her body with good foods after exercise, she also started cooking healthier breakfasts. After three months of postural correction treatments and personal workouts, Felicia felt like a new person and had lost 10 pounds; she had changed completely. The life transformation came from a single emotionally driven habit: her postural correction appointments.

Help your patients make life transformations by teaching them how to create and follow through with keystone posture habits. Explain to them the results they can have if they are committed to improving their posture. For example, an emotionally driven reward for many people would be to receive more praise at work for being more productive. Productivity is directly correlated with proper posture of the human body.

In order to change the keystone habit of being unproductive to being productive, have your patients try this sequence: place a posture reminder on their computer as the cue for good posture while working, which is the behavior. The behavior then produces higher levels of productivity, which lead to the reward of more praise. Once the patient experiences the reward of recognition for increased productivity, this keystone habit will change how they view productivity for the rest of their life. It will also help them achieve better results at work.

POSTURE HABIT RE-EDUCATION: COMMUNICATION

Kelly et al. (1991) discuss the dimensions of health beliefs that influence patients in making changes to their lifestyle habits. The most significant dimensions of health that influence the motivation for patients to make lifestyle changes include the perceived risk of continuing the lifestyle behavior that should be changed, the benefit of changing the lifestyle behavior, the social support that the patient receives from their family, friends, and colleagues, and the magnitude of self-efficacy that the patient will achieve when they change that lifestyle habit.

Each of these dimensions is important in lasting habit changes. The two dimensions that were demonstrated by Kelly et al. (1991) to have the most profound effect on motivation for changing lifestyle habits are the perceived benefits that the patient will experience with the changed habit and the magnitude of self-efficacy that they will achieve. In addition to these factors, extrinsic rewards are also shown to increase patients' level of motivation in making lifestyle changes.

It is very important to consider the psychosocial aspect of habit creation, and utilize this information when conversing with patients. Recognize what motivates your patients, and discuss the benefits of having proper posture with them.

As Teutsch (2003) explains, effective healthcare encompasses the art of human interaction. The challenges of doctor to patient communication include understanding how the patient's condition is affecting their quality of life, and then empowering the patient to make appropriate choices on personal health issues. The ability to communicate effectively is crucial to bringing the benefits of postural correction to patients, and is important to the professional satisfaction that patients get from doctor to patient interactions.

Once the need for posture habit re-education is determined and the patient is motivated to take action, then be ready to suggest successful posture habit interventions to re-educate their postural patterns.

POSTURE HABIT RE-EDUCATION: POSTURE REMINDERS

Mindfulness is postural awareness. At any given moment we are either elongating and opening the posture system or shortening and compressing it. For long-term postural correction, the patient needs to be mindful and intentional with their movements. They should perform movements that work with the natural design of the body, not against it. To create mindfulness, the patient should utilize "posture reminders".

A posture reminder can be a sticker that they place in the areas where they spend the most amount of time, or it could be an alarm set on the clock to go off multiple times throughout the day, or even a bracelet that the patient wears. When the patient sees the posture reminder, they will be prompted to be mindful of their bodily position and make necessary corrections for proper posture. For example, if the patient is at their desk at work and they see their posture sticker on their computer, they will be reminded to check their posture. This brings posture back into their consciousness so they can modify their working posture in that moment if necessary. Posture reminders help patients succeed in changing their posture.

Neuroplasticity occurs though consistency with posture habit re-education to create neural pathways that support sustained postural health. When beginning to create new habits or muscle memory patterns, the patient engages the conscious mind. Complex postural positions, such as the postural rehabilitation exercises that were explained earlier, require mechanical self-talk.

Mechanical self-talk is when the patient thinks about how to do the movement with proper posture step by step. Mechanical self-talk assists the patient in being aware of their body throughout each movement sequence of the activity. When they are beginning new, complex posture exercises, have your patients talk themselves through the process prior to performing the activity so that when it is performed, the patient is building their postural fitness.

Endurance postural habits are different from complex postural positions that require mechanical self-talk. Endurance posture activities, such as sitting at a desk for multiple hours at a time with proper posture, require motivational self-talk. The purpose of motivational self-talk is to increase performance over a long period of time. This is not step-by-step self-talk like mechanical self-talk where the patient needs to think of how to perform the activity. Endurance activities require motivation not to have postural collapse during a sustained or repetitive activity.

POSTURE HABIT RE-EDUCATION: POSTURE MAPPING

To support the process of changing postural habits, also encourage your patients to do posture mapping. Posture mapping identifies the points in your patients' lives where they are more likely to experience postural collapse. Have them make a posture map to identify these points, then determine what the cue is that causes postural collapse. Once the cue is identified, then determine a healthier behavior that will support good posture, and how they can reward themselves for that change in postural behavior. Mapping out their day in this manner creates a much higher level of mindfulness and intentional living. Mindless movements are habitual, mindful actions are intentional.

To set up a posture map, have the patient first identify where they experience postural collapse. If the answer is sitting at their desk, for example, have the patient then identify the principal cause at their desk of poor posture. Is it the chair, is it the computer placement, or is it the amount of time they spend seated? Maybe it is a combination of the aforementioned? Have the patient identify the primary factor of postural collapse. They will then make a plan to change that primary factor. If they cannot change it, they will train themselves to be mindful during that part of the day to avoid poor postural patterns.

If the amount of time they spend seated is identified as the primary factor associated with postural collapse, the patient can place a posture reminder sticker at their desk as a prompt to take frequent posture breaks. Because their desk is on their posture map, their attention will be drawn to this aspect of their day so they can consciously create lasting postural changes.

POSTURE HABIT RE-EDUCATION: POSTURE TAPING

An effective strategy for posture habit re-education is posture taping. From a clinical perspective, posture taping has multiple functions, and can be viewed as a form of posture habit re-education or seen as a form of posture rehabilitation as it is an effective modality in helping to correct postural presentation.

Posture taping provides support and stability to muscles and joints without restricting the body's range of motion. The tape provides extended soft tissue benefit of manual therapy administered within the clinical setting. It alleviates pain and facilitates lymphatic drainage by microscopically lifting the skin. This lifting effect forms convolutions in the skin, increasing the interstitial space and allowing for a decrease in inflammation of the affected areas.

Posture taping can be utilized for pain relief, but in this case (posture habit re-education), it is used to support proper postural design. Posture tape is considered functional as it is not restrictive in nature. Patients can perform their activities of daily living without being restricted by the tape.

Restrictive taping is widely used in the field of rehabilitation as both a means of treatment and prevention of sports-related injuries. The essential function of rigid tape is to provide support during movement. The most commonly used restrictive tape applications are done with non-stretch tape with the rationale of providing protection and support to a joint or a muscle (Thelen et al., 2008).

In recent years, the use of Kinesio tape (and other brands of functional tape) has become increasingly popular. Kinesio tape, invented by Kenzo Kase in 1996, is a new application of adhesive taping. It is a thin and elastic tape, which has the capability of being stretched up to 120–140% of its original length, making it quite elastic and resulting in fewer mechanism constraints when compared with traditional tape.

Kinesio tape was designed to mimic the qualities of human skin with roughly the same thickness as the epidermis layer of the skin. The elasticity of Kinesio tape conforms to the body, allowing for movement. The tape is latex-free, very thin, and stretches in the longitudinal plane. Kase et al. (1996) have proposed several benefits of the utilization of Kinesio tape. Results vary depending on the amount of stretch applied to the tape and to the skin during application.

Proposed benefits of Kinesio tape (Kase et al., 1996):

- To provide a positional stimulus through the skin

- To align fascial tissues

- To create more space by lifting fascia and soft tissue above area of pain/inflammation

- To provide sensory stimulation to assist or limit motion

- To assist in the removal of edema by directing exudates toward a lymph duct

Kinesio tape is unique in several respects when compared to most commercial brands of tape. It is latex free and the adhesive is 100% acrylic and heat activated.

According to Huang et al. (2011), the beneficial effects of functional tape include physical corrections, fascia relaxation, space recuperation, ligament and tendon support, movement rectification, and lymphatic fluid circulation. Functional tape offloads fascia of injured tissues to decrease pain while facilitating an up-regulation of neurological control.

There are two main theories proposed to explain the reported effects of functional tape. The first is increased blood and lymphatic fluid circulation in the taped area due to a lifting effect, which creates a wider space between the skin and the muscle and interstitial space (Halseth et al., 2004). The second theory is that functional tape may apply pressure or continual stretching of the skin within the taped area, and this external activation of cutaneous mechanoreceptors would activate modulatory mechanisms within the central nervous system, demonstrated as an increase in muscle excitability and proprioception (Gomez-Soriano, 2013).

Multiple different research studies have demonstrated that functional taping is an effective postural correction strategy, immediately effective in making postural changes with common postural distortion patterns.

Consider the following examples that have been demonstrated through research studies:

- The forward head posture angle has been shown to significantly decrease during computer work performed with neck retraction posture tape as compared to without neck retraction tape (Yoo, 2013)

- Rounded shoulder posture taping with stretch has been shown to produce immediate mechanical correction of rounded shoulder posture in seated male workers (Han, Lee, and Yoon, 2015)

- Posture taping to retract the scapulae has been shown to maintain better posture and decrease perception of pain in patients (Murray)

- Researchers concluded that posture tape might increase the provision of feedback to the muscles that sustain the stability of the thoracic spine and scapula as well as the preferred postural alignment (Lee and Yoo, 2011)

- It has been suggested that application of anterior pelvic tilt tape can be applied as an auxiliary treatment method for preventing changes in pelvic inclination and musculoskeletal problems of low back area by abnormal sitting posture in seated workers (Lee and Yoo, 2011)

When applying posture tape, you are recommended to apply it with a tension of 25%. Tape at this tension will remain adhesive to the patient's skin for a longer amount of time than tape with a high amount of tension.

Patients who utilize posture tape should experience an immediate result in which they claim they feel it "working" or they feel "straighter" or "more upright." If the tape is applied to the cervical spine for reduction of forward head posture, the Posture Expert should see an immediate positive result. If the tape is applied to the scapulae for reduction of anterior shoulder displacement, the patient should feel that their shoulders are back and the Posture Expert should see a change.

Please note, when applying posture tape to the spine, always apply it bilaterally. If it is applied to one side of the spine, but not the other, it may cause postural distortion patterns.

Photos have been provided below of how to use posture tape to stimulate better postural correction results of common postural distortion patterns.

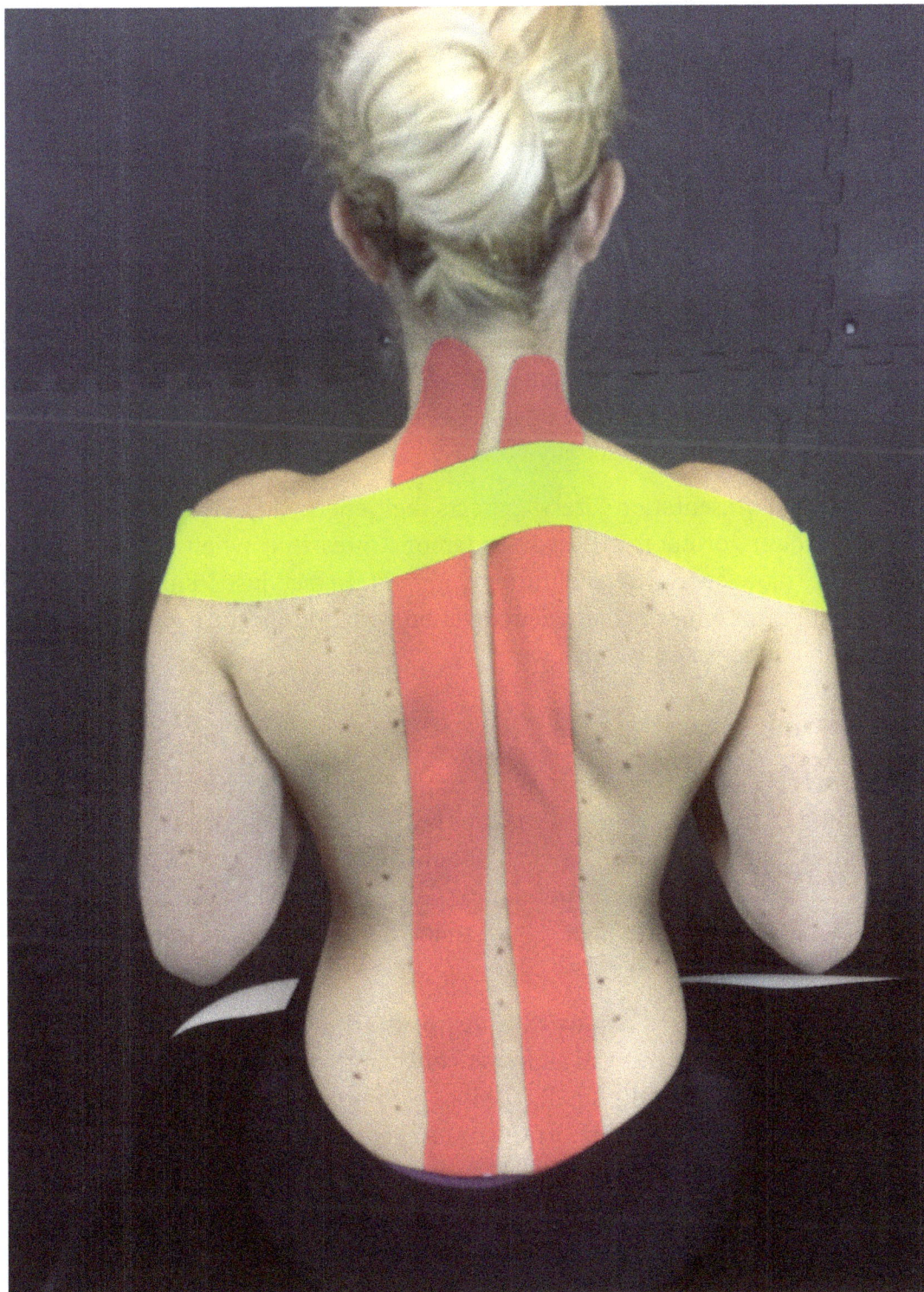

POSTURE HABIT RE-EDUCATION: PROPER POSTURE HABITS

Encourage your patients to utilize ergonomic lifestyle enhancements to support their new postural habits. By implementing the 10 ergonomic essentials into their daily lives, the patient will have a map for success for improved postural fitness. The ultimate design solutions for effective workspaces are a combination of ergonomics and human factors. This method considers the equipment that workers are using and the way in which they interact with it on a daily basis.

Patients' postural presentation directly affects their energy levels. Poor posture slowly decreases amounts of energy. Research demonstrates that when you slouch, your muscles utilize more energy to hold the body upright. In fact, just 15 minutes of reading or typing in an ergonomically inefficient position with poor posture exhausts the neck, shoulders, and upper-back muscles.

Ten ergonomic essentials

1. **Comfortable work chair with proper spinal support**. The chair should be designed so that employees can keep their backs straight and elongated comfortably. The chair should be height adjustable so the feet of the employee touch the ground and their knees are not restricted under the desk. If the employees' feet do not touch the ground, they should place a footrest under their feet.

2. **The spine should always be supported**. If necessary, the employee can insert lumbar and cervical supports between their chair and their spine (supports are generally small cushions). The purpose of the cervical and lumbar supports is to support the natural curve of the spine while seated. The spine should make a nice "S" curve, not a rounded "C" curve.

3. **Computer screens and reading materials should be placed at eye-level**. Having the material at eye-level, the employee is able to maintain a neutral cervical curve. If they are forced to look up, their neck is in

extension; if they are forced to look down, their neck is in flexion. Prolonged flexion or extension increases tension to the cervical spine and supporting musculature.

4. **Proper lighting and decreased noise pollution.** These allow the employee to concentrate and maintain a more deliberate focus. With limited visibility and/or a noisy environment, the employee must perform their job tasks in a highly distracting environment, stressing their system. In a workplace with inadequate lighting and/or noise pollution, the potential for human error, miscommunications, and injury is greater. The employee should be able to perform their work without squinting. If they are squinting, they are jutting their head forward, causing forward head posture. If they are unable to hear, they are leaning laterally toward the communication they are trying to hear.

5. **Comfortable mouse pad and keyboard placement.** The mouse and keyboard should be placed in a manner that does not strain the wrist and elbows. If they are placed too far forward, the employee is reaching for them with their upper extremity, whereas if they are too close, the employee is maintaining an awkward crunched posture. If the desk is too high, their wrists are in extension to type. Prolonged wrist extension can cause irritation to the median nerve, commonly seen as carpal tunnel syndrome (note: repetitive work activities performed with the hands, especially vibratory activities, increase the risk of carpal tunnel syndrome). Wrist rests are a good solution to prevent wrist pain. A wrist rest should be utilized with the keyboard and the mouse, allowing the employee to maintain neutral position of their wrists while working at their computer.

6. **Keep most commonly used items within an arm's reach away at elbow level.** Repetitive reaching causes strain to the upper extremity, can cause unnecessary rotation of the spine, and can compromise the important vasculature of the upper extremity. Repetitive reaching can cause uneven muscular development as individuals tend to reach forward with their dominant hand. Commonly used items that are too close to the body cause the employee to scrunch their body, and feel cramped and crowded. This results in a closed posture. If their arms are too close to their body, they may be repetitively hitting their elbows on their sides. Commonly used tools

should also be placed at elbow height. The arm then remains in a neutral position, not chronically flexed, extended, or stressed.

7. **Shoes with proper support**. Shoes with proper support are essential for employees, especially for employees who are on their feet for prolonged periods of time and who do a lot of walking, lifting, or physical activity. In certain high-risk jobs, protective shoes are necessary to protect the feet from injury. Proper shoe selection can help prevent foot pain and discomfort, as well as low back pain. Common foot problems due to hard floors and inadequate shoe support are blisters, callus formation, toe malformations, ankle sprains, fallen arches, bunions, shin splints, etc. Footwear should adequately support the natural design of the foot, and should fit properly. High heels cause unnatural muscular contraction of the lower leg muscles and shift the weight forward to the anterior aspect of the foot. Pointed shoes can cause strain to the toes; shoes with lack of adequate arch support can lead to fallen arches and common foot misalignments; shoes that are too tight can lead to blisters and calluses; shoes that are too loose can cause ankle sprains and instability on the job.

8. **Sitting on a posture cushion or exercise ball.** Posture cushions or exercise balls are the best option for sitting correctly at work. With an unstable surface, employees are constantly engaging their core muscles throughout the day to stay upright. The instability of the rounded surface doesn't allow you to be lazy and slouch, because if you do, you fall off. By engaging the inner core muscles to stay upright, employees are strengthening their postural muscles and supporting the natural alignment of their spine. Maintaining a "C" shaped curve of the spine is much more difficult on a wobble cushion or stability ball, thus maintaining proper posture becomes a natural habit. Movement is a key way to keep joints healthy and prevent degeneration. In addition, sitting on an uneven surface day in and day out improves balance and proprioceptive activation, both of which are important components of posture and wellbeing.

9. **Adjustable workstations.** These are the best option for employees of all size dimensions. Adjustable workstations are the innovative vision of businesses, recognizing that with office ergonomics it is not a "one size fits all" mentality. Businesses with proper ergonomic equipment recognize that

all employees have different body types, and they invest in adjustable equipment that meets the needs of the natural design of everyone's body type. Adjustable workstations allow the employee to perform their job-related tasks while sitting down or standing up. In this way, employees are prompted to stand up throughout the day and be more active. Being sedentary is not only contributing to back pain and lack of productivity of employees, but also the development of lifestyle related chronic diseases. An adjustable workstation allows employees to engage in good postural habits and stay productive.

10. **Posture breaks.** Posture breaks are another highly effective way of developing postural fitness at work. Posture breaks require little time but render healthy returns. They are effective because they engage the anti-gravity muscles that tend to be under-activated throughout the day. A posture break should be performed every hour for 20–30 seconds. The API Posture Break starts at the base of the spine. While seated at the edge of your chair, begin by engaging the transversus abdominis muscle by rolling your hips underneath you and flattening the lumbar curve. Elongate the spine, sitting tall. Roll the shoulders up, back, and down so they are not in a raised position. Straighten the upper extremity bringing your arms and hands wide. Arch your thoracic spine (keeping your core tight, don't collapse at the core), push your chest out, and bend back (at the point of the dorsal spine, not the lumbar spine). Arms stay wide. Feeling a stretch through the pectoral muscles and arms, bring the head back into extension. Hold the position for 15 seconds, or until you feel your proper posture collapse.

To remember to perform posture breaks, set a reminder at your workstation.

POSTURE HABIT RE-EDUCATION: ACTIVITIES OF DAILY LIVING

Proper posture is important during all activities of daily living. When patients recognize where they are most likely to experience postural collapse, and have the education of how to have proper posture, they begin the process of changing their lifestyle habits. Posture habit re-education is the responsibility of the patient. However, Posture Experts should be knowledgeable of how to change habits, so they can assist and motivate their patients in doing so.

Listed below are common examples of when patients experience postural collapse during their activities of daily living. These are important habits to change from postural collapse to postural fitness in order to achieve postural habit re-education.

Shoe support

Shoes with good support are necessary for maintaining good posture. The feet are the base of support for the body. When the feet are not properly supported, it affects the postural framework of the rest of the body. Proper shoes not only provide comfort to the low back and the lower body, but also help to prevent feet problems such as plantar fasciitis, fallen arches, hammertoes, and abnormal muscular strain.

Shoes should fit to the arch length of the foot with arch support. The overall length should be adequate to avoid cramming the toes or rubbing the heels. A shoe that is too narrow is uncomfortable and can cause blisters, whereas a wide shoe causes lack of support to the foot. Regarding the sole of the shoe, the thickness and flexibility are important factors. As well as the heel counter, consider the stiff material at the heel of the foot. The absence of a stiff counter in the heel allows the foot to deviate inward or outward, creating postural distortion patterns. High heels are directly associated with an anterior shift of weight. The higher the heel, the more weight is anteriorly distributed. High heels are not recommended for postural correction.

Many patients will ask if they need shoe supports or a heel lift. This will vary per patient. Some patients will benefit greatly from orthotics. Some patients, however, will not need orthotics if they are able to correct their posture with other postural correction strategies.

Shoes with adequate postural support should cover the following points:

- Shoes should provide arch support and not be flat

- Shoes should be flexible, lightweight, fit well but not be too tight, and be well-balanced

- If the soles of the shoes are worn out or are stretched out, consider buying a new pair of shoes

- Although it is not recommended to wear high heels, if the patient does choose to wear high heels, wide-based short heels are the best option

Texting without tech neck

Improper posture while utilizing technology, cell phones for example, is a very common factor contributing to poor posture. In fact, postural decline is advancing at the speed of technology. Technology is recognized as one of the principal causes of the modern day posture epidemic. Poor posture due to looking down at a cell phone is so common that a new medical diagnosis has been created to explain the phenomenon: "tech neck". This habit must be addressed with your patients to provide them the highest level of care.

Next time your patients send a text message or make a phone call, have them consider the damage to their neck they are creating if they are doing it with improper posture. Instead of the patient looking down while sending a text message or while checking their email or social media, have them bring the phone to eye level to avoid strain to their neck and back. The device should be close enough for the patient to see it clearly without jutting their head forward into forward head posture.

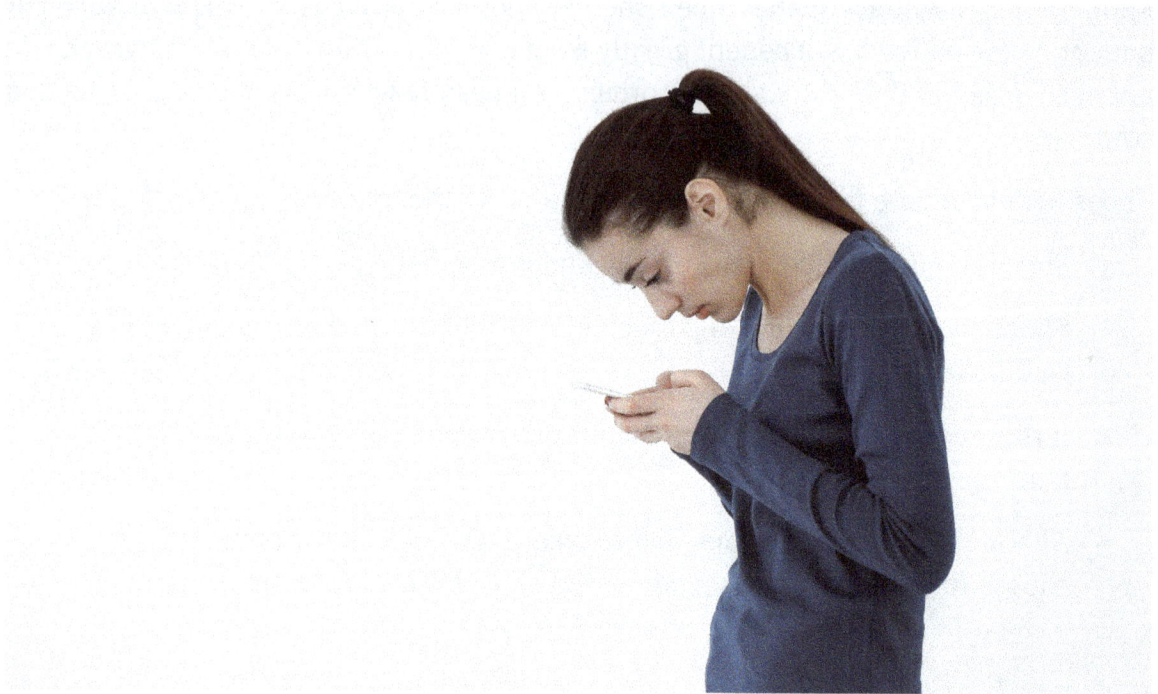

For proper posture while the patient is utilizing a cell phone or iPad, consider giving them the following posture tips to promote postural fitness while they are interacting with technology:

- Bring cell phone or iPad to eye level when sending a message or searching the Internet

- When they are talking on the phone, have the patient hold the phone to their ear instead of bending the cervical spine laterally to hold the phone

- If the patient makes regular phone calls, they can utilize a headset with earphones and a microphone so they do not have to hold the phone to their ear for extended periods of time

- When they are playing videogames, have your patients look straight ahead at the TV, computer, or other gaming device. Also have them position themselves with proper posture while seated to reduce spinal strain

- Explain the importance of patients not using their cell phones while driving, whether to talk or send a message. Both activities draw attention away from the road, increasing the likelihood of traumatic accidents

Healthy sitting

Healthy sitting is a fundamental lifestyle habit contributing to proper posture. When sitting is done properly, the posture system is supported and less strain is placed on the spinal discs and articulations. Maintaining proper posture while seated relies greatly on the quality of the chair selected by the patient. Have your patients review the ergonomic essentials to design their workplace in a way that promotes supported sitting.

Proper posture while seated is not only important at work, it is important throughout the lifespan of the patient. Consider the effect that poor posture while seated has on school-aged children. This is the period in which they begin developing lifestyle habits. If they learn to sit with proper posture, this will become a norm in their daily life. If they are seated for nearly 8 hours per day with poor posture, the health effects are debilitating and can greatly affect their performance at school.

While they are seated, it is important that patients do not have their wallet in their back pocket. Sitting on a wallet creates an uneven balance of the hips. Simply placing the wallet in the front pocket can improve posture and prevent symptoms associated with sciatica.

For healthy sitting, have your patients implement the following recommendations:

- Choose a chair that allows them to rest both feet flat on the floor while keeping their knees level with the hips. If necessary, prop up the feet with a footstool or other support

- Sit back in the chair. If the chair doesn't support the lumbar curve, place a rolled towel or small pillow behind the lumbar spine

- Have the patient roll their hips forward from a slouched posture so that approximately 60% of their body weight is distributed through the pelvis and about 40% through the legs and feet

- Maintain tone of the inner corset core musculature. This will keep the spine upright to prevent slouching

- Stretch the top of the head toward the ceiling, and tuck the chin in slightly, drawing the neck back so the ear and shoulder are aligned properly

- Keep the upper back and neck comfortably straight, without allowing the shoulders to roll forward

- Keep the shoulders relaxed, not elevated toward the ears

- Utilize an ergonomic chair, an exercise ball, or a posture cushion for prolonged sitting to support the spine and to engage the core musculature. If the patient does not contract their core muscles, they risk falling off the ball or being unable to move around. The feeling of falling off the ball but catching themselves is good as it stimulates neural plasticity to balance the body

Also consider the importance of active sitting. With the amount of hours that modern day employees are seated, it is important to maintain activity. Examples of active sitting are sitting on an exercise ball or a posture cushion, performing leg extensions or swinging the legs, performing regular breaks, and performing arm stretches.

Standing with confidence

Standing with proper posture exudes a higher level of confidence and physical appeal. It also distributes the weight of the body evenly among the articulations and muscles to avoid excessive strain of the lower back, the hips, the knees, or the feet. Patients who have occupations requiring them to be on their feet for prolonged periods of time should focus on improving their static standing posture so as to avoid unnecessary injury.

While standing, the patient should align themselves symmetrically around their center of gravity and maintain contraction of the core musculature so the hips and the stomach do not jut forward. They should pull their chin back so the neck does not jut forward. Once in this position, the patient should focus on keeping their eyes level with the horizon without looking down. They should also be mindful of keeping the weight evenly distributed over both feet, and avoid shifting the weight from one hip to the other.

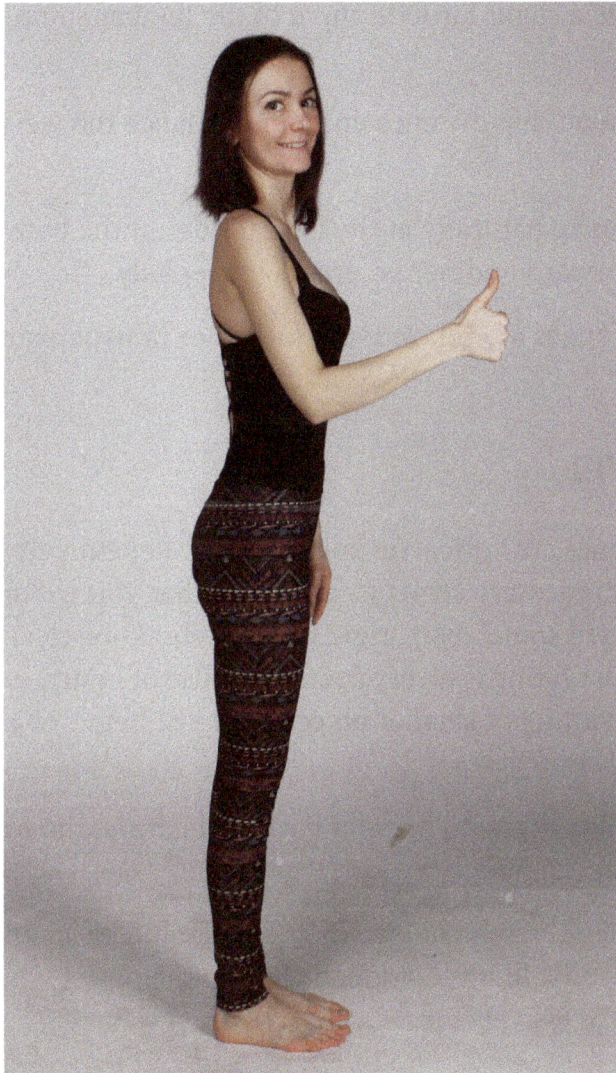

Standing with confidence requires the following steps:

- Pull the chin back so the ears are aligned over the shoulders. Keep eyes parallel to the horizon without neck flexion or extension

- Keep the shoulders back and relaxed; avoid drawing the shoulders up or rounding them anteriorly

- Pull in the abdomen so that the core muscles are strong and support the lower back. The hips and stomach should not jut forward

- There should be a slight lordotic curve of the lumbar spine, but not excessive

- Keep the feet about hip distance apart and balance the weight evenly on both feet

- Let the hands hang naturally at the lateral sides of the body; the thumbs should point forward and not be drawn in medially

- Make sure the knees are relaxed, not locked or in hyperextension

Intelligent lifting

Proper lifting techniques are critical for spinal health. Repetitively lifting heavy objects incorrectly causes unnecessary stress to the spine that will eventually lead to spinal degeneration, herniated spinal discs, rigid paravertebral muscles, and postural distortion patterns. Improper lifting is a very common cause of injury. Remember, injury can occur from repetitive lifting of smaller objects, not just heavy objects, when it is done with improper lifting strategies.

Pay attention now when lifting to prevent back problems in the future. Teach patients how to lift objects intelligently.

- Before the patient lifts the object, their feet should be shoulder width apart and the patient should be positioned close to the object where they don't need to reach excessively far forward

- They contract the core musculature by drawing the umbilicus toward the lumbar spine

- Keeping the spine straight while bending, they draw the shoulders back and avoid jutting the neck forward

- They bend with the knees to lift the object. Performing a squat to lift the object is indicated to shift the load from the spine to the legs

- They must never bend forward at the waist with the legs straight. This causes great strain to the lower back

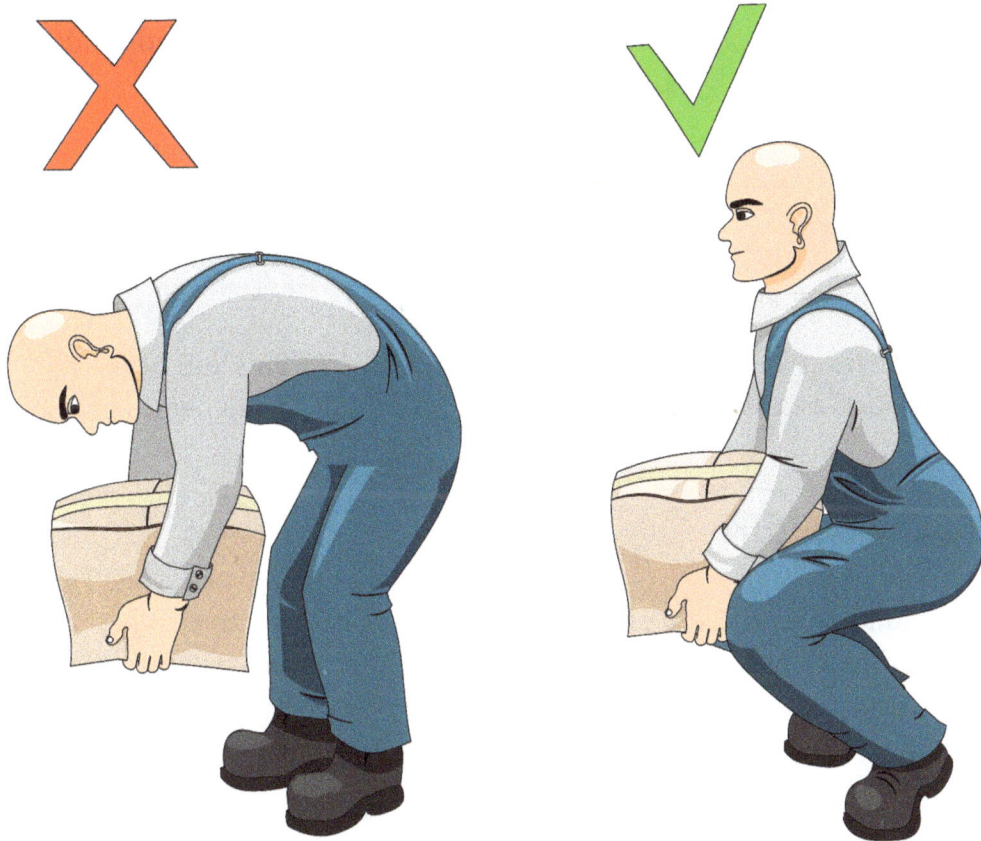

Better posture while walking and running

Proper walking and running posture will increase efficiency of respiration and circulation and improve stride length. Proper alignment is a critical component to improving running or walking form.

Provided below are tips that your patients can implement immediately to improve their posture while walking and running:

- Hold the head high by pulling the chin back to center the head between the shoulders and keeping the neck and back straight. Have the patient focus their gaze ahead of them instead of looking straight down at the ground. Have them relax their jaw and neck, keeping their shoulders relaxed and parallel to the ground

- Have the patient bend their arms, keeping the wrists loose. The elbows should bend at approximately a 90-degree angle with the hands gliding past the waistline.

- Proper breathing during walking and running is very important. Diaphragmatic breathing is ideal

- Engage the core musculature and feel the transerversus abdominis activate before, during, and after walking or running

- The foot-strike of the patient should be heel to toe. This will help prevent injury, such as a sprained ankle, or over pronation or supination of the foot

Purses and posture

Purses should not exceed 10% of the body weight of the person carrying them. If the load is excessive, the head and neck jut forward rather than staying over the shoulders, which can lead to headaches, neck tension, and back pain. Patients have a tendency of carrying purses or bags over the same shoulder each day, causing repetitive stresses.

Long-strapped shoulder bags are not ideal because they tug on one shoulder, creating asymmetric distribution of weight among the posture system. If the strap slips, patients will naturally hunch their shoulder superior to prevent the bag from falling, creating tension of the trapezius muscle. It is better to utilize purses with short handles for this reason.

Educate your patients on these ways to carry purses and handbags properly:

- Check the weight of the purse before leaving the house. If the weight is excessive, it is better to bring fewer items, or to carry two bags, one over each shoulder with equal weight distribution

- The best positions for a short-handled bag are over the shoulder and tucked under the arm close to the body or held in the hand close to the body

- When they are carrying a bag over the shoulder, tell patients to switch shoulders to evenly distribute the weight

- When patients are carrying a purse with a long strap, it is better to have the strap over the opposite shoulder to the purse. When the strap is worn over the opposite shoulder, the shoulders are relaxed and do not need to contract to prevent the purse from falling

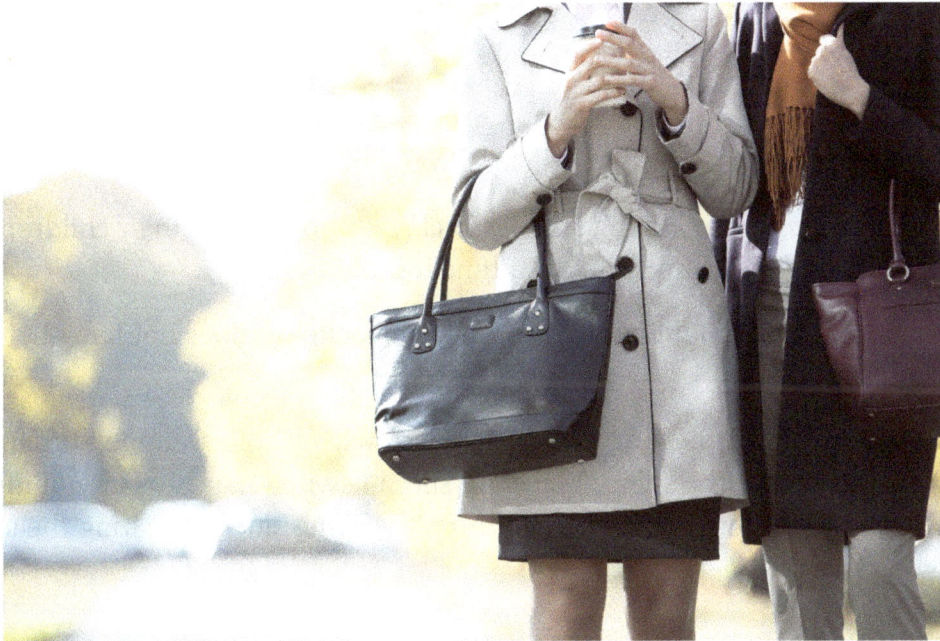

Backpack hygiene

According to the American Academy of Orthopedic Surgeons (AAOS), 70% of orthopedic surgeons believe that heavy backpacks are responsible for the development of back pain in children (Reneman et al., 2006). Heavy backpacks are contributing to the worldwide epidemic of postural decline.

Backpacks should not weigh more than 5–10% of the child's body weight. When the backpack exceeds this weight, it affects the child's posture. For example, when the weight of the backpack exceeds 15% of the child's body weight, the child will have a tendency to lean forward. Over time this causes strain of the musculature of the low back. Also, when backpacks exceed 15% of the child's body weight, the child experiences an increased frequency of short breaths due to the overloaded weight on their back. When backpack straps are only worn over one shoulder, another problem occurs. Due to the uneven weight distribution, children present with postural abnormalities of the head and neck affecting their spinal development (Brackley and Stevenson 2004).

To prevent unnecessary pain for children, educate your pediatric patients and their parents to follow the steps listed below for proper backpack hygiene:

- Always have the child carry the backpack over two shoulders

- They should pack the heaviest books or items in the backpack closest to the body for better support

- The backpack should be carried close to the body

- Parents can consider buying smaller backpacks to prevent their children from carrying too many items at a time

- Backpack straps should be tight so that the backpack does not hang below the hips

- Consider using a trolley or a backpack with wheels to lessen the burden of heavy weights on the spine. The child should switch hands when pulling the trolley, avoiding always pulling from the same side or rotating the spine

Supported sleeping

Human beings spend almost 1/3 of their lives in bed. Having a proper sleeping position is critical to protect the alignment of the posture system. It is optimal to sleep with the back in a neutral position, not arched a lot, but not flat either. This takes pressure off the spine. Also, tell patients to avoid bending and twisting their cervical spine during the night. Select a pillow that is not too thick to allow the cervical spine to be in a relaxed position without contracting the musculature or bending the spine during the night.

Recommended sleeping positions:

Sleeping on your side. When sleeping on your side, place a pillow between the knees. Try to keep the top leg from falling over the bottom leg creating a twist of the spine. You can also put a small pillow or a rolled-up towel under the waist.

Sleeping on your back. When sleeping on your back, place a pillow under the knees to relieve pressure of the lumbar spine. If the pillow provides inadequate cervical support, put a small rolled-up towel under the curve of the back.

Educate patients not to sleep on their stomachs. Sleeping on the stomach causes the cervical spine to be turned in one direction or the other with prolonged lumbar extension. Poor postural habits while sleeping can cause constant mechanical stress to the spine.

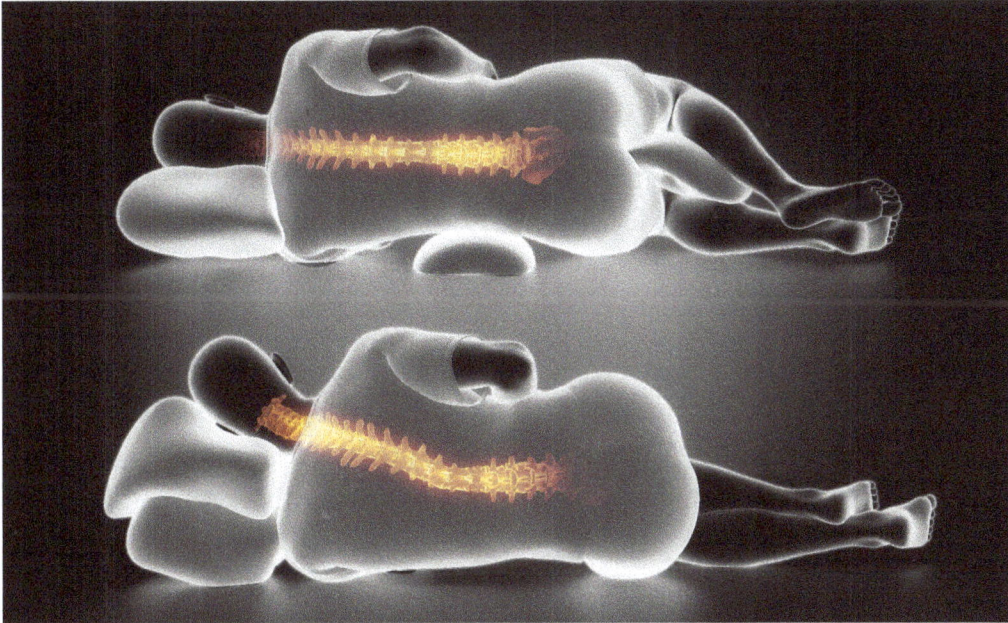

Mattress recommendations. The condition of a mattress can often dictate the sleeping position that your patients choose. With an old, worn-out mattress that sags in the middle, patients find it more difficult to sleep on their side. The mattress should be firm, but comfortable.

Many patients who present with low back pain will say that they feel more stiffness in the morning. Educate them on how to rise from bed in the best position:

- They should begin the process near the edge of the bed, making it easier to stand up

- Have them roll onto their side and bend both knees

- Drop their feet over the side of the bed while pushing with both arms to sit up

- The feet should be positioned under the buttocks

- Stand up, keeping the spine in a neutral position

For patients who experience pain and stiffness of the lumbar spine in the mornings, they can also utilize the posture cushion to warm up their back. Utilizing the posture cushion will help to relax the paravertebral musculature, eliminate strain to the articulations, while opening the disc space to assist in reduction of pain associated with a herniated disc.

Posture and pregnancy

Good postural habits during pregnancy play an exceptionally important role in preparing the pregnant mother's body for labor. Loosened ligaments, heightened emotions, and additional weight of the pregnant body can lead to back pain and even injury if patients do not learn correct postural habits during pregnancy.

To allow adequate growth space for the developing fetus, the mother's body will naturally compensate by tipping the pelvis backward. This is why pregnant women tend to have a greater lumbar curve. With the accentuated lumbar curve, many expectant mothers experience back pain and fatigue standing for prolonged periods of time.

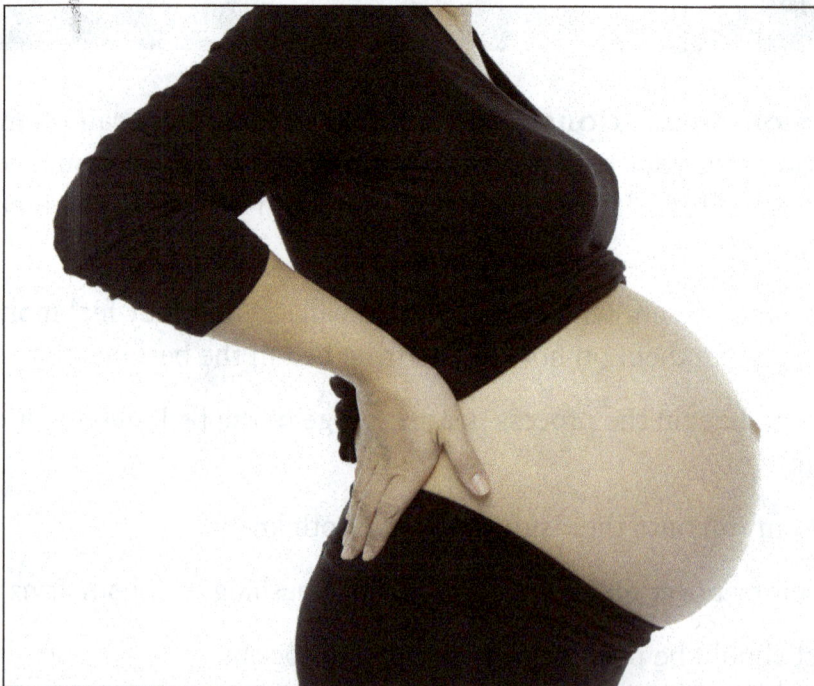

Pregnant mothers should consider these important tips during pregnancy, so they can live with more comfort and better postural design.

While seated, pregnant women should avoid crossing their legs. When women cross their legs, it can contribute to pelvic misalignments that are commonly felt for pregnant patients as lower back pain or sciatica. If the patient experiences difficulty sitting up straight with her back against the chair, she should place a lumbar support (or small pillow) behind the lumbar spine to support the natural lumbar curve.

During pregnancy, sleeping on the side with a small pillow between the legs is best. In particular, the mother sleeping on her left side may benefit the baby by improving blood flow and nutrient delivery to the placenta.

Avoid the common swayback postural presentation of pregnant women. Instead of having an incorrect swayback posture, focus on gently pulling in the abdomen and buttocks, relieving the lumbar spine of stress. It seems natural to compensate for the additional abdominal weight with a swayback posture, but this causes excessive strain to the joints, ligaments, and muscles of your low back.

Posture on the road

Patients who drive long distances each day commonly present with lower back pain. Even a long road trip can affect a seemingly healthy patient's posture. Although patients may experience difficulty in maintaining proper posture while seated in the seats of the car, it is important to do so. Refer to the recommendations regarding healthy sitting for how to maintain the proper posture while seated.

In addition, consider recommending the following advice to your patients to maintain proper posture while driving:

Patients should take frequent breaks during long road trips. During the break the patient should get out of the car and walk for a few minutes. They should also perform the posture break exercise explained earlier to open the chest cavity. During prolonged sitting, patients commonly experience trunk flexion and anterior displacement of the shoulders in the direction of gravity. To prevent this, patients should take posture breaks frequently when driving.

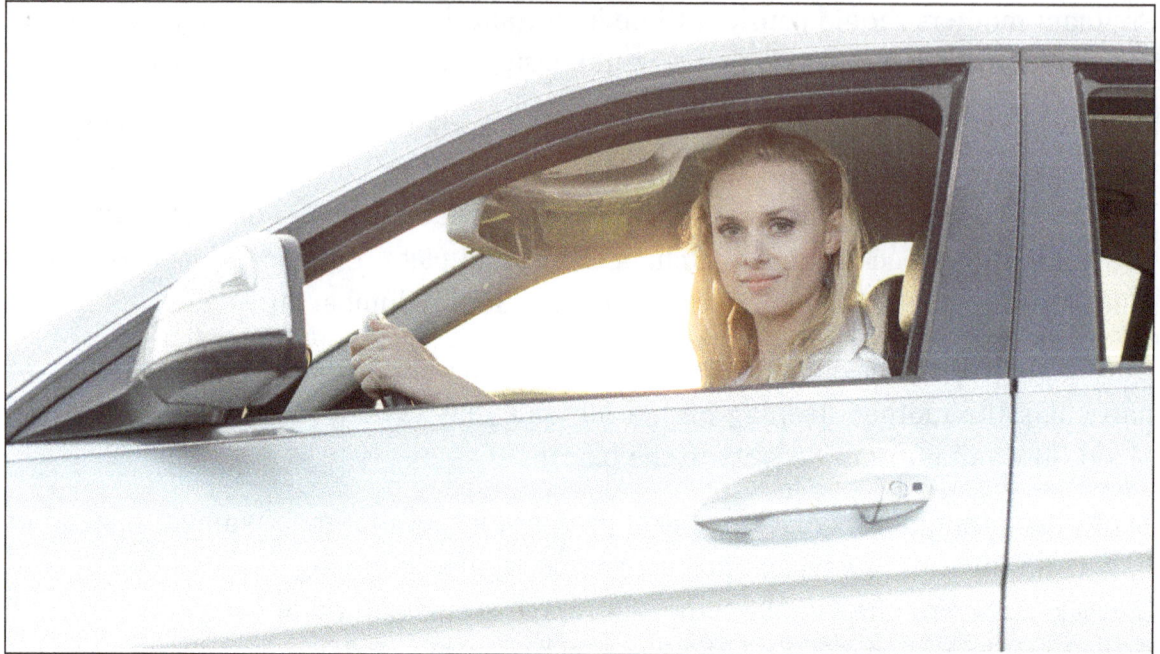

Place a small cushion behind the neck and lower back in the lumbar curve to support the spine and to keep the back straight while driving. If they don't have a cushion, they can roll up a towel. This will help patients maintain proper spinal posture while seated.

The position of the hands is important when driving long distances. Hold the arms close to the body with the elbows bent at a 90-degree angle to hold the steering wheel. Position the seat close enough to the steering wheel for the patient to grip the steering wheel comfortably without drawing the shoulders forward.

Community impact

Educating patients on the vital significance of having a healthy posture system is of utmost importance to Posture Experts. By correcting postural distortion patterns and teaching patients how to live healthier lives with proper postural design, Posture Experts truly make lasting changes in the lives of their patients. With more Posture Experts impacting their communities, together a shift toward the posture paradigm is possible. Patients do not need to be victims of their environment; rather, they should be empowered to live a life of optimal human function.

Postural hygiene programs are the difference that can change society's posture epidemic. It is not just the work that is done in your office that is important, but also the impact that you make outside of the office to educate your community. Why wait until adults come to your office with pain to begin the process of postural correction and postural education?

Wouldn't it be more impactful if we could reach the community before they were suffering? Healthy lifestyle habits are a choice, and yet the majority of society has no idea that the choices they are making on a daily basis are supporting postural decline.

A societal shift begins with the children and the parents of children. By educating children and parents of the importance of proper posture as a lifestyle choice, we will impact them and empower them to educate future generations. The best healthcare is prevention. Structure and function of the body are directly correlated. With an unbalanced posture system, the patient loses the ability to thrive in the environment in which they live.

To monitor the patients in your community, you are recommended to encourage all individuals to have a yearly posture image taken, beginning at the age of 6 years old. In this manner, Posture Experts can evaluate the presence of postural distortion patterns before the patient presents with pain. Stop postural decline before it begins and support the patient in obtaining optimal human performance.

Specializing in postural correction is a blue ocean market of opportunity for healthcare professionals. Patients need you; your community needs you. The quality of their life depends upon the knowledge that you possess.

With the implementation of the postural correction strategies explained in this book, improved clinical results and healthy patients are the outcome. In the world of healthcare, public health strategies to improve human function are a win-win.

Patients want to look better, move better, and feel better. Help them achieve this through the implementation of postural correction. To change lives, to impact communities, to optimize human performance, it's always "Posture by Design, Not by Circumstance".

REFERENCES

Aguilar, Naudi (2013) *The Power of Posture* Ebook. Functional Patterns Certification © 2013.

American Academy of Orthopedic Surgeons (2009) Ortho Info: The Effects of Aging. Retrieved from http://orthoinfo.aaos.org/topic.cfm?topic=A00191.

American Chiropractic Association (2014) Back Pain Facts and Statistics. Retrieved from http://www.acatoday.org/level2_css.cfm?T1ID=13&T2ID=68.

American Chiropractic Association (2015) Backpack Misuse Leads to Chronic Back Pain, Doctors of Chiropractic Say. Retrieved from https://www.acatoday.org/content_css.cfm?CID=65.

Amos, J. (2012) Acid Reflux (GERD) Statistics and Facts. Published on June 30, 2012. Medically Reviewed by George Krucik, MD http://www.healthline.com/health/gerd/statistics

Apkarian, A. et al. (2004) Chronic back pain is associated with decreased prefrontal and thalamic gray matter density. *Journal of Neuroscience* 24(46).

Arnette, S. & Pettijohn, T. (2012) The Effects of Posture on Self-Perceived Leadership. *International Journal of Business and Social Science*, 3(14) 8-13.

Ayub, E., Glasheen-Wray, M., Kraus, S. (1984) Head posture: a case study of the effects on rest position of the mandible. *Journal of Orthopaedics and Sport Physical Therapy*, 5, pp. 179–183

Baechle, T., & Earle, R. (2008) "Human Kinetics" *Essentials of Strength Training and Conditioning*. NSCA—National Strength & Conditioning Association 3rd Edition. ©2008.

Barham-Floreani, J. (2005) *Well Adjusted Babies* Vitality Productions Pty LTD © 2005.

Bond, M. (2007) *The New Rules of Posture: How to sit, stand, and move.* Healing Arts Press © 2007.

Boyle, K., Olinick, J., & Lewis, C. (2010) The Value of Blowing up a Balloon. *North American Journal of Sports Physical Therapy,* 5(3) p. 179–188.

Brackley, H, & Stevenson, J. (2004). Are Children's Backpack Weight Limits Enough? A critical review of the relevant literature. *Spine,* 29, 2184–2190.

Brace, T. (2005). Office Ergonomics Do They Work?. *Professional Safety, 50*(9), 51–55.

Brink, Y., Louw, Q., Grimmer, K., & Jordaan, E. (2014). The spinal posture of

computing adolescents in a real-life setting. *BMC Musculoskeletal Disorders, 15*(1), 2–21.

Brinol, P. et al. (2009) Body posture effects on self-evaluation: a self-validation approach. *European Journal of Self Psychology,* 39 1,053–1,064.

Cailliet R & Gross L, (1987) Rejuvenation Strategy. New York, Doubleday Co.

Carney et al. (2010) Power posing, brief non-verbal displays affect neuroendocrine levels and risk tolerance. *Psychological Science,* 21(10) 1,363–1,368.

Chestnut, J. (2003) Evaluating the quality of clinical practice guidelines *Journal of Manipulalive and Physiological Therapeutics* March/April.

Cheung, C. et al. (2010) The 14 Foundational Premises for the Scientific and Philosophical Validation of the Chiropractic Wellness Paradigm. Chestnut Wellness Chiropractic Corporation.

Chiropractor's Association of Australia (2010) "Forward Head Posture" Retrieved from http://whatsyourposture.com.au/posture-health/posture-problems/forward-head-posture/.

Cholewicki, J., Silfles, S., Shah, R., Greene, H., Reeves, N., Alvi, K., & Goldberg, B. (2005) Delayed trunk muscle reflex responses increase the risk of low back injuries. *Spine,* 30(23) p. 2,614–20.

Cote, P., Cassidy, D., Carroll, L. (1998) The prevalence of neck pain and related disability in Saskatchewan adults. *Spine.* 23, 1,689–1,698.

Critchley, D. (2002) Instructing pelvic floor contraction facilitates transversus abdominis thickness increase during low-abdominal hollowing. *Physiotherapy Research International,* 7(2) p. 65–75.

Crow, W. & Willis, D. (2009) Estimating Cost of Care for Patients With Acute Low Back Pain: A Retrospective Review of Patient Records. *The Journal of the American Osteopathic Association,* (109) 229–233.

Deuchars, J., Edwards, I. (2007). Bad posture could raise your blood pressure. *Journal of Neuroscience* 0638–07.

Drexler, H., Schafer, E., Petersen, J. (2014) Impacts of chair mechanics, sitting postures and sitting concepts of office chairs on back health; a systematic review. Institute and Policlinic for Occupational, Social and Environmental Medicine (IPASUM) of the Friedrich-Alexander University Erlangen-Nürnberg. DOI: 10.17147/ASUI.2014-09-01-02.

Dorland (2007) Dorland's Illustrated Medical Dictionary 28th edition.

Duhigg, C. (2012) *The Power of Habit: Why we do what we do in life and business.*

Fallon, J. (1990) Chiropractic and Pregnancy, a partnership of the future. ICA Review Nov/Dec 1990 p. 39–42.

Fernandez-de-las penas, C., Alonso-Bianco, C., San-Roman, J., Maingolarra-Page, J. (2006) Methodological quality of randomized controlled trials of spinal manipulation and mobilization in tension-type headache, migraine, and cervicogenic headache. *Journal of Orthopaedic & Sports Physical Therapy,* 36(3) p. 160-9.

Ferris, T. K. (2013). Evidence-Based Design and the Fields of Human Factors and Ergonomics: Complementary Systems-Oriented Approaches to Healthcare Design. *Health Environments Research & Design Journal (HERD),* 6(3), 3–5.

Fejer, R., Kyvik, K., & Hartvigsen, J. (2006) The prevalence of neck pain in the world population: a systematic critical review of the literature. *European Spine Journal,* 15(6): 834–48.

Forjuoh S, Little D, Schuchmann J, & Lane, B. (2003) Parental knowledge of school backpack weight and contents. *Archives of Disease in Childhood* 88(1) doi:10.1136/adc.88.1.18.

Fortin, C. et al. (2011) Clinical methods for quantifying body segment posture: a literature review. *Disability and Rehabilitation*, 33(5) 367–383.

Freburger, J. et al. (2009) Exercise Prescription for Chronic Back or Neck Pain: Who Prescribes It? Who Gets It? What Is Prescribed? *Arthritis Care and Research*, February.

Friberg O. (1983) Clinical Symptoms and in leg length inequality. Spine 8(6): 643-651.

Frietag (1987) Expert testimony comparing the results of two neighboring hospitals. US District Court Northern Illinois Eastern Division No. 76C 3777.

Fryman, V. & Springall, P. (1992) Effect of Osteopathic Medical Management on Neurologic Development in Children *JAOA* 92(729).

Fukuda, T. (1984) Statokinetic reflexes in equilibrium and movement. U. Tokyo Press.

Gardner, B., Lally, P., & Wardle, J. (2012) Making health habitual: the psychology of 'habit-formation' and general practice. *The British Journal of General Practice,* 62(605) 664–666.

Gaskin, D. & Richard, P. (2011) Relieving Pain in America: A Blueprint for Transforming Prevention, Care, Education, and Research. Institute of Medicine (US) Committee on Advancing Pain Research, Care, and Education.

Gelb H, Gelb M. (1994) An Orthopedic Approach to the Diagnosis and Treatment of Craniocervical Mandibular Disorders. In: New Concepts in Craniomandibular and Chronic Pain Management. Gelb H. ed. London: Mosby-Wolf. Pg. 215-253.

Giles, L. &Taylor, J. (1981) Low-back Pain Associated With Leg Length Inequity. *Spine*, 6(5) p. 510- 21.

Goggins, R. (2008) Cost Benefit measurement of Ergonomic Programs. *Journal of Safety Research*, 39: 339-344.

Goodgold, S. & Nielsen D. (2003). Effectiveness of a School-Based Backpack Health Promotion Program: Backpack Intelligence. *Work* 2, 113–123

Goldstein, L & Makofsky H. (2005) TMD/Facial Pain and Forward Head Posture. Pract Pain Manag. Jul/Aug 2005. 5(5) 36-39.

Green, B. N. (2008). A literature review of neck pain associated with computer use: public health implications. *Journal Of The Canadian Chiropractic Association, 52*(3), 161–167.

Griffeth, D. (2014) From the Ground Up Global Posture Patterns of the Human Body. Parker University CE course.

Gutmann, G. (1987) The atlas fixation syndrome in the baby and infant. Manuelle Medizin, 25 pp. 5–10. Retrieved from http://www.chiro.org/LINKS/FULL/The_VSC_3.shtml.

Guyton A. Textbook of Medical Physiology, 8th Edit. Philadelphia: W.B. Sanders Co. pp. 1991.

Haavik, H. (2014) *Reality Check* Haavik Research ©2014.

Hansraj, K. (2015) Assessment of Stresses in the Cervical Spine Caused by Posture and the Position of the Head. *Neuro and Spine Surgery*, Surgical and Technology International. 593 p. 1–3.

Harrison, DE., Cailliet, R., Harrison, DD., Janik, TJ., & Holland, B. (2002) A new 3-point

bending traction method for restoring cervical lordosis and cervical manipulation:

a nonrandomized clinical controlled trial. *Arch Phys Med Rehabil.* 2002;83(4): 447–453.

Harrison, DD., Harrison, DE., Janik, TJ., Caillet, R., Ferrantelli, JR., & Haas, JW. (2004)

Modeling of the sagittal cervical spine as a method to discriminate hypolordosis. *Spine*, 29(22) 2,485–2,492.

Harrison, D., Harrison, D., Haas, J. (2002) *CBP Structural Rehabilitation of the Cervical Spine*. Harrison CBP Seminars, Incorporated, 2002.

Harte, K., Mahieu, K., Mallett, D., Norville, J., & VanderWerf, S. (2011). Improving Workplace Productivity—It Isn't Just About Reducing Absence. *Benefits Quarterly, 27*(3), 13–26.

Hausswirth, C., Bigard, A., Guezennec, C. (1997) Relationship between running mechanics and energy cost of running at the end of a triathlon and marathon. *International Journal of Sports Medicine,* 18(5) p. 330–9.

Henderson, I. (1987) American Medical Association records released in US District Court Northern Illinois Eastern Division, No. 76C 3777.

Ho Ting Yip, C., Tai Wing Chiu, T., Tung Kuen Poon., A. (2008) The relationship between head posture and severity and disability of patients with neck pain. *Manual Therapy,* 13(2) 148–154.

Hodges, P., & Richardson, C. (1996) Inefficient muscular stabilization of the lumbar spine associated with low back pain. A motor control evaluation of transversus abdominis. *Spine,* 21(22) p. 2640–50.

Hodges, P., & Richardson, C. (1998) Delayed postural contraction of transversus abdominis in low back pain associated with movement of the lower limb. *Journal of Spinal Disorders,* 11(1) p. 46-56.

Holt, A., Shaw, N., Shetty, A., Greenough, C. (2002) The reliability of the Low Back Outcome Score for back pain. *Spine,* 27(2) p. 206–10.

Hooshmand, H. (1993) *Chronic Pain: Reflex Sympathetic Dystrophy, Prevention, and Management.* CRC Press ©1993 ISBN 0849386675.

Huggare J, et al. (1991) Head posture and dentofacial morphology in subjects treated for scoliosis. Proceedings of the Finnish Dental Society. Vol 87(1) p.151–8.

Irvin R. (2000) A philosophic basis for the alleviation of common, chronic pain by the optimization of posture. Annual AOA convention.

Janda, V. (1996) *Evaluations of Muscular Imbalance.* Rehabilitation of the Spine Ed. Liebenson. G. Williams & Wilkins, Baltimore pp. 97–112.

Jin, J., Sklar, G., Oh, V., & Li, S. (2008) Factors affecting therapeutic compliance: A review from the patient's perspective. *Ther Clin Risk Manag.,* 4(1) 269–286.

Jones, S. et al. (2011) Individuals with non-specific low back pain use a trunk stiffening strategy to maintain upright posture. *Journal of Electromyography and Kinesiology* 22(1) 13–20.

Jung-Ho Kang et al. (2012) The Effect of Forward Head Posture on Postural Balance in Long Time Computer Based Workers. Annals of Rehabilitation Medicine 36(1).

Kado, D., Huang, M., Barrett-Connor, E., & Greendale, G. (2005) Hyperkyphotic Posture and Poor Physical Functional Ability in Older Community-Dwelling Men and Women: The Rancho Bernardo Study. *Journals of Gerontology: Biological Sciences.* 60(5), 633–637

Kado, Prenovost, and Crandall (2007) Hyperkyphotic posture and risk of injurious falls in older persons: The Rancho Bernardo Study. *Journal of Gerontology: Medical Sciences,* 62(6) 652–657.

Kado, D. et al. (2009) Hyperkyphosis predicts mortality independent of vertebral osteoporosis in older women. *Annals of Internal Medicine* 150:681–687.

Kase K. 1994. Illustrated Kinesio Taping®, 3rd Ed., Ken'I Kai, Tokyo, pp.90–91.

Kase, K., Tatsuyuki, H., & Tomoko, O. (1996) Development of Kinesio tape. Kinesio Taping Perfect Manual. Kinesio Taping Association.

Katzman, W., Wanek, L., Shepher, J., and Sellmeyer, D. (2010) Age-Related Hyperkyphosis: Its Causes, Consequences, and Management. J Orthop Sports Phys Ther, 40(6) 352-360.

Kelby, J. (2014). Nuts & Bolts of Effective Ergonomics Programs. *Professional Safety,* 59(8), 53–54.

Kelly, R., Zyanski, S., & Alemagno, S. (1991) Prediction of motivation and behavior change following health promotion: Role of health beliefs, social support, and self-efficacy. *Social Science and Medicine,* 32(3) 311–320.

Kendall, F., McCreary, E., Provance, P., Rodgers, M., & Romani, W. (2005) *Muscles Testing and Function with Posture and Pain.* 5th Edition Lippincott Williams and Wilkins © 2005.

Kendall, R., Schwartz, J., & Jessel, T. (1991) *Principles of neural science,* third edition. Appleton & Lange, 1991. ISBN 0-8385-8068-8.

Kjaer, P., Leboeuf-Yde, C., Sorensen, J., Bendix, T. (2005) An Epidemiologic Study of MRI and Low Back Pain in 13-Year-Old Children. *Spine* 30(7) 798-806.

Knutson, G. (2005) Anatomic and functional leg-length inequality: A review and recommendation for clinical decision-making. Part I, anatomic leg-length inequality: prevalence, magnitude, effects and clinical significance. *Chiropractic and Osteopathy,* 13(11).

Laeser, K. L., Maxwell, L. E., & Hedge, A. (1998). The effect of computer workstation design on student posture. *Journal Of Research On Computing In Education, 31*(2), 173.

La Touche, R. et al. (2011) The influence of craniocervical posture on maximal mouth opening and pressure pain threshold in patients with myofascial temporomandibular pain disorders. Clinical Journal of Pain 27(1).

Lentrell., G., Kruse, M., Chock, B., Wilson, K., Iwamoto, M., Martin, R. (2002) Dimensions of the Cervical Neural Foramina in Resting and Retracted Positions Using Magnetic Resonance Imaging. *Journal of Orthopaedic & Sports Physical Therapy,* 32(8) p. 380-390.

Levine, J. (2013). Ergotran JustStand Survey and Index Report.

Retrieved from www.juststand.org.

Lewit, K. (1993) *Manipulative Therapy in Rehabilitation of the Locomotor System*, 2nd Edit. Oxford: Butterworth-Heinemann. p. 18–21.

Lopes, E. et al. (2006) Assessment of muscle shortening and static posture in children with persistent asthma. *European Journal of Pediatrics,* 166(7) 715–721.

Lotz, C. (2012). One-on-One Office Ergonomics Assessment. *Professional Safety, 57*(9), 58–59.

Ludwig, Leibsohn, Academy of General Dentistry, spokesperson.

MacLeod, D. (2006) 25 Ways Ergonomics can save you money, *The Ergonomics Kit for General Industry,* Taylor and Francis 2nd Edition.

MacLeod, D. (2009). Ergonomics, Productivity, and Safety *The Ergonomics Kit for General Industry*, 1–8.

McGill, S. (2007) "Lumbar Spine Stability: Mechanism of Injury and Restabilization" *Rehabilitation of the Spine, a Practitioner's Manual* Liebenson, C. © 2007.

McGill, S. (2010) Core Training: Evidence Translating to Better Performance and Injury Prevention. *Strength and Conditioning Journal,* 32(3) 33-46.

McKeon, P. & Hertel, J. (2008) Systematic Review of Postural Control and Lateral Ankle Instability, Part II: Is Balance Training Clinically Effective. *Journal of Athletic Training,* 43(3) p. 305–315.

Mendez, F. et al. (2001). Postural hygiene program to prevent low back pain. *Spine* 26(11) 1280-1286.

Michaelson P, Michaelson M, Jaric S, Latash ML, Sjolander P, Djupsjobacka M. (2003) Vertical posture and head stability in patients with chronic neck pain. *J Rehabil Med,* 35 p.229-35.

Morscher, E. (1972) Etiology and Pathophysiology of Leg Length Discrepancies, Eng. trans. from Der Orthopade © Springer-Verlag. Vol. 1, pp. 1–8.

Moustafa, I. & Diab, A. (2012) The efficacy of forward head correction on nerve root function and pain in cervical spondylotic radiculopathy: a randomized trial. *Clinical Rehabilitation,* 26(4) p. 351–61.

Munhoz, W. et al. (2004) Radiographic Evaluation of Cervical Spine of Subjects with Temporomandibular Joint Internal Disorder. Brazilian Oral Research 18(4).

National Institute of Neurological Disorders and Stroke (2014) Carpal Tunnel Syndrome Fact Sheet. Retrieved from http://www.ninds.nih.gov/disorders/carpal_tunnel/detail_carpal_tunnel.htm.

National Scoliosis Foundation (2007) Information and Support. Retrieved from http://www.scoliosis.org/info.php.

Neal D, Wood , Labrecque J, & Lally P. (2012) How do habits guide behavior? Perceived and actual triggers of habits in daily life. *J Exp Soc Psychol.,* 48 492–498.

Negrini, S., Carabalona, R., & Sililla, P. (1999) Backpack as a daily load for school-children. *Lancet* 354(9194).

Nikolakis, P et al. (2001) An Investigation of the Effectiveness of Exercise and Manual Therapy in Treating Symptoms of TMJ Osteoarthritis. Journal of Craniomandibular Practice.

Norton, P., Baker, J. (1994) Postural changes can reduce leakage in women with stress urinary incontinence. *Obstetrics and Gynecology,* 84(5) p. 770–4.

Oakley, P. A., Harrison, D. D., Harrison, D. E., & Haas, J. W. (2005). Evidence-based protocol for structural rehabilitation of the spine and posture: review of clinical biomechanics of posture (CBP®) publications. *The Journal of the Canadian Chiropractic Association, 49*(4), 270–296.

O'Brien M, & Newman, P, (2008) "Nonsurgical Treatment of Idiopathic Scoliosis," *Surgery of the Pediatric Spine,* ed. Daniel H. Kim et al. Thieme Medical Publishers, 580.

O'Sullivan, P., & Beales, D. (2007) Diagnosis and classification of pelvic girdle pain disorders- Part 1: A mechanism based approach within a biopsychosocial framework. *Manual Therapy,* 12 p. 86–97

O'Sullivan et al. (2002) Posture and Low Back Pain *Spine* 27 1,238–1,244.

Perry, L. S. (2012). Standing Up: Redesigning the Workplace to Address Obesity. *Professional Safety, 57*(6), 77–84.

Pettorossi, V. & Schieppati, M. (2014) Neck proprioception shapes body orientation and perception of motion. *Frontiers in Human Neuroscience,* 8:895.

Physiopedia (2014) Phases of the Gait Cycle. Retrieved from http://www.physiopedia.com/Gait#Phases_of_the_Gait_Cycle.

Plouvier S, Renahy E, Chastang JF, Bonenfant S, et al. (2008). Biomechanical strains and low back disorders: Quantifying the effects of the number of years of exposure on various types of pain. *Occupational and Environmental Medicine 65*(4): 268-274.

Porter, K. (2006) *Natural Posture for Pain Free Living: The practice of mindful alignment* Healing Arts Press © 2006.

Pool-Goudzwaard, A., Hoek van Dijke, G., Van Gurp, M., Mulder, P., Snijders, C, & Stoeckart, R. (2004) Contribution of pelvic floor muscles to stiffness of the pelvic ring. *Clinical Biomechanics,* 19 p. 564–571.

Pope R. (1990) Reversal of Residual Somatic Dysfunction via Postural Balancing and OMT: Workshop. AOA Convention.

Pope, R. (2003) The common compensatory pattern: its origin and relationship to the postural model. AAOJ 14(4) p. 19–40.

Porter, K. (2006) *Natural Posture for Pain-Free Living*: The practice of Mindful Alignment. Inner Traditions Bear and Company ©2006.

Posture. (2015) In *Merriam-Webster.com*. Retrieved July, 2015 http://www.merriam-webster.com/dictionary/posture

Posture. (2015) *Oxford Dictionary.com* Retrieved July, 2015 http://www.oxforddictionaries.com/definition/english/posture

Posture Committee of the American Academy of Orthopedic Surgeons (1967) Retrieved July, 2014 http://www.aaos.org/home.asp

Previc F. (1991) A General Theory Concerning the Prenatal Origins of Cerebral Lateralization in Humans. *Psychological Review*. Vol 98(3) 299–334.

Proctor & Cantu (2000) Head and Neck Injuries in Young Athletes. Journal of Clinic in Sports Medicine 19(4).

Raine, S. & Twomey, LT. (1997) Head and shoulder posture variations in 160 asymptomatic women and men. *Arch Phys Med Rehabil*, 78(11):1,215–1,223.

Riddle, J., & Purvis, L. (2004). 10 WAYS TO BOOST YOUR ENERGY. *Essence (Time Inc.)*, *35*(2), 93–97.

Reneman, M., Poels, B., Geertzen, J., Dijkstra, P. (2006). Back Packs and Back Pain in Children: Biomedical or Biopsychosocial model. *Disability and Rehabilitation*, 28(20) 1,293–1,297.

Robinson, M. (1996) The influence of head position on temporomandibular joint dysfunction.J Prosthet Dent. Vol 1:169–172.

Rodríguez-Oviedo, P., Ruano-Ravina, A., Perez-Rios, M., Garcia, F., Gomez-Fernandez, D., Fernandez, Alonso, A., Carriera-Nunez, I., Garcia-Pacios, P., Turiso, J. (2012) School children's backpacks, back pain and back pathologies. *Archives of Disease in Childhood*. doi:10.1136/archdischild-2011-301253

Rolf, I (1990) *Rolfing and Physical Reality*. Healing Arts Press © 1978, 1990 ISBN 0-89281-380-6.

Saal, J., Saal, J., & Yurth, E. (1996) Nonoperative management of herniated cervical intervertebral disc with radiculopathy. *Spine,* 21(16) p. 1877–83.

Sackett, D. (1976) Compliance with therapeutic regimens. Baltimore: *Johns Hopkins University Press*, 1–6.

Saha, D., Gard, S., Fatone, S., Ondra, S. (2007) The Effect of Trunk-Flexed Postures on Balance and Metabolic Energy Expenditure During Standing. *Spine,* 32(15) p. 1605-1611.

Salminen J (1984) The Adolescent Back: A field Survey of 270 Finnish School Children. *Acta Paediatrica Scandinavica,* 315: 1–122

Salminen, J., Pentti, J. and Terho, P. (1992), Low back pain and disability in 14-year-old schoolchildren. Acta Paediatrica, 81:1035–1039. doi: 10.1111/j.1651-2227.1992.tb12170.x

Sapsford, R., Hodges, P., Pengel, L. (2007) Postural and respiratory functions of the pelvic floor muscles. *Urology and Neurodynamics,* 26(3) p. 362–71.

Scheib JE, Gangestad SW, Thornhill R. Facial attractiveness, symmetry and cues of good genes. *Proceedings of the Royal Society B: Biological Sciences.* 1999;266(1431):1,913–1,917.

Schilling, D. et al (2003) Classroom seating for children with attention deficit hyperactivity disorder: therapy balls versus chairs. *Journal of Occupational Therapy,* 57(5) 534–541

Schilling, D. & Schwartz, I. (2004). Alternative seating for young children with autism spectrum disorder: effects on classroom behavior. *Journal of Autism and Developmental Disorders* 34(4) 423–432.

Shimizu, M., Tanaka, S., Takamagari, H., Honda, K., Shimizu. H. & Nakamura S (1994) Optimal positioning for an adult athetoid cerebral palsy patient in a wheelchair. *Hiroshoma Journal of Medical Science,* 43, 69-72.

Shahraki S, Bakar N. THE ROLE OF ERGONOMICS IN WORKFORCE PRODUCTIVITY IN SERVICES COMPANIES. *International Journal Of Academic Research* [serial online]. September 2011;3(5):204–210. Available from: Academic Search Premier, Ipswich, MA. Accessed August 25, 2014.

Shapiro-Mendoza, C., Colson, E., Willinger, M., Rybin, D., Camperlengo, L., Corwin, M. (2014) Trends in Infant Bedding Use: National Infant Sleep Position Study, 1993–2010. *Pediatrics*, doi: 10.1542/peds.2014-1793.

Silfies, S., Mehta, R., Smith, S., & Karduna, A. (2009) Differences in feedforward trunk muscle activity in subgroups of patients with mechanical low back pain. *Archives of Physical Medicine and Rehabilitation,* 90(7) p. 1,159–69.

Silva, A., Punt, T., Sharples, P., Vilas-Boas, JP., & Johnson, MI. (2009) Head posture and neck pain of chronic nontraumatic origin: a comparison between patients and pain-free persons. *Arch Phys Med Rehabil*, 90(4):669–674.

Silva, A., Punt, T., Sharples, P., Vilas-Boas, JP., & Johnson, MI. (2009) Head posture assessment for patients with neck pain, is it useful? *International Journal of Therapy and Rehabilitation*, 16(1).

Smith, (2003) page 7 visible X-ray degeneration kids

Sohn, M., Lee, S., Song, H. (2013) Effects of acute low back pain on postural control. *Annals of Rehabilitative Medicine,* 37(1) p. 17–25.

Speck, 2013 – Nursing home mortality (in resources)

Spiegel, T., Fried, H., Hubert, C., Peikin, S., Siegel, J., and Zeiger, L. (2000) Effects of posture on gastric emptying and satiety ratings after a nutritive liquid and solid meal. *American Journal of Physiology – Regulatory, Integrative and Comparative Physiology,* 279.

Starrett, K & Cordoza, G. (2013) *Becoming a Supple Leopard*. Victory Belt Publishing Inc. ©2013.

Stichler, J. (2013). Considering Human Factors When Designing for Safety. *Health Environments Research & Design Journal (HERD)*. pp. 6–8.

Strachan F, Robinson M. (1965) Short leg linked to malocclusion. *Osteopathic News*, Apr.1965.

Stolinski, L., & Kotwicki, T. (2012). Self-correction of posture: assessment of the quality of the movement accomplished by non-instructed school children. *Scoliosis*, 7(Suppl 1), O66. doi:10.1186/1748-7161-7-S1-O66.

Suter E, McMorland G, Herzog W, Bray R. (1999) Decrease in quadriceps inhibition after sacroiliac joint manipulation in patients with anterior knee pain. *Journal of Manipulative Physio Therapy*, 22 p. 149–153.

Szeto, G., Straker, L., Raine, S. (2002) A field comparison of neck and shoulder postures in symptomatic and asymptomatic office workers. *Applied Ergonomics*, 33(1) 75-84.

Tetsuya, N. (2003) Computers Put Workers at Risk for Mental Illness. *The Telegraph*, January, 2003.

Teutsch, C. (2003) Patient-Doctor Communication. *Med CLin N Am*, 87 1,115–45.

Teychenne, M., Ball, K., & Salmon, J. (2010) Sedentary Behavior and Depression Among Adults: A Review. *International Journal of Behavioral Medicine*, 17(4) 246–254.

Thomas, McCullen, & Yuan (1999) Cervical Spine Injuries in Football Players. American Academy of Orthopedic Surgeons 7(5).

Travell, J. & Simmons, D. (1993) Myofascial Pain and Dysfunction: The Trigger Point Manual. Baltimore: Williams and Wilkins. Vol. 1, pp. 104–109.

US Department of Labor, OSHA (2013) https://www.osha.gov/dsg/topics/safety-health/

Uthaikhup, S., Jull, G., Sungkarat, S., Treleaven, J. (2012) The influence of neck pain on sensorimotor function in the elderly. *Archives of Gerontology and Geriatrics*, 55(3) p. 667-72.

van Uffelen JG, Wong J, Chau JY, van der Ploeg HP, Riphagen I, Healy GH, et al. (2010) Occupational sitting and health risks: a systematic review. Am J Prev Med 39: 379–388.

Vera-garcia, F., Elvira, J., Brown, S., & McGill, S. (2007) Effects of abdominal stabilization maneuvers on the control of spine motion and stability against sudden trunk perturbations. *Journal of Electromyography and Kinesiology*, 17(5) p. 556–567.

Vernikos, J. (2011) Sitting Kills, Moving Heals. Quill Driver Books.

Walker, M., Whincup, P., & Shaper, A. (2004) British Regional Heart Study (1975-2004). *International Journal of Epidemiology*, 33(6) 1,185–1,192.

Wannamethee, S., Shaper, A., Lennon, L. & Whincup, P. (2006) Height loss in older men: associations with total mortality and incidence of cardiovascular disease. *Archives of Internal Medicine,* 166 (22) 2,546–2,552.

Waterman, B., Owens, B., & Davey, S. (2010) The epidemiology of ankle sprains in the United States. *Journal of Bone and Joint Surgery*, 92 p. 2279–2284.

Watson, D. & Trott, P. (1993) Cervical headache: an investigation of natural head posture and upper cervical flexor muscle performance. *Cephalgia,* 13(4) p. 272–84.

Weiniger, S. (2008) Stand Taller, Live Longer Bodyzone LLC © 2008.

Woodhull-McNeal (1992) Changes in Posture and Balance with Age. Aging Clinical and Experimental Research 4(3).

Wright, E. et al (2000) Usefulness of Posture Training for Patients With Temporomandibular Disorder. Journal of the American Dental Association 131(2).

Zink, G. & Lawson, W. (1979) An Osteopathic Structural Examination and Functional Interpretation of the Soma. *Osteopathic Annals,* 7 p. 12–19.

ACKNOWLEDGEMENTS

First and foremost, I would like to acknowledge all of the students of the Certified Posture Expert program. Their dedication to changing the world by getting better results with their patients is admirable. Next, I'd like to thank our patients who have been committed to their treatment plans to take control of their lives and live healthier with better posture. Their success stories have made all of this worth it.

I'd like to acknowledge Dr. Mark Wade's persistence and dedication to our core value at the American Posture Institute that "Your Success is Our Priority." The whole American Posture Institute team deserves considerable recognition for their contributions to the API community, excellence in education, and customer experience. And finally, my mom, dad, and sister for their continual support to go big and achieve my dreams! Their level of support and encouragement is unparalleled.

THE AUTHORS

Dr. Krista Burns

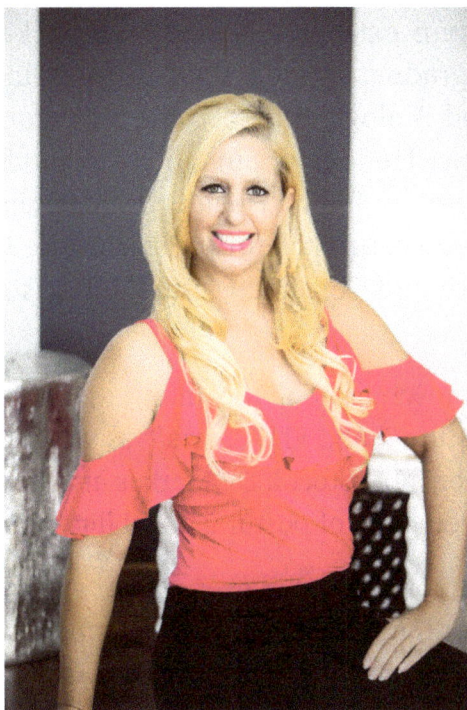

Dr. Krista Burns, co-founder of the American Posture Institute, graduated with honors as a Doctor of Chiropractic from Palmer College of Chiropractic. To increase her clinical expertise, she completed certifications as a Certified Postural Neurologist, Certified Posture Expert, Certified Posture Exercise Professional, and is Board Eligible in Functional Chiropractic Neurology.

Dr. Krista is an inspiring public speaker and has been a featured presenter at seminars around the world including the World Congress of Neurology and Neurologic Disorders. She is also a contributing expert on the media. She has contributed to Fox News Radio and was featured in *Global Woman Magazine* as a successful entrepreneur and doctor.

Beyond her professional accomplishments, Dr. Krista has always had a love for fitness. She was a competitive member of the United States Freestyle Development Ski Team, competing at the US National Ski Championships. She is also a nationally recognized fitness competitor in the category of Bikini Bodybuilding, and finished 3rd overall in the IBFA Bodybuilding World Championships.

Dr. Mark Wade

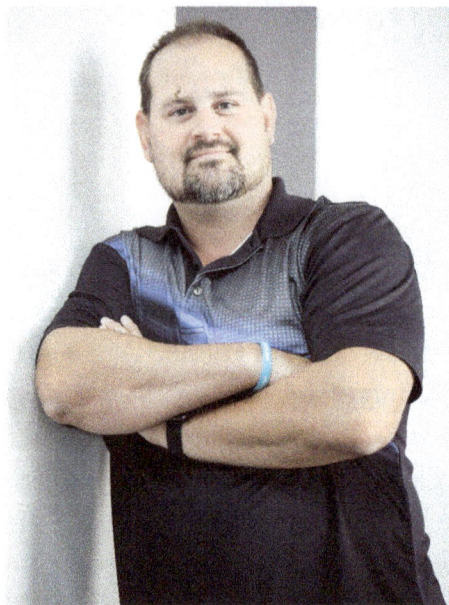

Dr. Mark Wade is the CEO of the American Posture Institute. He is a born leader and veteran of the United States army. He is the president of the Council on Human Function and a Board Member of the International Posture Association.

Dr. Mark has an extensive educational background. He graduated with dual degrees in Chemistry and Biology, then became a Doctor in Chiropractic. He is now pursuing a second doctorate degree in Public Health. Dr. Mark is also a Certified Postural Neurologist, Certified Posture Expert, and Certified Postural Exercise Professional.

Dr. Mark is the creator of the internationally renowned posture programs, 12 Weeks To Better Posture™ and FITPosture™ as well as the developer of the CPC (Complete Posture Correction™) Protocol. Dr. Mark is also the inventor of the 'Spinal Push Test', which is used for detection of postural instability.

Dr. Mark has worked with professional athletes and sports teams in every major sports arena and has served as the official Posture Expert for the 4-time National Champions, the Parma Panthers. Dr. Mark is the creator and host of the #1 Health Podcast on ITunes, the Council on Human Function.

To learn more about the American Posture Institute and how you can become a Certified Posture Expert, please visit our website at AmericanPostureInstitute.com. For on-going posture information, we invite you to follow us on social media at Facebook.com/AmericanPostureInstitute.